ACUTE ISCHEMIC STROKE

R.G. Gonzalez, J.A. Hirsch,
W.J. Koroshetz, M.H. Lev,
P. Schaefer
(Eds.)

Acute Ischemic Stroke

Imaging and Intervention

With 107 Figures and 59 Tables

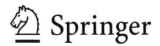 Springer

Library of Congress
Control Number 2005928382
ISBN-10 3-540-25264-9
Springer Berlin Heidelberg New York
ISBN-13 978-3-540-25264-9
Springer Berlin Heidelberg New York

R. Gilberto González
Neuroradiology Division
Massachusetts General Hospital
and Harvard Medical School
Boston, Mass., USA

Joshua A. Hirsch
Interventional Neuroradiology
and Endovascular Neurosugery Service
Massachusetts General Hospital
Harvard Medical School
Boston, Mass., USA

W.J. Koroshetz
Acute Stroke Service
Massachusetts General Hospital
Fruit Street, Boston, MA 02114, USA

Michael H. Lev
Neuroradiology Division
Massachusetts General Hospital
Harvard Medical School
Boston, Mass., USA

Pamela W. Schaefer
Neuroradiology
GRB 285, Fruit Street
Massachusetts General Hospital
Boston, MA 02114-2696

Springer is a part of Springer Science + Business Media

springeronline.com

© Springer-Verlag Berlin Heidelberg 2006
Printed in Germany

Medical Editor: Dr. Ute Heilmann, Heidelberg, Germany
Desk Editor: Wilma McHugh, Heidelberg, Germany
Cover design: Frido Steinen-Broo, Estudio Calamar, Spain
Layout: Bernd Wieland, Heidelberg, Germany
Production: LE-TEX Jelonek, Schmidt & Vöckler GbR, Leipzig, Germany
Reproduction and typesetting: AM-productions GmbH, Wiesloch, Germany

21/3151 – 5 4 3 2 1 0
Printed on acid-free paper

Preface

Acute ischemic stroke is treatable. Rapidly evolving imaging technology is revolutionizing the management of the acute stroke patient, and the field of acute stroke therapy is undergoing positive change. This book is intended as a guide for a wide variety of clinicians who are involved in the care of acute stroke patients, and is a compendium on how acute stroke patients are imaged and managed at the Massachusetts General Hospital (MGH). The approaches delineated in this book derive from the published experiences of many groups, and the crucible of caring for thousands of acute stroke patients at the MGH. It is the result of the clinical experiences of the emergency department physicians, neurologists, neuroradiologists, and interventional neuroradiologists that comprise the acute stroke team.

This book focuses on *hyperacute* ischemic stroke, which we define operationally as that early period after stroke onset when a significant portion of threatened brain is potentially salvageable. The time period this encompasses will depend on many factors; it may only be a few minutes in some individuals or greater than 12 hours in others. In most people, this hyperacute period will encompass less than 6 hours when intervention is usually most effective.

The authors believe that patients with acute ischemic stroke can benefit most from the earliest possible definitive diagnosis and rapid, appropriate treatment. In the setting of hyperacute stroke, imaging plays a vital role in the assessment of patients. The most recent advances in imaging can identify the precise location of the occluded vessel, estimate the age of the infarcted core, and estimate the area at risk or the 'ischemic penumbra'. This book will cover these modern imaging modalities; advanced computed tomography and magnetic resonance methods are considered in detail. These two modalities are emphasized because of their widespread availability and the rapid development of their capacities in the diagnosis of stroke. Only brief mention is made of other modalities because they are less widely available and less commonly used in the evaluation of hyperacute stroke patients.

Another major aspect of this book is the use of standard and developing interventions that aim to limit the size of a cerebral infarct and prevent its growth. With the approval of intravenous therapy using recombinant tissue plasminogen activator (rt-PA), this treatment is now in use throughout the United States, Canada, and Europe. Although this is a major advance in the treatment of acute stroke, the 3-hour 'window' for rt-PA makes this therapy suitable for only a minority of patients. Studies have indicated that intra-arterial thrombolysis is also effective in patients in a wider window up to 6 hour. More recently, phase II clinical studies have shown that intravenous therapy with a new fibrinolytic agent may be effective up to 9 hours after ischemic stroke onset in patients selected using imaging criteria. Thus, this approach is potentially available to many more individuals. Finally, a wide variety of novel and innovative new devices are being developed to mechanically recanalize the occluded vessel. It is likely that these devices will come into clinical use in the near future. The authors hope that their experiences as summarized in these pages are of value to the reader and, ultimately, the acute stroke patient.

R. Gilberto González

Contents

7   Diffusion MR of Acute Stroke
Pamela W. Schaefer, A. Kiruluta,
R. Gilberto González

8   Perfusion MRI of Acute Stroke
Pamela W. Schaefer, William A. Copen,
R. Gilberto González

9   Acute Stroke Imaging
with SPECT, PET, Xenon-CT,
and MR Spectroscopy
Mark E. Mullins

PART III

Intervention in Acute Ischemic Stroke

Contributors

Erica C.S. Camargo
Neuroradiology Division
Massachusetts General Hospital
Harvard Medical School
Boston, Mass., USA

William A. Copen
Neuroradiology Division
Massachusetts General Hospital
and Harvard Medical School
Boston, Mass., USA

Turgay Dalkara
Department of Neurology
Faculty of Medicine Hacettepe University
Ankara, Turkey

Guido González
Neuroradiology Division
Massachusetts General Hospital
Harvard Medical School
Boston, Mass., USA

R. Gilberto González
Neuroradiology Division
Massachusetts General Hospital
and Harvard Medical School
Boston, Mass., USA

Joshua A. Hirsch
Interventional Neuroradiology
and Endovascular Neurosugery Service
Massachusetts General Hospital
Harvard Medical School
Boston, Mass., USA

Andrew Kiruluta
Neuroradiology Division
Massachusetts General Hospital
and Harvard Medical School
Boston, Mass., USA

W. J. Koroshetz
Acute Stroke Service
Massachusetts General Hospital
Fruit Street, Boston, MA 02114, USA

Michael H. Lev
Neuroradiology Division
Massachusetts General Hospital
Harvard Medical School
Boston, Mass., USA

Eng H. Lo
Neuroprotection Research Laboratory
Departments of Radiology and Neurology
Massachusetts General Hospital
Harvard Medical School
Charlestown, Mass., USA

Michael A. Moskowitz
Stroke and Neurovascular Regulation Laboratory
Neuroscience Center
Departments of Radiology and Neurology
Massachusetts General Hospital
and Harvard Medical School
Charlestown, Mass., USA

Mark E. Mullins
Neuroradiology Division
Massachusetts General Hospital
Harvard Medical School
Boston, Mass., USA

Raul G. Nogueira
Interventional Neuroradiology
and Endovascular Neurosugery Service
Massachusetts General Hospital
Harvard Medical School
Boston, Mass., USA

Johnny C. Pryor
Interventional Neuroradiology
and Endovascular Neurosugery Service
Massachusetts General Hospital
Harvard Medical School
Boston, Mass., USA

James D. Rabinov
Interventional Neuroradiology
and Endovascular Neurosugery Service
Massachusetts General Hospital
Harvard Medical School
Boston, Mass., USA

Pamela W. Schaefer
Neuroradiology
GRB 285, Fruit Street
Massachusetts General Hospital
Boston, MA 02114-2696

L.H. Schwamm
Acute Stroke Service
Massachusetts General Hospital
Harvard Medical School
Boston, Mass., USA

Shams Sheikh
Neuroradiology Division
Massachusetts General Hospital
Harvard Medical School
Boston, Mass., USA

Sanjay K. Shetty
Neuroradiology Division
Massachusetts General Hospital
Harvard Medical School
Boston, Mass., USA

Aneesh B. Singhal
Stroke Service, Department of Neurology
and Neuroprotection Research Laboratory
Massachusetts General Hospital
Harvard Medical School
Boston, Mass., USA

David Vu
Neuroradiology Division
Massachusetts General Hospital
and Harvard Medical School
Boston, Mass., USA

Albert Yoo
Interventional Neuroradiology
and Endovascular Neurosugery Service
Massachusetts General Hospital
Harvard Medical School
Boston, Mass., USA

PART I
Fundamentals of Acute Ischemic Stroke

Ischemic Stroke: Basic Pathophysiology and Neuroprotective Strategies

Aneesh B. Singhal, Eng H. Lo, Turgay Dalkara, Michael A. Moskowitz

1.1 Introduction

Since the late 1980s, basic science research in the field of stroke has elucidated multiple pathways of cellular injury and repair after cerebral ischemia, resulting in the identification of several promising targets for neuroprotection. A large number of neuroprotective agents have been shown to reduce stoke-related damage in animal models. To date, however, no single agent has achieved success in clinical trials. Nevertheless, analysis of the reasons behind the failure of recent drug trials, combined with the success of clot-lysing drugs in improving clinical outcome, has revealed new potential therapeutic opportunities and raised expectations that successful stroke treatment will be achieved in the near future. In this chapter we first highlight the major mechanisms of neuronal injury, emphasizing those that are promising targets for stroke therapy. We then discuss the influence of these pathways on white matter injury, and briefly review the emerging concept of the neurovascular unit. Finally, we review emerging strategies for treatment of acute ischemic stroke.

1.2 Mechanisms of Ischemic Cell Death

Ischemic stroke compromises blood flow and energy supply to the brain, which triggers at least five fundamental mechanisms that lead to cell death: excitotoxicity and ionic imbalance, oxidative/nitrative stress, inflammation, apoptosis, and peri-infarct depolarization (Fig. 1.1). These pathophysiological processes evolve in a series of complex spatial and temporal events spread out over hours or even days

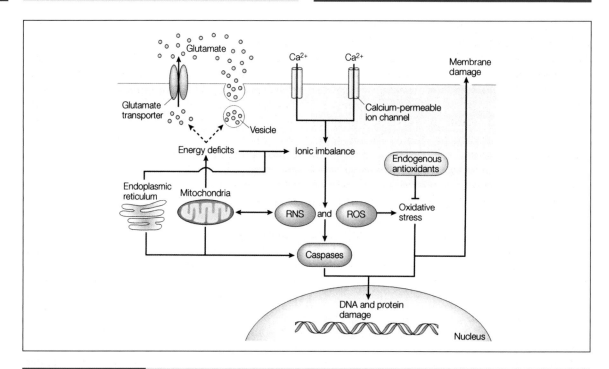

Figure 1.1

Major pathways implicated in ischemic cell death: excitotoxicity, ionic imbalance, oxidative and nitrative stresses, and apoptotic-like mechanisms. There is extensive interaction and overlap between multiple mediators of cell injury and cell death. After ischemic onset, loss of energy substrates leads to mitochondrial dysfunction and the generation of reactive oxygen species (*ROS*) and reactive nitrogen species (*RNS*). Additionally, energy deficits lead to ionic imbalance, and excitotoxic glutamate efflux and build up of intracellular calcium. Downstream pathways ultimately include direct free radical damage to membrane lipids, cellular proteins, and DNA, as well as calcium-activated proteases, plus caspase cascades that dismantle a wide range of homeostatic, reparative, and cytoskeletal proteins. (From Lo et al., *Nat Rev Neurosci* 2003, 4: 399–415)

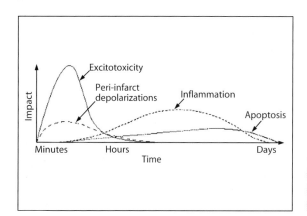

Fig. 1.2

Putative cascade of damaging events in focal cerebral ischemia. Very early after the onset of the focal perfusion deficit, excitotoxic mechanisms can damage neurons and glia lethally. In addition, excitotoxicity triggers a number of events that can further contribute to the demise of the tissue. Such events include peri-infarct depolarizations and the more-delayed mechanisms of inflammation and programmed cell death. The *x*-axis reflects the evolution of the cascade over time, while the *y*-axis aims to illustrate the impact of each element of the cascade on the final outcome. (From Dirnagel et al., *Trends Neurosci* 1999; 22: 391–397)

(Fig. 1.2), have overlapping and redundant features, and mediate injury within neurons, glial cells, and vascular elements [1]. The relative contribution of each process to the net stroke-related injury is graphically depicted in Fig. 1.2. Within areas of severely reduced blood flow – the "core" of the ischemic territory – excitotoxic and necrotic cell death occurs within minutes, and tissue undergoes irreversible damage in the absence of prompt and adequate reperfusion. However, cells in the peripheral zones are supported by collateral circulation, and their fate is determined by several factors including the degree of ischemia and timing of reperfusion. In this peripheral region, termed the "ischemic penumbra," cell death occurs relatively slowly via the active cell death mechanisms noted above; targeting these mechanisms provides promising therapeutic opportunities.

1.2.1 Excitotoxicity and Ionic Imbalance

Ischemic stroke results in impaired cellular energy metabolism and failure of energy-dependent processes such as the sodium-potassium ATPase. Loss of energy stores results in ionic imbalance, neurotransmitter release, and inhibition of the reuptake of excitatory neurotransmitters such as glutamate. Glutamate binding to ionotropic *N*-methyl-D-aspartate (NMDA) and α-amino-3-hydroxy-5-methyl-4-isoxazolepropionic acid (AMPA) receptors promotes excessive calcium influx that triggers a wide array of downstream phospholipases and proteases, which in turn degrade membranes and proteins essential for cellular integrity. In experimental models of stroke, extracellular glutamate levels increase in the microdialysate [2, 3], and glutamate receptor blockade attenuates stroke lesion volumes. NMDA receptor antagonists prevent the expansion of stroke lesions in part by blocking spontaneous and spreading depolarizations of neurons and glia (cortical spreading depression) [4]. More recently, activation of the metabotropic subfamily of receptors has been implicated in glutamate excitotoxicity [5].

Up- and downregulation of specific glutamate receptor subunits contribute to stroke pathophysiology in different ways [6]. For example, after global cerebral ischemia, there is a relative reduction of calcium-impermeable GluR2 subunits in AMPA-type receptors, which makes these receptors more permeable to deleterious calcium influx [7]. Antisense knockdown of calcium-impermeable GluR2 subunits significantly increased hippocampal injury in a rat model of transient global cerebral ischemia, confirming the importance of these regulatory subunits in mediating neuronal vulnerability [8]. Variations in NMDA receptor subunit composition can also have an impact on tissue outcome. Knockout mice deficient in the NR2A subunit show decreased cortical infarction after focal stroke [9]. Medium spiny striatal neurons, which are selectively vulnerable to ischemia and excitotoxicity, preferentially express NR2B subunits [10]. Depending upon the subtype, metabotropic glutamate receptors can trigger either pro-survival or pro-death signals in ischemic neurons [5]. Understanding how the expression of specific glutamate receptor subunits modifies cell survival should stimulate the search for stroke neuroprotective drugs that selectively target specific subunits.

Ionotropic glutamate receptors also promote perturbations in ionic homeostasis that play a critical role in cerebral ischemia. For example, L-, P/Q-, and N-type calcium channel receptors mediate excessive calcium influx, and calcium channel antagonists reduce ischemic brain injury in preclinical studies [11–13]. Zinc is stored in vesicles of excitatory neurons and co-released upon depolarization after focal cerebral ischemia, resulting in neuronal death [14, 15]. Recently, imbalances in potassium have also been implicated in ischemic cell death. Compounds that selectively modulate a class of calcium-sensitive high-conductance potassium (maxi-K) channels protect the brain against stroke in animal models [16].

1.2.2 Oxidative and Nitrative Stress

Reactive oxygen species (ROS) such as superoxide and hydroxyl radicals are known to mediate reperfusion-related tissue damage in several organ systems including the brain, heart, and kidneys [17]. Oxygen free radicals are normally produced by the mitochondria during electron transport, and, after ischemia, high levels of intracellular Ca^{2+}, Na^+, and

ADP stimulate excessive mitochondrial oxygen radical production. Oxygen radical production may be especially harmful to the injured brain because levels of endogenous antioxidant enzymes [including superoxide dismutase (SOD), catalase, glutathione], and antioxidant vitamins (e.g., alpha-tocopherol, and ascorbic acid) are normally not high enough to match excess radical formation. After ischemia-reperfusion, enhanced production of ROS overwhelms endogenous scavenging mechanisms and directly damages lipids, proteins, nucleic acids, and carbohydrates. Importantly, oxygen radicals and oxidative stress facilitate mitochondrial transition pore (MTP) formation, which dissipates the proton motive force required for oxidative phosphorylation and ATP generation [18]. As a result, mitochondria release apoptosis-related proteins and other constituents within the inner and outer mitochondrial membranes [19]. Upon reperfusion and renewed tissue oxygenation, dysfunctional mitochondria may generate oxidative stress and MTP formation. Oxygen radicals are also produced during enzymatic conversions such as the cyclooxygenase-dependent conversion of arachidonic acid to prostanoids and degradation of hypoxanthine, especially upon reperfusion. Furthermore, free radicals are also generated during the inflammatory response after ischemia (see below). Not surprisingly then, oxidative stress, excitotoxicity, energy failure, and ionic imbalances are inextricably linked and contribute to ischemic cell death.

Oxidative and nitrative stresses are modulated by enzyme systems such as SOD and the nitric oxide synthase (NOS) family. The important role of SOD in cerebral ischemia is demonstrated in studies showing that mice with enhanced SOD expression show reduced injury after cerebral ischemia whereas those with a deficiency show increased injury [20–23]. Similarly, in the case of NOS, stroke-induced injury is attenuated in mice with deficient expression of the neuronal and inducible NOS isoforms [24, 25]. NOS activation during ischemia increases the generation of NO production, which combines with superoxide to produce peroxynitrite, a potent oxidant [26]. The generation of NO and oxidative stress is also linked to DNA damage and activation of poly(ADP-ribose) polymerase-1 (PARP-1), a nuclear enzyme that facilitates DNA repair and regulates transcription [27]. PARP-1 catalyzes the transformation of β-nicotinamide adenine dinucleotide (NAD+) into nicotinamide and poly(ADP-ribose). In response to DNA strand breaks, PARP-1 activity becomes excessive and depletes the cell of NAD+ and possibly ATP. Inhibiting PARP-1 activity or deleting the *parp-1* gene reduces apoptotic and necrotic cell death [28, 29], pointing to the possible relevance of this enzyme as a target for stroke therapy.

1.2.3 Apoptosis

Apoptosis, or programmed cell death [30], is characterized histologically by cells positive for terminal-deoxynucleotidyl-transferase-mediated dUTP nick end labeling (TUNEL) that exhibit DNA laddering. Necrotic cells, in contrast, show mitochondrial and nuclear swelling, dissolution of organelles, nuclear chromatin condensation, followed by rupture of nuclear and cytoplasmic membranes, and the degradation of DNA by random enzymatic cuts. Cell type, cell age, and brain location render cells more or less resistant to apoptosis or necrosis. Mild ischemic injury preferentially induces cell death via an apoptotic-like process rather than necrosis, although "aponecrosis" more accurately describes the pathology.

Apoptosis occurs via caspase-dependent as well as caspase-independent mechanisms (Fig. 1.3). Caspases are protein-cleaving enzymes (zymogens) that belong to a family of cysteine aspartases constitutively expressed in both adult and especially newborn brain cells, particularly neurons. Since caspase-dependent cell death requires energy in the form of ATP, apoptosis predominantly occurs in the ischemic penumbra (which sustains milder injury) rather than in the ischemic core, where ATP levels are rapidly depleted [31]. The mechanisms of cleavage and activation of caspases in human brain are believed to be similar to those documented in experimental models of stroke, trauma, and neurodegeneration [32]. Apoptogenic triggers [33] include oxygen free radicals [34], Bcl2, death receptor ligation [35], DNA damage, and possibly lysosomal protease activation [36]. Several mediators facilitate cross communication between

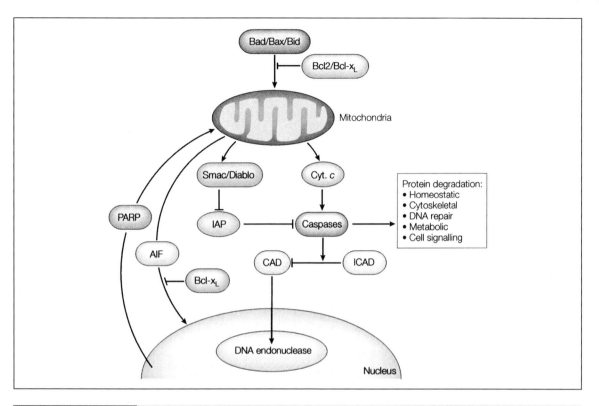

Figure 1.3

Cell death pathways relevant to an apoptotic-like mechanism in cerebral ischemia. Release of cytochrome *c* (*Cyt. c*) from the mitochondria is modulated by pro- as well as anti-apoptotic Bcl2 family members. Cytochrome *c* release activates downstream caspases through apoptosome formation (not shown) and caspase activation can be modulated by secondary mitochondria-derived activator of caspase (*Smac/Diablo*) indirectly through suppressing protein inhibitors of apoptosis (*IAP*). Effector caspases (caspases 3 and 7) target several substrates, which dismantle the cell by cleaving homeostatic, cytoskeletal, repair, metabolic, and cell signaling proteins. Caspases also activate caspase-activated deoxyribonuclease (*CAD*) by cleavage of an inhibitor protein (*ICAD*). Caspase-independent cell death may also be important. One mechanism proposes that poly-ADP(ribose)polymerase activation (*PARP*) promotes the release of apoptosis-inducing factor (*AIF*), which translocates to the nucleus, binds to DNA, and promotes cell death through a mechanism that awaits clarification. (From Lo et al., *Nat Rev Neurosci* 2003, 4: 399–415)

cell death pathways [37, 38], including the calpains, cathepsin B [39], nitric oxide [40, 41], and PARP [42]. Ionic imbalances, and mechanisms such as NMDA receptor-mediated K^+ efflux, can also trigger apoptotic-like cell death under certain conditions [43, 44]. This inter-relationship between glutamate excitotoxicity and apoptosis presents an opportunity for combination stroke therapy targeting multiple pathways.

The normal human brain expresses caspases-1, -3, -8, and -9, apoptosis protease-activating factor 1 (APAF-1), death receptors, P53, and a number of Bcl2 family members, all of which are implicated in apoptosis. In addition, the tumor necrosis factor (TNF) superfamily of death receptors powerfully regulates upstream caspase processes. For example, ligation of Fas induces apoptosis involving a series of caspases, particularly procaspase-8 and caspase-3 [45]. Caspase-3 has a pivotal role in ischemic cell death. Caspase-3 cleavage occurs acutely in neurons and it appears in the ischemic core as well as penumbra early during reperfusion [46]. A second wave of caspase cleavage usually follows hours to days later, and probably participates in delayed ischemic cell death. Emerging data suggest that the nucleus – traditionally believed to be simply the target of apoptosis – is involved in releasing signals for apoptosis. However, the mitochondrion plays a central role in mediating apoptosis [47, 48]. Mitochondria possess membrane recognition elements for upstream proapoptotic signaling molecules such as Bid, Bax, and Bad. Four mitochondrial molecules mediate downstream cell-death pathways: cytochrome c, secondary mitochondria-derived activator of caspase (Smac/Diablo), apoptosis-inducing factor, and endonuclease G [49]. Apoptosis-inducing factor and endonuclease G mediate *caspase-independent* apoptosis, which is discussed below. Cytochrome c and Smac/Diablo mediate *caspase-dependent* apoptosis. Cytochrome c binds to Apaf-1, which, together with procaspase-9, forms the "apoptosome," which activates caspase-9. In turn, caspase-9 activates caspase-3. Smac/Diablo binds to inhibitors of activated caspases and causes further caspase activation. Upon activation, executioner caspases (caspase-3 and -7) target and degrade numerous substrate proteins including gelsolin, actin, PARP-1, caspase-activated deoxyribonuclease inhibitor protein (ICAD), and other caspases, ultimately leading to DNA fragmentation and cell death (Fig. 1.3).

Caspase-independent apoptosis was recently recognized to play an important role in cell death and probably deserves careful scrutiny as a novel therapeutic target for stroke. NMDA receptor perturbations activate PARP-1, which promotes apoptosis-inducing factor (AIF) release from the mitochondria [42]. AIF then relocates to the nucleus, binds DNA, promotes chromatin condensation, and kills cells by a complex series of events. Cell death by AIF appears resistant to treatment with pan-caspase inhibitors but can be suppressed by neutralizing AIF before its nuclear translocation.

A number of experimental studies have shown that caspase inhibition reduces ischemic injury [50].

Caspase-3 inhibitors [51], gene deletions of Bid or caspase-3 [52], and the use of peptide inhibitors, viral vector-mediated gene transfer, and antisense oligonucleotides that suppress the expression and activity of apoptosis genes have all been found to be neuroprotective [50]. However, caspase inhibitors do not reduce infarct size in all brain ischemia models, perhaps related to the greater severity of ischemia, limited potency or inability of the agent to cross the blood–brain barrier, relatively minor impact of apoptosis on stroke outcome, and upregulation of caspase-independent or redundant cell death pathways. Ultimately, it may be necessary to combine caspase inhibitors and other inhibitors of apoptosis with therapies directed towards other pathways, for successful neuroprotection.

1.2.4 Inflammation

Inflammation is intricately related to the onset of stroke, and to subsequent stroke-related tissue damage. Inflammation within the arterial wall plays a vital role in promoting atherosclerosis [53, 54]. Arterial thrombosis (usually associated with ulcerated plaques) is triggered by multiple processes involving endothelial activation, as well as pro-inflammatory and pro-thrombotic interactions between the vessel wall and circulating blood elements. Elevated stroke risk has been linked to high levels of serologic markers of inflammation such as C-reactive protein [55], erythrocyte sedimentation rate (ESR), interleukin-6, TNF-α and soluble intercellular adhesion molecule (sICAM) [56]. These events are promoted in part by the binding of cell adhesion molecules from the selectin and immunoglobulin gene families expressed on endothelial cells to glycoprotein receptors expressed on the neutrophil surface. As evidence, reduced ischemic infarction is observed in ICAM-1 knockout mice, and infarction volumes are increased in mice that overexpress P-selectin [57, 58]. The pro-inflammatory molecule P-selectin is expressed on vascular endothelium within 90 min after cerebral ischemia, ICAM-1 by 4 h, and E-selectin by 24 h [59]. Inhibiting both selectin adhesion molecules and activation of complement reduces brain injury and suppresses neutrophil and platelet accumulation after focal ischemia in mice [60]. In humans, neutrophil and complement activation significantly worsened outcomes in a clinical trial using humanized mouse antibodies directed against ICAM (Enlimomab) [61]. Hence, the complexities of interactions between multiple pathways will have to be carefully considered for optimal translation to the clinic.

Ischemic stroke-related brain injury itself triggers inflammatory cascades within the parenchyma that further amplify tissue damage [1, 59]. As reactive microglia, macrophages, and leukocytes are recruited into ischemic brain, inflammatory mediators are generated by these cells as well as by neurons and astrocytes. Inducible nitric oxide synthase (iNOS), cyclooxygenase-2 (COX-2), interleukin-1 (IL-1), and monocyte chemoattractant protein-1 (MCP-1) are key inflammatory mediators, as evidenced by attenuated ischemic injury in mutant mice with targeted disruption of their genes [1, 62–65]. Initially after occlusion, there is a transient upregulation of immediate early genes encoding transcription factors (e.g., c-*fos*, c-*jun*) that occurs within minutes. This is followed by a second wave of heat shock genes (e.g., *HSP70*, *HSP72*) that increase within 1–2 h and then decrease by 1–2 days. Approximately 12–24 h after a stroke, a third wave comprised of chemokines and cytokines is expressed (e.g., IL-1, IL-6, IL-8, TNF-α, MCP-1, etc.). It is not known whether these three waves are causally related. Nevertheless, therapies that seek to target these pathways need to be carefully timed to match the complex temporal evolution of tissue injury.

Inflammatory cascades stimulate both detrimental and potentially beneficial pathways after ischemia. For example, administering TNF-α-neutralizing antibodies reduces brain injury after focal ischemia in rats [66], whereas ischemic injury increases in TNF receptor knockout mice [67]. In part, these contrasting results may reflect signal transduction cascades activated by TNF-R1 and TNF-R2; with TNF-R1 augmenting cell death and TNF-R2 mediating neuroprotection [68]. Similarly, the peptide vascular endothelial growth factor (VEGF) exacerbates edema in the acute phase of cerebral ischemia but promotes vascular remodeling during stroke recovery [69]. Ultimately, the net effect of these mediators depends upon the

stage of tissue injury or the predominance of a single signaling cascade among multiple divergent pathways.

1.2.5 Peri-infarct Depolarizations

Brain tissue depolarizations after ischemic stroke are believed to play a vital role in recruiting adjacent penumbral regions of reversible injury into the core area of infarction. Cortical spreading depression (CSD) is a self-propagating wave of electrochemical activity that advances through neural tissues at a rate of 2–5 mm/min, causing prolonged (1–5 min) cellular depolarization, depressed neuro-electrical activity, potassium and glutamate release into adjacent tissue and reversible loss of membrane ionic gradients. CSD is associated with a change in the levels of numerous factors including immediate early genes, growth factors, and inflammatory mediators such as interleukin-1β and TNF-α [70]. CSD is a reversible phenomenon, and, while implicated in conditions such as migraine, reportedly does not cause permanent tissue injury in humans. In severely ischemic regions, energy failure is so profound that ionic disturbances and simultaneous depolarizations become permanent, a process termed anoxic depolarization [71]. In penumbral regions after stroke, where blood supply is compromised, spreading depression exacerbates tissue damage, perhaps due to the increased energy requirements for reestablishing ionic equilibrium in the metabolically compromised ischemic tissues. In this context, spreading depression waves are referred to as peri-infarct depolarizations (PIDs) [4], reflecting their pathogenic role and similarity to anoxic depolarization.

PIDs have been demonstrated in mice, rat, and cat stroke models [72, 73]; however, their relevance to human stroke pathophysiology remains unclear. In the initial 2–6 h after experimental stroke, PIDs result in a step-wise increase in the region of core-infarcted tissue into adjacent penumbral regions [74, 75], and the incidence and total duration of spreading depression is shown to correlate with infarct size [76]. Recent evidence suggests that PIDs contribute to the expansion of the infarct core throughout the period of infarct maturation [77]. Inhibition of spreading depression using pharmaceutical agents such as NMDA or glycine antagonists [77, 78], or physiological approaches such as hypothermia [79], could be an important strategy to suppress the expansion of an ischemic lesion.

1.3 Grey Matter Versus White Matter Ischemia

In addition to the size of the stroke, its location, and the relative involvement of gray versus white matter are key determinants of outcome. For example, small white matter strokes often cause extensive neurologic deficits by interrupting the passage of large axonal bundles such as those within the internal capsule. Blood flow in white matter is lower than in gray matter, and white matter ischemia is typically severe, with rapid cell swelling and tissue edema because there is little collateral blood supply in deep white matter. Moreover, cells within the gray and white matter have different susceptibilities to ischemic injury. Amongst the neuronal population, well-defined subsets (the CA1 hippocampal pyramidal neurons, cortical projection neurons in layer 3, neurons in dorsolateral striatum, and cerebellar Purkinje cells) are particularly susceptible and undergo selective death after transient global cerebral ischemia [80]. The major cell types composing the neurovascular module within white matter include the endothelial cell, perinodal astrocyte, axon, oligodendrocyte, and myelin. In general, oligodendrocytes are more vulnerable than astroglial or endothelial cells.

There are important differences in the pathophysiology of white matter ischemia as compared to that of gray matter, which have implications for therapy [81]. In the case of excitotoxicity, since the white matter lacks synapses, neurotransmitter release from vesicles does not occur despite energy depletion and neurotransmitter accumulation. Instead, there is reversal of Na^+-dependent glutamate transport [82], resulting in glutamate toxicity with subsequent AMPA receptor activation, and excessive accumulation of calcium, which in turn activates calcium-dependent enzymes such as calpain, phospholipases, and protein kinase C, resulting in irreversible injury. The distinct lack of AMPA receptors expressing calci-

um-impermeable GluR2 subunits may make oligodendroglia particularly vulnerable to excitotoxic injury [83]. In the case of oxidative stress-induced white matter injury, the severity of injury appears to be greater in large axons as compared to small axons [80], although the mechanisms underlying these differences need further study. Despite these differences between gray and white matter injury, several common cascades of injury do exist. Damaged oligodendrocytes express death signals such as TNF and Fas ligand, and recruit caspase-mediated apoptotic-like pathways [84]. Degradation of myelin basic protein by matrix metalloproteinases (MMPs) [85], and upregulation of MMPs in autopsied samples from patients with vascular dementia [86] suggest that proteolytic pathways are also recruited in white matter. These pathways might serve as common targets for stroke therapy.

1.4 The Neurovascular Unit

In July 2001, the National Institutes of Neurological Disorders and Stroke convened the Stroke Program Review Group (SPRG) [87] to advise on directions for basic and clinical stroke research for the following decade. Although much progress had been made in dissecting the molecular pathways of ischemic cell death, focusing therapy to a single intracellular pathway or cell type had not yielded clinically effective stroke treatment. Integrative approaches were felt to be mandatory for successful stroke therapy. This meeting emphasized the relevance of dynamic interactions between endothelial cells, vascular smooth muscle, astro- and microglia, neurons, and associated tissue matrix proteins, and gave rise to the concept of the "neurovascular unit." This modular concept emphasized the dynamics of vascular, cellular, and matrix signaling in maintaining the integrity of brain tissue within both the gray and white matter, and its importance to the pathophysiology of conditions such as stroke, vascular dementia, migraine, trauma, multiple sclerosis, and possibly the aging brain (Fig. 1.4).

The neurovascular unit places stroke in the context of an integrative tissue response in which all cel-

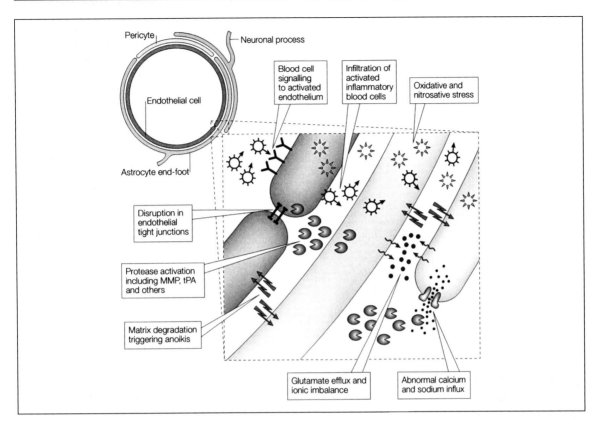

Figure 1.4

Schematic view of the neurovascular unit or module, and some of its components. Circulating blood elements, endothelial cells, astrocytes, extracellular matrix, basal lamina, adjacent neurons, and pericytes. After ischemia, perturbations in neurovascular functional integrity initiate multiple cascades of injury. Upstream signals such as oxidative stress together with neutrophil and/or platelet interactions with activated endothelium upregulate matrix metalloproteinases (*MMPs*), plasminogen activators and other proteases which degrade matrix and lead to blood–brain barrier leakage. Inflammatory infiltrates through the damaged blood–brain barrier amplify brain tissue injury. Additionally, disruption of cell-matrix homeostasis may also trigger anoikis-like cell death in both vascular and parenchymal compartments. Overlaps with excitotoxicity have also been documented via t-PA-mediated interactions with the NMDA receptor that augment ionic imbalance and cell death. (*t-PA* Tissue plasminogen activator)

lular and matrix elements, not just neurons or blood vessels, are players in the evolution of tissue injury. For example, efficacy of the blood–brain barrier is critically dependent upon endothelial–astrocyte–matrix interactions [88]. Disruption of the neurovascular matrix, which includes basement membrane components such as type IV collagen, heparan sulfate proteoglycan, laminin, and fibronectin, upsets the cell–matrix and cell–cell signaling that maintains neurovascular homeostasis. Although many proteases including cathepsins and heparanases contribute to extracellular matrix proteolysis, in the context of stroke, plasminogen activator (PA) and MMP are probably the two most important. This is because tissue plasminogen activator (t-PA) has been used successfully as a stroke therapy, and because emerging data show important linkages between t-PA, MMPs, edema, and hemorrhage after stroke.

The MMPs are zinc endopeptidases produced by all cell types of the neurovascular unit [89], that are secreted as zymogens requiring cleavage for enzymatic activation. MMPs can be classified into gelatinases (MMP-2 and -9), collagenases (MMP-1, -8, -13), stromelysins (MMP-3, -10, -11), membrane-type MMPs (MMP-14, -15, -16, -17), and others (e.g., MMP-7 and -12) [90]. Together with the PA system, MMPs play a central role in brain development and plasticity as they modulate extracellular matrix to allow neurite outgrowth and cell migration [91]. Upstream triggers of MMP include MAP kinase pathways [92] and oxidative stress [93]. MMP signaling is intricately linked to other well-recognized pathways after stroke, including oxidative and nitrative stress [94], caspase-mediated cell death [95], excitotoxicity, and neuro-inflammation [96, 97]. Several experimental as well as human studies provide evidence for a major role of MMPs (particularly MMP-9) in ischemic stroke, primary brain hemorrhage, blood–brain barrier disruption and post-ischemic or reperfusion hemorrhage [98–106]. For example, MMP levels have been correlated with the extent of stroke as measured by diffusion- and perfusion-weighted MRI [107]. Unlike MMPs, however, there is controversy surrounding the role of the PA axis (the other major proteolytic system in mammalian brain, comprising t-PA and urokinase PA, and their inhibitors plasminogen activator inhibitor-1 and neuroserpin) in stroke. Primary neuronal cultures genetically deficient in t-PA are resistant to oxygen-glucose deprivation [108] and t-PA knockout mice are protected against excitotoxic injury [109]. In a mouse focal ischemia model, treatment with neuroserpin reduces infarction [110]. In contrast, the responses are variable in t-PA knockouts, which are protected against focal stroke in some [111] but not other studies [112]. In part, these inconsistencies may reflect genetic differences and perhaps more importantly the balance between the clot-lysing beneficial effects of t-PA and its neurotoxic properties [113]. Emerging data suggest that administered t-PA upregulates MMP-9 via the low-density lipoprotein receptor-related protein (LRP), which avidly binds t-PA and possesses signaling properties [114]. Targeting the t-PA–LRP–MMP pathway may offer new therapeutic approaches for improving the safety profile of t-PA in patients with stroke.

1.5 Neuroprotection

Neuroprotection can be defined as the protection of cell bodies and neuronal and glial processes by strategies that impede the development of irreversible ischemic injury by effects on the cellular processes involved. Neuroprotection can be achieved using pharmaceutical or physiological therapies that directly inhibit the biochemical, metabolic, and cellular consequences of ischemic injury, or by using indirect approaches such as t-PA and mechanical devices to restore tissue perfusion. The complex and overlapping pathways involving excitotoxicity, ionic imbalance, oxidative and nitrative stress, and apoptotic-like mechanisms have been reviewed above. Each of these pathways offers several potential therapeutic targets, several of which have proved successful in reducing ischemic injury in animal models. However, the successful translation of experimental results into clinical practice remains elusive.

1.6 Stroke Neuroprotective Clinical Trials: Lessons from Past Failures

Various classes of neuroprotective agents have been tested in humans, with some showing promising phase II results. However, with the exception of the National Institute of Neurological Disorders and Stroke (NINDS) rt-PA trial [115], none has been proven efficacious on the basis of a positive phase III trial. Notable failures include trials of the lipid peroxidation inhibitor tirilazad mesylate [116], the ICAM-1 antibody enlimomab [61], the calcium channel blocker nimodipine [117], the γ-aminobutyric acid (GABA) agonist clomethiazole [118, 119], the glutamate antagonist and sodium channel blocker lubeluzole [120], the competitive NMDA antagonist selfotel [121], and several noncompetitive NMDA antagonists (dextrorphan, gavestinel, aptiganel and eliprodil) [122–124]. The high financial costs of these trials have raised questions about the commercial viability of continued neuroprotective drug development. How can we explain this apparent discrepancy between bench and bedside studies [125, 126]? The lack of efficacy can be related to several factors, some relating to the preclinical stage of drug development, and others to clinical trial design and methodology.

In the preclinical stage, therapies are often tested on healthy, young animals under rigorously controlled laboratory conditions, and, most often, the treatment is not adequately tested (for example, by multiple investigators in different stroke models) before it is brought to clinical trial. Whereas experimental animals are bred for genetic homogeneity, genetic differences and factors such as advanced age and co-morbidities (hypertension, diabetes) in patients may alter their therapeutic response. Moreover, despite similarities in the basic pathophysiology of stroke between species, there are important differences in brain structure, function, and vascular anatomy. The human brain is gyrated, has greater neuronal and glial densities, and is larger than the rodent brain. Some rodents (gerbils) lack a complete circle of Willis (gerbils), while others (rats) have highly effective collaterals between large cerebral vessels. As a result, there are important differences in the size, spatial distribution, and temporal evolution of the ischemic lesions between experimental models and humans. This is important, because the infarct volume is the standard outcome measure in animal models, whereas success in clinical trials is typically defined by clinical improvement. Finally, outcomes in animal models are usually assessed within days to weeks, whereas in humans, functional scores [National Institutes of Health Stroke Scale (NIHSS), Barthel index, etc.] are typically assessed after 3–6 months.

In the clinical trial stage, major problems include the relatively short therapeutic time window of most drugs; the difficulties in transporting patients quickly to the hospital; the imprecise correlation between symptom onset and the actual onset of cerebral ischemia; the high cost of enrolling patients for an adequately powered study; and the use of nonstandardized and relatively insensitive outcome measures. A recent review showed that of 88 stroke neuroprotective trials, the mean sample size was only 186 patients, and the median time window for recent (1995–1999) neuroprotective trials was as late as 12 h [127]. Another major factor accounting for past failures is that patients with different stroke pathophysiology and subtype are often combined in a trial, whereas the drug being tested might be more effective in a certain stroke subtype (e.g., strokes with predominant gray matter involvement).

In addition to the above, delivery of the drug to target ischemic tissues poses unique challenges [128]. Pharmacokinetic properties of the drug, and alterations in cerebral blood flow after stroke need to be taken into account. Blood flow can drop to below 5–10% of normal levels in the infarct core, and to 30–40% of baseline in the surrounding penumbra [129]. In addition, the blood–brain barrier restricts direct exchange between the vascular compartment and the cerebral parenchyma, and post-stroke edema and raised intracranial pressure further impair efficient delivery. Strategies that have been explored to penetrate the blood–brain barrier include intracerebral and intraventricular delivery, use of hyperosmolar substances (e.g., mannitol, arabinose) and pharmacological agents (bradykinin, mannitol, nitric oxide) to facilitate osmolar opening, and the development of carrier-mediated transport systems. These strategies appear promising; however, they remain limited by the prohibitively narrow time windows for effective stroke treatment.

Given these past failures, the focus has shifted towards expanding the therapeutic time window, improved patient selection, the use of brain imaging as a selection criterion, combination acute stroke drug treatments, use of validated rating scales to assess functional end points, and improved stroke trial design and organization [127, 130]. A number of new neuroprotection trials are currently underway or in the planning stages. These include trials of the free radical spin trap agent NXY-059 (now in phase III trials), intravenous magnesium, the antioxidant ebselen, the AMPA antagonist YM872, and the serotonin antagonist repinotan [131–133]. With the insights gained from prior neuroprotective trials, it is anticipated that one or more of the impending trials will prove successful.

1.7 Identifying the Ischemic Penumbra

As discussed above, although irreversible cell death begins within minutes after stroke onset within regions of maximally reduced blood flow (the infarct "core"), for several hours there exists a surrounding "penumbra" of ischemic but noninfarcted tissue that is potentially salvageable [134–137]. The concept of an "ischemic penumbra" provides a rationale for the use of neuroprotective drugs and reperfusion techniques to improve outcome after acute ischemic stroke. However, the extent of penumbral tissue is thought to diminish rapidly with time, hence the therapeutic time window is narrow. With intravenous t-PA [the only stroke therapy approved by the Food and Drug Administration (FDA)] the window is 3 h, which severely limits its use [138]; delayed therapy increases the risk of hemorrhage [115]. Similarly, administering therapy outside of the therapeutic window is considered one of the most important factors leading to the failure of neuroprotective drug trials. Developing methods to rapidly and accurately identify the ischemic penumbra is therefore an important area of current stroke research.

Imaging studies have validated the concept that tissue viability is heterogeneous distal to an occluded brain blood vessel. In animal models, the ischemic penumbra can be visualized by autoradiographic techniques that compare regions of reduced blood flow to regions of actively metabolizing tissue (2-deoxyglucose), or larger regions of suppressed protein synthesis to core areas with complete loss of ATP. In humans, imaging and biochemical studies similarly suggest that the window for efficacy may be prolonged in select individuals. Positron emission tomography (PET) [139, 140] can detect oxygen-utilizing tissue (oxygen extraction fraction) within regions of low blood flow, as well as locate ^{11}C-flumazenil recognition sites on viable neurons within underperfused brain areas. While PET is arguably the most accurate method, the greatest promise and experience appear to lie with multimodal magnetic resonance imaging (MRI) and multimodal CT because of their widespread availability, lower cost, technical ease, and shorter imaging times. With MRI, there is often a volume mismatch between tissue showing reduced water molecule diffusion (a signature for cell swelling and ischemic tissue) and a larger area of compromised tissue perfusion early after stroke onset – the so-called diffusion–perfusion mismatch. The difference, at least for all practical purposes, is believed to reflect the ischemic penumbra [129, 141–144]. Perfusion MRI currently affords a relative, rather than absolute, quantitative measure of cerebral tissue perfusion. Recent studies indicate that perfusion-CT can also be used to identify regions of ischemic, noninfarcted tissue after stroke, and that perfusion-CT may be comparable to MRI for this purpose [145–147]. The main advantage of perfusion-CT is that it allows rapid data acquisition and postprocessing, and can be performed in conjunction with CT angiography to complete the initial evaluation of stroke [148]. Xenon-enhanced CT is a more accurate technique than perfusion-CT and provides quantitative measurements of cerebral blood flow within 10–15 min; however, it requires the use of specialized equipment and at present its use is restricted to only a few centers [149]. Imaging methods such as these can optimize the selection of candidates for thrombolytic therapy or for adjunctive therapy many hours after stroke onset. Importantly, imaging may also provide quantitative surrogate endpoints for clinical trials. Several clinical trials employing imaging to select patients who might benefit from delayed therapy are now in progress. The Desmoteplase in Acute Ischemic Stroke Trial (DIAS) is the first published acute stroke thrombolysis trial using MRI both for patient selection and as a primary efficacy endpoint [150]. In this trial, patients were selected on the basis of perfusion–diffusion mismatch on the admission MRI and treated as late as 3–9 h after stroke symptom onset with intravenous (i.v.) desmoteplase, a newer plasminogen activator with high fibrin specificity. Desmoteplase-treated patients had significantly higher rates of reperfusion, as defined by MR-perfusion, and improved 90-day clinical outcome. These results support the utility of MRI in improving patient selection and as a surrogate outcome measure.

1.8 Combination Neuroprotective Therapy

Considering that several pathways leading to cell death are activated in cerebral ischemia, effective neuroprotection may require combining or adding drugs in series that target distinct pathways during the evolution of ischemic injury. Although seemingly independent treatments may not always yield additive results [151], various neuroprotective combinations have been used with some success in animal models. These include the co-administration of an NMDA receptor antagonist with GABA receptor agonists [152], free radical scavengers [153], cytidine-5′-diphosphocholine (Citicholine®) [154], the protein synthesis inhibitor cyclohexamide [155], caspase inhibitors [156] or growth factors such as basic fibroblast growth factor (bFGF) [157]. Synergy is also observed with 2 different antioxidants [158], and cytidine-5′-diphosphocholine plus bFGF [159]. Caspase inhibitors given with bFGF or an NMDA receptor antagonist extend the therapeutic window and lower effective doses [160].

Neuroprotective drugs may have a role in increasing the efficacy and safety of thrombolysis. Because the risk of hemorrhage increases with time, treatment with intravenous t-PA is currently limited to 3 h after vascular occlusion [161]. However, because ischemic but noninfarcted, potentially salvageable tissue exists for several hours after stroke in rats [162] and probably also in humans [134–137], clot lysis may be therapeutically useful at later times. Results from the PROACT II study, in which recombinant pro-urokinase was administered intra-arterially until 8 h post-stroke to patients with middle cerebral artery (MCA) occlusion, and a pooled analysis of the ATLANTIS, ECASS, and NINDS rt-PA stroke trials [163], support the contention that potential benefit exists beyond the 3-h time window. However, the use of thrombolysis must be weighed against the risk of intracerebral hemorrhage and brain edema after 3 h. Most preclinical observations suggest that treatment is suboptimal without combining neuroprotective therapy with clot-lysing drugs. This combination reduces reperfusion injury and inhibits downstream targets in cell death cascades. Synergistic or additive effects have been reported when thrombolysis was used with neuroprotectants such as oxygen radical scavengers [164], AMPA [165] and NMDA [166] receptor antagonists, MMP inhibitors [103], cytidine-5′-diphosphocholine [167], topiramate [168], antileukocytic adhesion antibodies [169], and antithrombotics [170]. Combination therapies may decrease dosages for each agent, thereby reducing the occurrence of adverse events. Two recent clinical trials have reported the feasibility and safety of treating with intravenous t-PA followed by neuroprotectants, clomethiazole [171] or lubeluzole [172]. Rational therapy based on inhibiting multiple cell death mechanisms may ultimately prove as useful for stroke as for cancer chemotherapy.

1.9 Ischemic Pre-conditioning

Transient, nondamaging ischemic/hypoxic brain insults are known to protect against subsequent prolonged, potentially detrimental episodes by upregulating powerful endogenous pathways that increase the resistance to injury [173]. The tolerance induced by ischemic preconditioning can be acute (within minutes), or delayed by several hours. Acute protective effects are short lasting and are mediated by posttranslational protein modifications; delayed tolerance is sustained for days to weeks and results from changes in gene expression and new protein synthesis [for example, of heat shock protein, Bcl2, hypoxia-inducible factor, and mitogen-activated protein (MAP) kinases] [174, 175]. Emerging human data indicate that preceding transient ischemic attacks (TIAs) reduce the severity of subsequent stroke, perhaps from a preconditioning effect [176–178]. In a study of 65 patients studied by diffusion and perfusion MRI, those with a prior history of TIA ($n=16$) were found to have smaller initial diffusion lesions and final infarct volumes, as well as milder clinical deficits, despite a similar size and severity of the perfusion deficit [176]. Preconditioning may offer novel insights into molecular mechanisms responsible for endogenous neuroprotection, and thus provide new strategies for making brain cells more resistant to ischemic injury [179].

1.10 Nonpharmaceutical Strategies for Neuroprotection

1.10.1 Magnesium

Magnesium is involved in multiple processes relevant to cerebral ischemia, including inhibition of presynaptic glutamate release [180], NMDA receptor blockade [181], calcium channel antagonism, and maintenance of cerebral blood flow [182]. In animal models of stroke, administration of intravenous magnesium as late as 6 h after stroke onset, in doses that double its physiological serum concentration, was found to reduce infarct volumes [183, 184]. In pilot clinical studies, magnesium was found to reduce death and disability from stroke, raising expectations that magnesium could be a safe and inexpensive treatment [185]. However, in a large multicenter trial involving 2589 patients, magnesium given within 12 h after acute stroke did not significantly reduce the risk of death or disability, although some benefit was documented in lacunar strokes [131]. Further studies are ongoing to determine whether paramedic initiation of magnesium, by reducing the time to treatment, yields benefit in stroke patients [186].

1.10.2 Albumin Infusion

Albumin infusion enhances red cell perfusion and suppresses thrombosis and leukocyte adhesion within the brain microcirculation, particularly during the early reperfusion phase after experimental focal ischemia [187]. Albumin also significantly lowers the hematocrit and by so doing improves microcirculatory flow, viscosity of plasma and cell deformability, as well as oxygen transport capacity. Albumin reduces infarct size, improves neurological scores, and reduces cerebral edema in experimental animals [188]. These effects may reflect a combination of therapeutic properties including its antioxidant effects, antiapoptotic effects on the endothelium, and effects on reducing blood stasis within the microcirculation. Clinical trials to test the effects of albumin are now being organized.

1.10.3 Hypothermia

Nearly all ischemic events are modulated by temperature, and cerebroprotection from hypothermia is believed to increase resistance against multiple deleterious pathways including oxidative stress and inflammation [189–195]. Generally, most biological processes exhibit a Q_{10} of approximately 2.5, which means that a 1°C reduction in temperature reduces the rate of cellular respiration, oxygen demand, and carbon dioxide production by approximately 10% [196]. Reduced temperature also slows the rate of pathological processes such as lipid peroxidation, as well as the activity of certain cysteine or serine proteases. However, detoxification and repair processes are also slowed, so the net outcome may be complex. Hence, hypothermia appears to be an attractive therapy that targets multiple injury mechanisms.

Brain cooling can be achieved more rapidly (and spontaneously) when blood flow to the entire brain ceases following cardiac arrest, and thermoregulation may be abnormal due to hypothalamic dysfunction. If only a segment of brain is ischemic, noninjured brain remains a metabolically active heat source. While moderate hypothermia (28–32 °C) is technically difficult and fraught with complications, recent experimental studies have shown that small decreases in core temperature (from normothermia to 33–36 °C) are sufficient to reduce neuronal death. The consensus from preclinical data suggests that the opportunity to treat does not extend beyond minutes after reversible MCA occlusion when hypothermia is maintained for a short duration (a few hours) [197]. In a global model of hippocampal ischemia, hypothermia is beneficial if begun 30 min before but not 10 min after stroke onset [198]. However, if cooling is prolonged (12–48 h), protection against injury is substantial following focal as well as global cerebral ischemia [199, 200]. In humans, encouraging positive results were recently reported in two randomized clinical trials of mild hypothermia in survivors of out-of-hospital cardiac arrest [201, 202]. Cooling significantly improved outcomes despite a relatively delayed interval (105 min) from ischemic onset until the initiation of cooling. Based on these results, additional controlled trials are now underway to test the therapeutic impact of hypothermia in focal ischemia and embolic stroke when combined with thrombolysis. Preliminary data justify enthusiasm. In a study of 25 patients with acute, large, complete MCA infarction, mild hypothermia (33°C maintained for 48–72 h) significantly reduced morbidity and improved long-term neurologic outcome [203]. The results of a recent trial [Cooling for Acute Ischemic Brain Damage (COOL-AID)] [204] suggest that the combination of intra-arterial thrombolysis plus mild hypothermia is safe; however, complications such as cardiac arrhythmia, deep vein thrombosis, and pneumonia have been reported previously [205]. Several single and multicenter randomized trials are underway in patients with ischemic and hemorrhagic stroke.

1.10.4 Induced Hypertension

The ischemic penumbra shows impaired autoregulation, and appears to be particularly sensitive to blood pressure manipulation. The rationale for using induced hypertension as a stroke therapy is provided by early studies showing that raising mean arterial pressure results in improved cerebral perfusion within the penumbra, and a concomitant return of electrical activity. In animal models of focal cerebral ischemia, induced hypertension therapy was found to augment cerebral blood flow, attenuate brain injury, and improve neurological function [206, 207]. In humans with acute ischemic stroke, a spontaneous increase in blood pressure is common, and neurological deterioration can occur with "excessive" antihypertensive therapy [208]. Furthermore, a paradigm for induced hypertension for cerebral ischemia exists in the treatment of vasospasm after subarachnoid hemorrhage [209].

Based upon this rationale, recent trials have studied the effect of induced hypertension (using intravenous phenylephrine) on clinical and imaging outcomes in patients with acute stroke [210–212]. Patients with significant diffusion–perfusion "mismatch" on MRI, large vessel occlusive disease, and fluctuating neurological deficits were found to be more likely to respond, and improvement in tests of cortical function correlated with improved perfusion of corresponding cortical regions [213, 214]. A multi-

center randomized trial of induced hypertension is ongoing. The main concerns with induced hypertension therapy include the risk of precipitating intracerebral hemorrhage and worsening cerebral edema, particularly in patients with reperfusion, as well as systemic complications such as myocardial ischemia, cardiac arrhythmias, and ischemia from phenylephrine-induced vasoconstriction. Ultimately, this treatment might be more applicable to stroke patients who are not candidates for thrombolytic therapy.

1.10.5 Hyperoxia

Tissue hypoxia plays a critical role in the primary and secondary events leading to cell death after ischemic stroke [215]; therefore, increasing brain oxygenation has long been considered a logical stroke treatment strategy. Theoretically, oxygen should be an excellent drug for treating stroke since it has distinct advantages over pharmaceutical agents: it easily diffuses across the blood–brain barrier, has multiple beneficial biochemical, molecular, and hemodynamic effects, it is well tolerated, and can be delivered in high doses without dose-limiting side-effects (except in patients with chronic obstructive pulmonary disease). Experimental studies have shown that supplemental oxygen favorably alters the levels of glutamate, lactate, bcl2, manganese superoxide dismutase, cyclooxygenase-2, and inhibits cell-death mechanisms such as apoptosis [216–222]. Because the rationale for oxygen in stroke is so compelling, numerous groups have focused on it as a potential therapy. Hyperbaric oxygen therapy (HBO) has been widely studied because it significantly raises brain tissue partial pressure of oxygen (brain $p_{ti}O_2$), a factor believed critical for effective neuroprotection. Clinical improvement during exposure to HBO was observed nearly 40 years ago [223]. HBO proved effective in animal stroke studies [224–232]; however, it failed three clinical trials [233–235], resulting in reduced interest in HBO. There is now growing recognition that factors such as barotrauma from excessive chamber pressures, delayed time to therapy (2–5 days after stroke), and poor patient selection may have led to the failure of previous HBO clinical trials, and the therapeutic potential of HBO in acute stroke is being re-examined.

In light of the difficulties of HBO, several groups have begun to investigate the therapeutic potential of normobaric hyperoxia therapy (NBO) [236–241]. NBO has several advantages: it is simple to administer, well tolerated, inexpensive, widely available, can be started very quickly after stroke onset (e.g., by paramedics), and is noninvasive. In animal studies, NBO has been shown to reduce infarct volumes, improve neurobehavioral deficits, improve diffusion and perfusion MRI parameters of ischemia, and increase brain interstitial pO_2 in penumbral tissues [236–238, 241]. In a small pilot clinical study of patients with acute ischemic stroke and diffusion–perfusion "mismatch" on MRI, NBO improved clinical deficits and reversed diffusion-MRI abnormalities, suggesting that similar beneficial effects can be obtained in humans [239]. As compared to HBO, NBO is relatively ineffective in raising brain $p_{ti}O_2$, and the mechanism of neuroprotection remains unclear. An indirect hemodynamic mechanism ("reverse steal") has been suggested, but further studies are needed to elucidate the precise mechanism(s) of action. Further studies are also warranted to investigate the safety of this therapy. Theoretically, increasing oxygen delivery can increase oxygen free radicals, which could theoretically worsen injury by promoting processes such as lipid peroxidation, inflammation, apoptosis, and glutamate excitotoxicity [17, 242–244]. Existing data suggest that the benefit of oxygen is transient, and cannot be sustained without timely reperfusion. Ultimately, oxygen therapy may be most useful if combined with reperfusion therapy, or used as a strategy to extend time windows for therapies such as t-PA.

1.11 Prophylactic and Long-term Neuroprotection

While the above discussion concerned neuroprotection in the hyperacute and acute stages after stroke, there is a rationale for using neuroprotective agents *before* stroke, in high-risk populations such as patients undergoing carotid endarterectomy, carotid

angioplasty or stent placement, coronary artery bypass grafting, cardiac valvular surgery, repair of aortic dissections, and heart transplant. Similarly, drugs such as aspirin, clopidogrel (Plavix®), aggrenox, and warfarin, which reduce the actual risk for stroke, can be considered long-term neuroprotective agents. Newer agents that target the vascular endothelium and cerebral microcirculation – notably thiazide diuretics, angiotensin-converting enzyme inhibitors and hydroxy-3-methylglutaryl-CoA (HMG-CoA) reductase inhibitors (statins) – have been shown to reduce the risk for stroke as well as improve outcomes after stroke [245–248]. Statins act by enhancing the endothelial release of nitric oxide, which relaxes vascular smooth muscle and raises cerebral blood flow, and exhibits additional beneficial effects by limiting platelet aggregation and the adhesivity of white blood cells, both of which impede microvascular flow during stroke [249, 250]. These effects are independent of their cholesterol-lowering effects [251]. Other pleiotropic statin effects, such as suppression of pro-thrombotic activity (upregulating endogenous t-PA and inhibiting plasminogen inhibitor-1), or protein-C serum levels and inflammation in the atheromatous plaque, may all contribute to stroke mitigation. Numerous clinical trials targeting the microcirculation are in various stages of completion for acute stroke and for stroke prophylaxis.

1.12 Conclusion

Several complex and overlapping pathways underlie the pathophysiology of cell death after ischemic stoke. While pharmaceutical agents can inhibit these pathways at various levels, resulting in effective neuroprotection in experimental models, no single agent intended for neuroprotection has been shown to improve outcome in clinical stroke trials. Refinements in patient selection, brain imaging, and methods of drug delivery, as well as the use of more clinically relevant animal stroke models and use of combination therapies that target the entire neurovascular unit are warranted to make stroke neuroprotection an achievable goal. Ongoing trials assessing the efficacy of thrombolysis with neuroprotective agents, and strategies aimed at extending the therapeutic window for reperfusion therapy promise to enhance the known benefits of reperfusion therapy. Most investigators agree that genomics and proteomics are the most promising recent developments impacting the future of stroke prevention, diagnosis, treatment, and outcome. Although many challenges lie ahead, an attitude of cautious optimism seems justified at this time.

References

1. Barone FC, Feuerstein GZ (1999) Inflammatory mediators and stroke: new opportunities for novel therapeutics. J Cereb Blood Flow Metab 19:819–834
2. Shimizu-Sasamata M, Bosque-Hamilton P, Huang PL, Moskowitz MA, Lo EH (1998) Attenuated neurotransmitter release and spreading depression-like depolarizations after focal ischemia in mutant mice with disrupted type I nitric oxide synthase gene. J Neurosci 18:9564–9571
3. Wang X, Shimizu-Sasamata M, Moskowitz MA, Newcomb R, Lo EH (2001) Profiles of glutamate and GABA efflux in core versus peripheral zones of focal cerebral ischemia in mice. Neurosci Lett 313:121–124
4. Hossmann KA (1996) Periinfarct depolarizations. Cerebrovasc Brain Metab Rev 8:195–208
5. Bruno V, Battaglia G, Copani A, D'Onofrio M, Di Iorio P, De Blasi A, Melchiorri D, Flor PJ, Nicoletti F (2001) Metabotropic glutamate receptor subtypes as targets for neuroprotective drugs. J Cereb Blood Flow Metab 21:1013–1033
6. Michaelis EK (1998) Molecular biology of glutamate receptors in the central nervous system and their role in excitotoxicity, oxidative stress and aging. Prog Neurobiol 54: 369–415
7. Pellegrini-Giampietro DE, Zukin RS, Bennett MV, Cho S, Pulsinelli WA (1992) Switch in glutamate receptor subunit gene expression in CA1 subfield of hippocampus following global ischemia in rats. Proc Natl Acad Sci USA 89:10499–10503
8. Oguro K, Oguro N, Kojima T, Grooms SY, Calderone A, Zheng X, Bennett MV, Zukin RS (1999) Knockdown of AMPA receptor GluR2 expression causes delayed neurodegeneration and increases damage by sublethal ischemia in hippocampal CA1 and CA3 neurons. J Neurosci 19:9218–9227
9. Morikawa E, Mori H, Kiyama Y, Mishina M, Asano T, Kirino T (1998) Attenuation of focal ischemic brain injury in mice deficient in the epsilon1 (NR2A) subunit of NMDA receptor. J Neurosci 18:9727–9732
10. Calabresi P, Centonze D, Gubellini P, Marfia GA, Pisani A, Sancesario G, Bernardi G (2000) Synaptic transmission in the striatum: from plasticity to neurodegeneration. Prog Neurobiol 61:231–265
11. Horn J, Limburg M (2001) Calcium antagonists for ischemic stroke: a systematic review. Stroke 32:570–576
12. Paschen W (2000) Role of calcium in neuronal cell injury: which subcellular compartment is involved? Brain Res Bull 53:409–413
13. Zipfel GJ, Lee JM, Choi DW (1999) Reducing calcium overload in the ischemic brain. N Engl J Med 341:1543–1544
14. Weiss JH, Hartley DM, Koh JY, Choi DW (1993) AMPA receptor activation potentiates zinc neurotoxicity. Neuron 10:43–49
15. Sorensen JC, Mattsson B, Andreasen A, Johansson BB (1998) Rapid disappearance of zinc positive terminals in focal brain ischemia. Brain Res 812:265–269
16. Gribkoff VK, Starrett JE Jr., Dworetzky SI, Hewawasam P, Boissard CG, Cook DA, Frantz SW, Heman K, Hibbard JR, Huston K, Johnson G, Krishnan BS, Kinney GG, Lombardo LA, Meanwell NA, Molinoff PB, Myers RA, Moon SL, Ortiz A, Pajor L, Pieschl RL, Post-Munson DJ, Signor LJ, Srinivas N, Taber MT, Thalody G, Trojnacki JT, Wiener H, Yeleswaram K, Yeola SW (2001) Targeting acute ischemic stroke with a calcium-sensitive opener of maxi-K potassium channels. Nat Med 7:471–477
17. Chan PH (2001) Reactive oxygen radicals in signaling and damage in the ischemic brain. J Cereb Blood Flow Metab 21:2–14
18. Kroemer G, Reed JC (2000) Mitochondrial control of cell death. Nat Med 6:513–519
19. Bernardi P, Petronilli V, Di Lisa F, Forte M (2001) A mitochondrial perspective on cell death. Trends Biochem Sci 26:112–117
20. Kondo T, Reaume AG, Huang TT, Carlson E, Murakami K, Chen SF, Hoffman EK, Scott RW, Epstein CJ, Chan PH (1997) Reduction of CuZn-superoxide dismutase activity exacerbates neuronal cell injury and edema formation after transient focal cerebral ischemia. J Neurosci 17:4180–4189
21. Kinouchi H, Epstein CJ, Mizui T, Carlson E, Chen SF, Chan PH (1991) Attenuation of focal cerebral ischemic injury in transgenic mice overexpressing CuZn superoxide dismutase. Proc Natl Acad Sci USA 88:11158–11162
22. Sheng H, Bart RD, Oury TD, Pearlstein RD, Crapo JD, Warner DS (1999) Mice overexpressing extracellular superoxide dismutase have increased resistance to focal cerebral ischemia. Neuroscience 88:185–191
23. Kim GW, Kondo T, Noshita N, Chan PH (2002) Manganese superoxide dismutase deficiency exacerbates cerebral infarction after focal cerebral ischemia/reperfusion in mice: implications for the production and role of superoxide radicals. Stroke 33:809–815

24. Huang Z, Huang PL, Panahian N, Dalkara T, Fishman MC, Moskowitz MA (1994) Effects of cerebral ischemia in mice deficient in neuronal nitric oxide synthase. Science 265:1883–1885

25. Iadecola C, Zhang F, Casey R, Nagayama M, Ross ME (1997) Delayed reduction of ischemic brain injury and neurological deficits in mice lacking the inducible nitric oxide synthase gene. J Neurosci 17:9157–9164

26. Beckman JS, Beckman TW, Chen J, Marshall PA, Freeman BA (1990) Apparent hydroxyl radical production by peroxynitrite: implications for endothelial injury from nitric oxide and superoxide. Proc Natl Acad Sci USA 87:1620–1624

27. Zhang J, Dawson VL, Dawson TM, Snyder SH (1994) Nitric oxide activation of poly(ADP-ribose) synthetase in neurotoxicity. Science 263:687–689

28. Eliasson MJ, Sampei K, Mandir AS, Hurn PD, Traystman RJ, Bao J, Pieper A, Wang ZQ, Dawson TM, Snyder SH, Dawson VL (1997) Poly(ADP-ribose) polymerase gene disruption renders mice resistant to cerebral ischemia. Nat Med 3:1089–1095

29. Endres M, Wang ZQ, Namura S, Waeber C, Moskowitz MA (1997) Ischemic brain injury is mediated by the activation of poly(ADP-ribose) polymerase. J Cereb Blood Flow Metab 17:1143–1151

30. Yuan J, Yankner BA (2000) Apoptosis in the nervous system. Nature 407:802–809

31. Nicotera P, Leist M, Fava E, Berliocchi L, Volbracht C (2000) Energy requirement for caspase activation and neuronal cell death. Brain Pathol 10:276–282

32. Chopp M, Chan PH, Hsu CY, Cheung ME, Jacobs TP (1996) DNA damage and repair in central nervous system injury: national institute of neurological disorders and stroke workshop summary. Stroke 27:363–369

33. Nicotera P, Lipton SA (1999) Excitotoxins in neuronal apoptosis and necrosis. J Cereb Blood Flow Metab 19:583–591

34. Budd SL, Tenneti L, Lishnak T, Lipton SA (2000) Mitochondrial and extramitochondrial apoptotic signaling pathways in cerebrocortical neurons. Proc Natl Acad Sci USA 97:6161–6166

35. Martin-Villalba A, Herr I, Jeremias I, Hahne M, Brandt R, Vogel J, Schenkel J, Herdegen T, Debatin KM (1999) CD95 ligand (fas-l/apo-1 l) and tumor necrosis factor-related apoptosis-inducing ligand mediate ischemia-induced apoptosis in neurons. J Neurosci 19:3809–3817

36. Salvesen GS (2001) A lysosomal protease enters the death scene. J Clin Invest 107:21–22

37. Digicaylioglu M, Lipton SA (2001) Erythropoietin-mediated neuroprotection involves cross-talk between Jak2 and NF-kappaB signalling cascades. Nature 412:641–647

38. Mannick JB, Hausladen A, Liu L, Hess DT, Zeng M, Miao QX, Kane LS, Gow AJ, Stamler JS (1999) Fas-induced caspase denitrosylation. Science 284:651–654

39. Yamashima T (2000) Implication of cysteine proteases calpain, cathepsin and caspase in ischemic neuronal death of primates. Prog Neurobiol 62:273–295

40. Mohr S, Stamler JS, Brune B (1994) Mechanism of covalent modification of glyceraldehyde-3-phosphate dehydrogenase at its active site thiol by nitric oxide, peroxynitrite and related nitrosating agents. FEBS Lett 348:223–227

41. Elibol B, Soylemezoglu F, Unal I, Fujii M, Hirt L, Huang PL, Moskowitz MA, Dalkara T (2001) Nitric oxide is involved in ischemia-induced apoptosis in brain: a study in neuronal nitric oxide synthase null mice. Neuroscience 105:79–86

42. Yu SW, Wang H, Poitras MF, Coombs C, Bowers WJ, Federoff HJ, Poirier GG, Dawson TM, Dawson VL (2002) Mediation of poly(ADP-ribose) polymerase-1-dependent cell death by apoptosis-inducing factor. Science 297:259–263

43. Yu SP, Choi DW (2000) Ions, cell volume, and apoptosis. Proc Natl Acad Sci USA 97:9360–9362

44. Yu SP, Yeh C, Strasser U, Tian M, Choi DW (1999) NMDA receptor-mediated K+ efflux and neuronal apoptosis. Science 284:336–339

45. Qiu J, Whalen MJ, Lowenstein P, Fiskum G, Fahy B, Darwish R, Aarabi B, Yuan J, Moskowitz MA (2002) Upregulation of the fas receptor death-inducing signaling complex after traumatic brain injury in mice and humans. J Neurosci 22:3504–3511

46. Namura S, Zhu J, Fink K, Endres M, Srinivasan A, Tomaselli KJ, Yuan J, Moskowitz MA (1998) Activation and cleavage of caspase-3 in apoptosis induced by experimental cerebral ischemia. J Neurosci 18:3659–3668

47. Fiskum G (2000) Mitochondrial participation in ischemic and traumatic neural cell death. J Neurotrauma 17:843–855

48. Leist M, Jaattela M (2001) Four deaths and a funeral: from caspases to alternative mechanisms. Nat Rev Mol Cell Biol 2:589–598

49. Friedlander RM (2003) Apoptosis and caspases in neurodegenerative diseases. N Engl J Med 348:1365–1375

50. Graham SH, Chen J (2001) Programmed cell death in cerebral ischemia. J Cereb Blood Flow Metab 21:99–109

51. Han BH, Xu D, Choi J, Han Y, Xanthoudakis S, Roy S, Tam J, Vaillancourt J, Colucci J, Siman R, Giroux A, Robertson GS, Zamboni R, Nicholson DW, Holtzman DM (2002) Selective, reversible caspase-3 inhibitor is neuroprotective and reveals distinct pathways of cell death after neonatal hypoxic-ischemic brain injury. J Biol Chem 277:30128–30136

52. Le DA, Wu Y, Huang Z, Matsushita K, Plesnila N, Augustinack JC, Hyman BT, Yuan J, Kuida K, Flavell RA, Moskowitz MA (2002) Caspase activation and neuroprotection in caspase-3- deficient mice after in vivo cerebral ischemia and in vitro oxygen glucose deprivation. Proc Natl Acad Sci USA 99:15188–15193

53. Chamorro A (2004) Role of inflammation in stroke and atherothrombosis. Cerebrovasc Dis 17 (Suppl 3):1–5

54. Elkind MS, Cheng J, Boden-Albala B, Rundek T, Thomas J, Chen H, Rabbani LE, Sacco RL (2002) Tumor necrosis factor receptor levels are associated with carotid atherosclerosis. Stroke 33:31–37

55. Ridker PM, Hennekens CH, Buring JE, Rifai N (2000) C-reactive protein and other markers of inflammation in the prediction of cardiovascular disease in women. N Engl J Med 342:836–843

56. Tanne D, Haim M, Boyko V, Goldbourt U, Reshef T, Matetzky S, Adler Y, Mekori YA, Behar S (2002) Soluble intercellular adhesion molecule-1 and risk of future ischemic stroke: a nested case-control study from the bezafibrate infarction prevention (BIP) study cohort. Stroke 33:2182–2186

57. Connolly ES Jr., Winfree CJ, Springer TA, Naka Y, Liao H, Yan SD, Stern DM, Solomon RA, Gutierrez-Ramos JC, Pinsky DJ (1996) Cerebral protection in homozygous null ICAM-1 mice after middle cerebral artery occlusion. Role of neutrophil adhesion in the pathogenesis of stroke. J Clin Invest 97:209–216

58. Connolly ES Jr., Winfree CJ, Prestigiacomo CJ, Kim SC, Choudhri TF, Hoh BL, Naka Y, Solomon RA, Pinsky DJ (1997) Exacerbation of cerebral injury in mice that express the p-selectin gene: Identification of p-selectin blockade as a new target for the treatment of stroke. Circ Res 81: 304–310

59. del Zoppo G, Ginis I, Hallenbeck JM, Iadecola C, Wang X, Feuerstein GZ (2000) Inflammation and stroke: putative role for cytokines, adhesion molecules and iNOS in brain response to ischemia. Brain Pathol 10:95–112

60. Huang J, Kim LJ, Mealey R, Marsh HC Jr., Zhang Y, Tenner AJ, Connolly ES Jr., Pinsky DJ (1999) Neuronal protection in stroke by an sLex-glycosylated complement inhibitory protein. Science 285:595–599

61. Enlimomab Acute Stroke Trial Investigators (2001) Use of anti-ICAM-1 therapy in ischemic stroke: results of the enlimomab acute stroke trial. Neurology 57:1428–1434

62. Hughes PM, Allegrini PR, Rudin M, Perry VH, Mir AK, Wiessner C (2002) Monocyte chemoattractant protein-1 deficiency is protective in a murine stroke model. J Cereb Blood Flow Metab 22:308–317

63. Iadecola C, Niwa K, Nogawa S, Zhao X, Nagayama M, Araki E, Morham S, Ross ME (2001) Reduced susceptibility to ischemic brain injury and N-methyl-D-aspartate-mediated neurotoxicity in cyclooxygenase-2-deficient mice. Proc Natl Acad Sci USA 98:1294–1299

64. Boutin H, LeFeuvre RA, Horai R, Asano M, Iwakura Y, Rothwell NJ (2001) Role of IL-1alpha and IL-1beta in ischemic brain damage. J Neurosci 21:5528–5534

65. Schielke GP, Yang GY, Shivers BD, Betz AL (1998) Reduced ischemic brain injury in interleukin-1 beta converting enzyme-deficient mice. J Cereb Blood Flow Metab 18:180–185

66. Nawashiro H, Tasaki K, Ruetzler CA, Hallenbeck JM (1997) TNF-alpha pretreatment induces protective effects against focal cerebral ischemia in mice. J Cereb Blood Flow Metab 17:483–490

67. Bruce AJ, Boling W, Kindy MS, Peschon J, Kraemer PJ, Carpenter MK, Holtsberg FW, Mattson MP (1996) Altered neuronal and microglial responses to excitotoxic and ischemic brain injury in mice lacking TNF receptors. Nat Med 2:788–794

68. Fontaine V, Mohand-Said S, Hanoteau N, Fuchs C, Pfizenmaier K, Eisel U (2002) Neurodegenerative and neuroprotective effects of tumor necrosis factor (TNF) in retinal ischemia: opposite roles of TNF receptor 1 and TNF receptor 2. J Neurosci 22:RC216

69. Zhang ZG, Zhang L, Jiang Q, Zhang R, Davies K, Powers C, Bruggen N, Chopp M (2000) VEGF enhances angiogenesis and promotes blood-brain barrier leakage in the ischemic brain. J Clin Invest 106:829–838

70. Jander S, Schroeter M, Peters O, Witte OW, Stoll G (2001) Cortical spreading depression induces proinflammatory cytokine gene expression in the rat brain. J Cereb Blood Flow Metab 21:218–225

71. Hansen AJ, Nedergaard M (1988) Brain ion homeostasis in cerebral ischemia. Neurochem Pathol 9:195–209

72. Strong AJ, Smith SE, Whittington DJ, Meldrum BS, Parsons AA, Krupinski J, Hunter AJ, Patel S, Robertson C (2000) Factors influencing the frequency of fluorescence transients as markers of peri-infarct depolarizations in focal cerebral ischemia. Stroke 31:214–222

73. Gill R, Andine P, Hillered L, Persson L, Hagberg H (1992) The effect of MK-801 on cortical spreading depression in the penumbral zone following focal ischaemia in the rat. J Cereb Blood Flow Metab 12:371–379

74. Iijima T, Mies G, Hossmann KA (1992) Repeated negative DC deflections in rat cortex following middle cerebral artery occlusion are abolished by MK-801: effect on volume of ischemic injury. J Cereb Blood Flow Metab 12:727–733

75. Busch E, Gyngell ML, Eis M, Hoehn-Berlage M, Hossmann KA (1996) Potassium-induced cortical spreading depressions during focal cerebral ischemia in rats: Contribution to lesion growth assessed by diffusion-weighted NMR and biochemical imaging. J Cereb Blood Flow Metab 16:1090–1099

76. Dijkhuizen RM, Beekwilder JP, van der Worp HB, Berkelbach van der Sprenkel JW, Tulleken KA, Nicolay K (1999) Correlation between tissue depolarizations and damage in focal ischemic rat brain. Brain Res 840:194–205

77. Hartings JA, Rolli ML, Lu XC, Tortella FC (2003) Delayed secondary phase of peri-infarct depolarizations after focal cerebral ischemia: relation to infarct growth and neuroprotection. J Neurosci 23:11602–11610

78. Tatlisumak T, Takano K, Meiler MR, Fisher M (1998) A glycine site antagonist, ZD9379, reduces number of spreading depressions and infarct size in rats with permanent middle cerebral artery occlusion. Stroke 29:190–195

79. Chen Q, Chopp M, Bodzin G, Chen H (1993) Temperature modulation of cerebral depolarization during focal cerebral ischemia in rats: correlation with ischemic injury. J Cereb Blood Flow Metab 13:389–394

80. Petty MA, Wettstein JG (1999) White matter ischaemia. Brain Res Brain Res Rev 31:58–64

81. Stys PK (1998) Anoxic and ischemic injury of myelinated axons in CNS white matter: From mechanistic concepts to therapeutics. J Cereb Blood Flow Metab 18:2–25

82. Li S, Mealing GA, Morley P, Stys PK (1999) Novel injury mechanism in anoxia and trauma of spinal cord white matter: glutamate release via reverse Na$^+$-dependent glutamate transport. J Neurosci 19:RC16

83. McDonald JW, Althomsons SP, Hyrc KL, Choi DW, Goldberg MP. (1998) Oligodendrocytes from forebrain are highly vulnerable to AMPA/kainate receptor-mediated excitotoxicity. Nat Med 4:291–297

84. Gu C, Casaccia-Bonnefil P, Srinivasan A, Chao MV (1999) Oligodendrocyte apoptosis mediated by caspase activation. J Neurosci 19:3043–3049

85. Chandler S, Coates R, Gearing A, Lury J, Wells G, Bone E (1995) Matrix metalloproteinases degrade myelin basic protein. Neurosci Lett 201:223–226

86. Rosenberg GA, Sullivan N, Esiri MM (2001) White matter damage is associated with matrix metalloproteinases in vascular dementia. Stroke 32:1162–1168

87. Stroke Progress Review Group (SPRG) (2002) Report of the Stroke Progress Review Group (SPRG) to the Director and the National Advisory Neurological Disorders and Stroke Council of the National Institute of Neurological Disorders and Stroke (NINDS), pp 1–116

88. Petty MA, Lo EH (2002) Junctional complexes of the blood–brain barrier: permeability changes in neuroinflammation. Prog Neurobiol 68:311–323

89. Yong VW, Krekoski CA, Forsyth PA, Bell R, Edwards DR (1998) Matrix metalloproteinases and diseases of the CNS. Trends Neurosci 21:75–80

90. Cuzner ML, Opdenakker G (1999) Plasminogen activators and matrix metalloproteases, mediators of extracellular proteolysis in inflammatory demyelination of the central nervous system. J Neuroimmunol 94:1–14

91. Yong VW, Power C, Forsyth P, Edwards DR (2001) Metalloproteinases in biology and pathology of the nervous system. Nat Rev Neurosci 2:502–511

92. Wang X, Mori T, Jung JC, Fini ME, Lo EH (2002) Secretion of matrix metalloproteinase-2 and -9 after mechanical trauma injury in rat cortical cultures and involvement of map kinase. J Neurotrauma 19:615–625

93. Gasche Y, Copin JC, Sugawara T, Fujimura M, Chan PH (2001) Matrix metalloproteinase inhibition prevents oxidative stress-associated blood–brain barrier disruption after transient focal cerebral ischemia. J Cereb Blood Flow Metab 21:1393–1400

94. Gu Z, Kaul M, Yan B, Kridel SJ, Cui J, Strongin A, Smith JW, Liddington RC, Lipton SA (2002) S-Nitrosylation of matrix metalloproteinases: signaling pathway to neuronal cell death. Science 297:1186–1190

95. Lee SR, Lo EH (2004) Induction of caspase-mediated cell death by matrix metalloproteinases in cerebral endothelial cells after hypoxia-reoxygenation. J Cereb Blood Flow Metab 24:720–727

96. Justicia C, Panes J, Sole S, Cervera A, Deulofeu R, Chamorro A, Planas AM (2003) Neutrophil infiltration increases matrix metalloproteinase-9 in the ischemic brain after occlusion/reperfusion of the middle cerebral artery in rats. J Cereb Blood Flow Metab 23:1430–1440

97. Campbell SJ, Finlay M, Clements JM, Wells G, Miller KM, Perry VH, Anthony DC (2004) Reduction of excitotoxicity and associated leukocyte recruitment by a broad-spectrum matrix metalloproteinase inhibitor. J Neurochem 89:1378–1386

98. Clark AW, Krekoski CA, Bou SS, Chapman KR, Edwards DR (1997) Increased gelatinase A (MMP-2) and gelatinase B (MMP-9) activities in human brain after focal ischemia. Neurosci Lett 238:53–56

99. Gasche Y, Fujimura M, Morita-Fujimura Y, Copin JC, Kawase M, Massengale J, Chan PH (1999) Early appearance of activated matrix metalloproteinase-9 after focal cerebral ischemia in mice: a possible role in blood–brain barrier dysfunction. J Cereb Blood Flow Metab 19:1020–1028

100. Heo JH, Lucero J, Abumiya T, Koziol JA, Copeland BR, del Zoppo GJ (1999) Matrix metalloproteinases increase very early during experimental focal cerebral ischemia. J Cereb Blood Flow Metab 19:624–633

101. Asahi M, Asahi K, Jung JC, del Zoppo GJ, Fini ME, Lo EH (2000) Role for matrix metalloproteinase 9 after focal cerebral ischemia: effects of gene knockout and enzyme inhibition with BB-94. J Cereb Blood Flow Metab 20:1681–1689

102. Montaner J, Alvarez-Sabin J, Molina C, Angles A, Abilleira S, Arenillas J, Gonzalez MA, Monasterio J (2001) Matrix metalloproteinase expression after human cardioembolic stroke: temporal profile and relation to neurological impairment. Stroke 32:1759–1766

103. Sumii T, Lo EH (2002) Involvement of matrix metalloproteinase in thrombolysis-associated hemorrhagic transformation after embolic focal ischemia in rats. Stroke 33:831–836

104. Abilleira S, Montaner J, Molina CA, Monasterio J, Castillo J, Alvarez-Sabin J (2003) Matrix metalloproteinase-9 concentration after spontaneous intracerebral hemorrhage. J Neurosurg 99:65–70

105. Fukuda S, Fini CA, Mabuchi T, Koziol JA, Eggleston LL Jr., del Zoppo GJ (2004) Focal cerebral ischemia induces active proteases that degrade microvascular matrix. Stroke 35:998–1004

106. Lo EH, Wang X, Cuzner ML (2002) Extracellular proteolysis in brain injury and inflammation: role for plasminogen activators and matrix metalloproteinases. J Neurosci Res 69:1–9

107. Montaner J, Rovira A, Molina CA, Arenillas JF, Ribo M, Chacon P, Monasterio J, Alvarez-Sabin J (2003) Plasmatic level of neuroinflammatory markers predict the extent of diffusion-weighted image lesions in hyperacute stroke. J Cereb Blood Flow Metab 23:1403–1407

108. Nagai N, Yamamoto S, Tsuboi T, Ihara H, Urano T, Takada Y, Terakawa S, Takada A. (2001) Tissue-type plasminogen activator is involved in the process of neuronal death induced by oxygen-glucose deprivation in culture. J Cereb Blood Flow Metab 21:631–634

109. Nicole O, Docagne F, Ali C, Margaill I, Carmeliet P, MacKenzie ET, Vivien D, Buisson A (2001) The proteolytic activity of tissue-plasminogen activator enhances NMDA receptor-mediated signaling. Nat Med 7:59–64

110. Yepes M, Sandkvist M, Wong MK, Coleman TA, Smith E, Cohan SL, Lawrence DA (2000) Neuroserpin reduces cerebral infarct volume and protects neurons from ischemia-induced apoptosis. Blood 96:569–576

111. Wang YF, Tsirka SE, Strickland S, Stieg PE, Soriano SG, Lipton SA (1998) Tissue plasminogen activator (tPA) increases neuronal damage after focal cerebral ischemia in wild-type and tPA-deficient mice. Nat Med 4:228–231

112. Tabrizi P, Wang L, Seeds N, McComb JG, Yamada S, Griffin JH, Carmeliet P, Weiss MH, Zlokovic BV (1999) Tissue plasminogen activator (tPA) deficiency exacerbates cerebrovascular fibrin deposition and brain injury in a murine stroke model: Studies in tPA-deficient mice and wild-type mice on a matched genetic background. Arterioscler Thromb Vasc Biol 19:2801–2806

113. Ginsberg MD (1999) On ischemic brain injury in genetically altered mice. Arterioscler Thromb Vasc Biol 19: 2581–2583

114. Wang X, Lee SR, Arai K, Tsuji K, Rebeck GW, Lo EH (2003) Lipoprotein receptor-mediated induction of matrix metalloproteinase by tissue plasminogen activator. Nat Med 9:1313–1317

115. Anonymous (1995) Tissue plasminogen activator for acute ischemic stroke. The national institute of neurological disorders and stroke rt-PA stroke study group. N Engl J Med 333:1581–1587

116. The RANTTAS Investigators (1996) A randomized trial of tirilazad mesylate in patients with acute stroke (RANTTAS). Stroke 27:1453–1458

117. (1992) Clinical trial of nimodipine in acute ischemic stroke. The American Nimodipine Study Group. Stroke 23:3–8

118. Wahlgren NG, Ranasinha KW, Rosolacci T, Franke CL, van Erven PM, Ashwood T, Claesson L (1999) Clomethiazole acute stroke study (CLASS): results of a randomized, controlled trial of clomethiazole versus placebo in 1360 acute stroke patients. Stroke 30:21–28

119. Lyden P, Shuaib A, Ng K, Levin K, Atkinson RP, Rajput A, Wechsler L, Ashwood T, Claesson L, Odergren T, Salazar-Grueso E (2002) Clomethiazole acute stroke study in ischemic stroke (class-I): final results. Stroke 33:122–128

120. Diener HC, Cortens M, Ford G, Grotta J, Hacke W, Kaste M, Koudstaal PJ, Wessel T (2000) Lubeluzole in acute ischemic stroke treatment: a double-blind study with an 8-hour inclusion window comparing a 10-mg daily dose of lubeluzole with placebo. Stroke 31:2543–2551

121. Davis SM, Lees KR, Albers GW, Diener HC, Markabi S, Karlsson G, Norris J (2000) Selfotel in acute ischemic stroke: possible neurotoxic effects of an NMDA antagonist. Stroke 31:347–354

122. Albers GW, Goldstein LB, Hall D, Lesko LM (2001) Aptiganel hydrochloride in acute ischemic stroke: a randomized controlled trial. J Am Med Assoc 286:2673–2682

123. Lees KR, Asplund K, Carolei A, Davis SM, Diener HC, Kaste M, Orgogozo JM, Whitehead J (2000) Glycine antagonist (gavestinel) in neuroprotection (gain international) in patients with acute stroke: a randomised controlled trial. Gain international investigators. Lancet 355:1949–1954

124. Sacco RL, DeRosa JT, Haley EC Jr., Levin B, Ordronneau P, Phillips SJ, Rundek T, Snipes RG, Thompson JL (2001) Glycine antagonist in neuroprotection for patients with acute stroke: GAIN Americas: a randomized controlled trial. J Am Med Assoc 285:1719–1728

125. Del Zoppo GJ (1995) Why do all drugs work in animals but none in stroke patients? 1. Drugs promoting cerebral blood flow. J Intern Med 237:79–88

126. Grotta J (1995) Why do all drugs work in animals but none in stroke patients? 2. Neuroprotective therapy. J Intern Med 237:89–94

127. Kidwell CS, Liebeskind DS, Starkman S, Saver JL (2001) Trends in acute ischemic stroke trials through the 20th century. Stroke 32:1349–1359

128. Lo EH, Singhal AB, Torchilin VP, Abbott NJ (2001) Drug delivery to damaged brain. Brain Res Brain Res Rev 38:140–148

129. Sorensen AG, Copen WA, Ostergaard L, Buonanno FS, Gonzalez RG, Rordorf G, Rosen BR, Schwamm LH, Weisskoff RM, Koroshetz WJ (1999) Hyperacute stroke: simultaneous measurement of relative cerebral blood volume, relative cerebral blood flow, and mean tissue transit time. Radiology 210:519–527

130. Fisher M (2003) Recommendations for advancing development of acute stroke therapies: stroke therapy academic industry roundtable 3. Stroke 34:1539–1546

131. Muir KW, Lees KR, Ford I, Davis S (2004) Magnesium for acute stroke (intravenous magnesium efficacy in stroke trial): randomised controlled trial. Lancet 363:439–445

132. Yamaguchi T, Sano K, Takakura K, Saito I, Shinohara Y, Asano T, Yasuhara H (1998) Ebselen in acute ischemic stroke: a placebo-controlled, double-blind clinical trial. Ebselen Study Group. Stroke 29:12–17

133. Lees KR, Barer D, Ford GA, Hacke W, Kostulas V, Sharma AK, Odergren T (2003) Tolerability of NXY-059 at higher target concentrations in patients with acute stroke. Stroke 34:482–487

134. Hossmann KA (1994) Viability thresholds and the penumbra of focal ischemia. Ann Neurol 36:557–565

135. Baron JC (2001) Perfusion thresholds in human cerebral ischemia: historical perspective and therapeutic implications. Cerebrovasc Dis 11 (Suppl. 1):2–8

136. Ginsberg MD, Pulsinelli WA (1994) The ischemic penumbra, injury thresholds, and the therapeutic window for acute stroke. Ann Neurol 36:553–554

137. Markus R, Reutens DC, Kazui S, Read S, Wright P, Pearce DC, Tochon-Danguy HJ, Sachinidis JI, Donnan GA (2004) Hypoxic tissue in ischaemic stroke: persistence and clinical consequences of spontaneous survival. Brain 127:1427–1436

138. Reed SD, Cramer SC, Blough DK, Meyer K, Jarvik JG (2001) Treatment with tissue plasminogen activator and inpatient mortality rates for patients with ischemic stroke treated in community hospitals. Stroke 32:1832–1840

139. Baron JC (2001) Mapping the ischaemic penumbra with PET: a new approach. Brain 124:2–4

140. Heiss WD, Kracht LW, Thiel A, Grond M, Pawlik G (2001) Penumbral probability thresholds of cortical flumazenil binding and blood flow predicting tissue outcome in patients with cerebral ischaemia. Brain 124:20–29

141. Baird AE, Warach S (1998) Magnetic resonance imaging of acute stroke. J Cereb Blood Flow Metab 18:583–609

142. Kidwell CS, Alger JR, Saver JL (2003) Beyond mismatch: evolving paradigms in imaging the ischemic penumbra with multimodal magnetic resonance imaging. Stroke 34:2729–2735

143. Schlaug G, Benfield A, Baird AE, Siewert B, Lovblad KO, Parker RA, Edelman RR, Warach S (1999) The ischemic penumbra: operationally defined by diffusion and perfusion MRI. Neurology 53:1528–1537

144. Schaefer PW, Ozsunar Y, He J, Hamberg LM, Hunter GJ, Sorensen AG, Koroshetz WJ, Gonzalez RG (2003) Assessing tissue viability with MR diffusion and perfusion imaging. Am J Neuroradiol 24:436–443

145. Lev MH, Segal AZ, Farkas J, Hossain ST, Putman C, Hunter GJ, Budzik R, Harris GJ, Buonanno FS, Ezzeddine MA, Chang Y, Koroshetz WJ, Gonzalez RG, Schwamm LH (2001) Utility of perfusion-weighted CT imaging in acute middle cerebral artery stroke treated with intra-arterial thrombolysis: prediction of final infarct volume and clinical outcome. Stroke 32:2021–2028

146. Wintermark M, Reichhart M, Thiran JP, Maeder P, Chalaron M, Schnyder P, Bogousslavsky J, Meuli R (2002) Prognostic accuracy of cerebral blood flow measurement by perfusion computed tomography, at the time of emergency room admission, in acute stroke patients. Ann Neurol 51:417–432

147. Wintermark M, Reichhart M, Cuisenaire O, Maeder P, Thiran JP, Schnyder P, Bogousslavsky J, Meuli R (2002) Comparison of admission perfusion computed tomography and qualitative diffusion- and perfusion-weighted magnetic resonance imaging in acute stroke patients. Stroke 33:2025–2031

148. Hunter GJ, Hamberg LM, Ponzo JA, Huang-Hellinger FR, Morris PP, Rabinov J, Farkas J, Lev MH, Schaefer PW, Ogilvy CS, Schwamm L, Buonanno FS, Koroshetz WJ, Wolf GL, Gonzalez RG (1998) Assessment of cerebral perfusion and arterial anatomy in hyperacute stroke with three-dimensional functional CT: early clinical results. Am J Neuroradiol 19:29–37

149. Jovin TG, Yonas H, Gebel JM, Kanal E, Chang YF, Grahovac SZ, Goldstein S, Wechsler LR (2003) The cortical ischemic core and not the consistently present penumbra is a determinant of clinical outcome in acute middle cerebral artery occlusion. Stroke 34:2426–2433

150. Hacke W, Albers G, Al-Rawi Y, Bogousslavsky J, Davalos A, Eliasziw M, Fischer M, Furlan A, Kaste M, Lees KR, Soehngen M, Warach S (2005) The desmoteplase in acute ischemic stroke trial (DIAS). A phase II MRI-based 9-hour window acute stroke thrombolysis trial with intravenous desmoteplase. Stroke (in press)

151. Nogawa S, Forster C, Zhang F, Nagayama M, Ross ME, Iadecola C. (1998) Interaction between inducible nitric oxide synthase and cyclooxygenase-2 after cerebral ischemia. Proc Natl Acad Sci USA 95:10966–10971

152. Lyden PD, Jackson-Friedman C, Shin C, Hassid S (2000) Synergistic combinatorial stroke therapy: a quantal bioassay of a GABA agonist and a glutamate antagonist. Exp Neurol 163:477–489

153. Barth A, Barth L, Newell DW (1996) Combination therapy with MK-801 and alpha-phenyl-tert-butyl-nitrone enhances protection against ischemic neuronal damage in organotypic hippocampal slice cultures. Exp Neurol 141:330–336

154. Onal MZ, Li F, Tatlisumak T, Locke KW, Sandage BW Jr., Fisher M (1997) Synergistic effects of citicoline and MK-801 in temporary experimental focal ischemia in rats. Stroke 28:1060–1065

155. Du C, Hu R, Csernansky CA, Liu XZ, Hsu CY, Choi DW (1996) Additive neuroprotective effects of dextrorphan and cycloheximide in rats subjected to transient focal cerebral ischemia. Brain Res 718:233–236

156. Ma J, Endres M, Moskowitz MA (1998) Synergistic effects of caspase inhibitors and MK-801 in brain injury after transient focal cerebral ischaemia in mice. Br J Pharmacol 124:756–762

157. Barth A, Barth L, Morrison RS, Newell DW (1996) bFGF enhances the protective effects of MK-801 against ischemic neuronal injury in vitro. Neuroreport 7:1461–1464

158. Schmid-Elsaesser R, Hungerhuber E, Zausinger S, Baethmann A, Reulen HJ (1999) Neuroprotective efficacy of combination therapy with two different antioxidants in rats subjected to transient focal ischemia. Brain Res 816:471–479

159. Schabitz WR, Li F, Irie K, Sandage BW Jr., Locke KW, Fisher M (1999) Synergistic effects of a combination of low-dose basic fibroblast growth factor and citicoline after temporary experimental focal ischemia. Stroke 30:427–431; discussion 431–422

160. Ma J, Qiu J, Hirt L, Dalkara T, Moskowitz MA (2001) Synergistic protective effect of caspase inhibitors and bFGF against brain injury induced by transient focal ischaemia. Br J Pharmacol 133:345–350

161. Hacke W, Brott T, Caplan L, Meier D, Fieschi C, von Kummer R, Donnan G, Heiss WD, Wahlgren NG, Spranger M, Boysen G, Marler JR (1999) Thrombolysis in acute ischemic stroke: controlled trials and clinical experience. Neurology 53:S3–14

162. Garcia JH, Liu KF, Ho KL (1995) Neuronal necrosis after middle cerebral artery occlusion in Wistar rats progresses at different time intervals in the caudoputamen and the cortex. Stroke 26:636–642; discussion 643

163. Hacke W, Donnan G, Fieschi C, Kaste M, von Kummer R, Broderick JP, Brott T, Frankel M, Grotta JC, Haley EC Jr., Kwiatkowski T, Levine SR, Lewandowski C, Lu M, Lyden P, Marler JR, Patel S, Tilley BC, Albers G (2004) Association of outcome with early stroke treatment: pooled analysis of ATLANTIS, ECASS, and NINDS rt-PA stroke trials. Lancet 363:768–774

164. Asahi M, Asahi K, Wang X, Lo EH (2000) Reduction of tissue plasminogen activator-induced hemorrhage and brain injury by free radical spin trapping after embolic focal cerebral ischemia in rats. J Cereb Blood Flow Metab 20:452–457

165. Meden P, Overgaard K, Sereghy T, Boysen G (1993) Enhancing the efficacy of thrombolysis by AMPA receptor blockade with NBQX in a rat embolic stroke model. J Neurol Sci 119:209–216

166. Zivin JA, Mazzarella V (1991) Tissue plasminogen activator plus glutamate antagonist improves outcome after embolic stroke. Arch Neurol 48:1235–1238

167. Andersen M, Overgaard K, Meden P, Boysen G, Choi SC (1999) Effects of citicoline combined with thrombolytic therapy in a rat embolic stroke model. Stroke 30:1464–1471

168. Yang Y, Li Q, Shuaib A (2000) Enhanced neuroprotection and reduced hemorrhagic incidence in focal cerebral ischemia of rat by low dose combination therapy of urokinase and topiramate. Neuropharmacology 39:881–888

169. Bowes MP, Rothlein R, Fagan SC, Zivin JA (1995) Monoclonal antibodies preventing leukocyte activation reduce experimental neurologic injury and enhance efficacy of thrombolytic therapy. Neurology 45:815–819

170. Shuaib A, Yang Y, Nakada MT, Li Q, Yang T (2002) Glycoprotein IIB/IIIA antagonist, murine 7e3 f(ab') 2, and tissue plasminogen activator in focal ischemia: evaluation of efficacy and risk of hemorrhage with combination therapy. J Cereb Blood Flow Metab 22:215–222

171. Lyden P, Jacoby M, Schim J, Albers G, Mazzeo P, Ashwood T, Nordlund A, Odergren T (2001) The clomethiazole acute stroke study in tissue-type plasminogen activator-treated stroke (class-T): final results. Neurology 57:1199–1205

172. Grotta J (2001) Combination therapy stroke trial: recombinant tissue-type plasminogen activator with/without lubeluzole. Cerebrovasc Dis 12:258–263

173. Kitagawa K, Matsumoto M, Tagaya M, Hata R, Ueda H, Niinobe M, Handa N, Fukunaga R, Kimura K, Mikoshiba K (1990) "Ischemic tolerance" phenomenon found in the brain. Brain Res 528:21–24

174. Kawahara N, Wang Y, Mukasa A, Furuya K, Shimizu T, Hamakubo T, Aburatani H, Kodama T, Kirino T (2004) Genome-wide gene expression analysis for induced ischemic tolerance and delayed neuronal death following transient global ischemia in rats. J Cereb Blood Flow Metab 24:212–223

175. Kirino T (2002) Ischemic tolerance. J Cereb Blood Flow Metab 22:1283–1296

176. Wegener S, Gottschalk B, Jovanovic V, Knab R, Fiebach JB, Schellinger PD, Kucinski T, Jungehulsing GJ, Brunecker P, Muller B, Banasik A, Amberger N, Wernecke KD, Siebler M, Rother J, Villringer A, Weih M (2004) Transient ischemic attacks before ischemic stroke: preconditioning the human brain? A multicenter magnetic resonance imaging study. Stroke 35:616–621

177. Weih M, Kallenberg K, Bergk A, Dirnagl U, Harms L, Wernecke KD, Einhaupl KM (1999) Attenuated stroke severity after prodromal TIA: a role for ischemic tolerance in the brain? Stroke 30:1851–1854

178. Moncayo J, de Freitas GR, Bogousslavsky J, Altieri M, van Melle G (2000) Do transient ischemic attacks have a neuroprotective effect? Neurology 54:2089–2094

179. Dirnagl U, Simon RP, Hallenbeck JM (2003) Ischemic tolerance and endogenous neuroprotection. Trends Neurosci 26:248–254

180. Lin JY, Chung SY, Lin MC, Cheng FC (2002) Effects of magnesium sulfate on energy metabolites and glutamate in the cortex during focal cerebral ischemia and reperfusion in the gerbil monitored by a dual-probe microdialysis technique. Life Sci 71:803–811

181. Nowak L, Bregestovski P, Ascher P, Herbet A, Prochiantz A (1984) Magnesium gates glutamate-activated channels in mouse central neurones. Nature 307:462–465

182. Chi OZ, Pollak P, Weiss HR (1990) Effects of magnesium sulfate and nifedipine on regional cerebral blood flow during middle cerebral artery ligation in the rat. Arch Int Pharmacodyn Ther 304:196–205

183. Izumi Y, Roussel S, Pinard E, Seylaz J (1991) Reduction of infarct volume by magnesium after middle cerebral artery occlusion in rats. J Cereb Blood Flow Metab 11:1025–1030

184. Marinov MB, Harbaugh KS, Hoopes PJ, Pikus HJ, Harbaugh RE (1996) Neuroprotective effects of preischemia intraarterial magnesium sulfate in reversible focal cerebral ischemia. J Neurosurg 85:117–124

185. Muir KW, Lees KR (1995) A randomized, double-blind, placebo-controlled pilot trial of intravenous magnesium sulfate in acute stroke. Stroke 26:1183–1188

186. Saver JL, Kidwell C, Eckstein M, Starkman S (2004) Pre-hospital neuroprotective therapy for acute stroke: results of the field administration of stroke therapy-magnesium (fast-Mag) pilot trial. Stroke 35:E106–E108

187. Belayev L, Pinard E, Nallet H, Seylaz J, Liu Y, Riyamongkol P, Zhao W, Busto R, Ginsberg MD (2002) Albumin therapy of transient focal cerebral ischemia: in vivo analysis of dynamic microvascular responses. Stroke 33:1077–1084

188. Belayev L, Liu Y, Zhao W, Busto R, Ginsberg MD (2001) Human albumin therapy of acute ischemic stroke: marked neuroprotective efficacy at moderate doses and with a broad therapeutic window. Stroke 32:553–560

189. Astrup J, Sorensen PM, Sorensen HR (1981) Inhibition of cerebral oxygen and glucose consumption in the dog by hypothermia, pentobarbital, and lidocaine. Anesthesiology 55:263–268

190. Cardell M, Boris-Moller F, Wieloch T (1991) Hypothermia prevents the ischemia-induced translocation and inhibition of protein kinase C in the rat striatum. J Neurochem 57:1814–1817

191. Globus MY, Busto R, Lin B, Schnippering H, Ginsberg MD (1995) Detection of free radical activity during transient global ischemia and recirculation: effects of intraischemic brain temperature modulation. J Neurochem 65:1250–1256

192. Krieger DW, Yenari MA (2004) Therapeutic hypothermia for acute ischemic stroke: what do laboratory studies teach us? Stroke 35:1482–1489

193. Han HS, Karabiyikoglu M, Kelly S, Sobel RA, Yenari MA (2003) Mild hypothermia inhibits nuclear factor-kappaB translocation in experimental stroke. J Cereb Blood Flow Metab 23:589–598

194. Wang GJ, Deng HY, Maier CM, Sun GH, Yenari MA (2002) Mild hypothermia reduces ICAM-1 expression, neutrophil infiltration and microglia/monocyte accumulation following experimental stroke. Neuroscience 114:1081–1090

195. Yenari MA, Iwayama S, Cheng D, Sun GH, Fujimura M, Morita-Fujimura Y, Chan PH, Steinberg GK (2002) Mild hypothermia attenuates cytochrome C release but does not alter bcl-2 expression or caspase activation after experimental stroke. J Cereb Blood Flow Metab 22:29–38

196. Prosser CL (1973) Temperature. In: Prosser CL (ed) Comparative animal physiology. Saunders, Philadelphia, Pa., pp 362–428

197. Markarian GZ, Lee JH, Stein DJ, Hong SC (1996) Mild hypothermia: therapeutic window after experimental cerebral ischemia. Neurosurgery 38:542–550; discussion 551

198. Welsh FA, Harris VA (1991) Postischemic hypothermia fails to reduce ischemic injury in gerbil hippocampus. J Cereb Blood Flow Metab 11:617–620

199. Ginsberg MD (1997) Hypothermic neuroprotection in cerebral ischemia. In: Welch KMA, Caplan LR, Reis DJ, Siesjo BK, Weir B (eds) Primer on cerebrovascular diseases. Academic Press, San Diego, Calif., pp 272–275

200. Corbett D, Hamilton M, Colbourne F (2000) Persistent neuroprotection with prolonged postischemic hypothermia in adult rats subjected to transient middle cerebral artery occlusion. Exp Neurol 163:200–206

201. The Hypothermia after Cardiac Arrest Study Group (2002) Mild therapeutic hypothermia to improve the neurologic outcome after cardiac arrest. N Engl J Med 346:549–556

202. Bernard SA, Gray TW, Buist MD, Jones BM, Silvester W, Gutteridge G, Smith K (2002) Treatment of comatose survivors of out-of-hospital cardiac arrest with induced hypothermia. N Engl J Med 346:557–563

203. Schwab S, Schwarz S, Spranger M, Keller E, Bertram M, Hacke W (1998) Moderate hypothermia in the treatment of patients with severe middle cerebral artery infarction. Stroke 29:2461–2466

204. Krieger DW, De Georgia MA, Abou-Chebl A, Andrefsky JC, Sila CA, Katzan IL, Mayberg MR, Furlan AJ (2001) Cooling for acute ischemic brain damage (cool aid): an open pilot study of induced hypothermia in acute ischemic stroke. Stroke 32:1847–1854

205. Kammersgaard LP, Rasmussen BH, Jorgensen HS, Reith J, Weber U, Olsen TS (2000) Feasibility and safety of inducing modest hypothermia in awake patients with acute stroke through surface cooling: a case–control study: The Copenhagen Stroke Study. Stroke 31:2251–2256

206. Hayashi S, Nehls DG, Kieck CF, Vielma J, DeGirolami U, Crowell RM (1984) Beneficial effects of induced hypertension on experimental stroke in awake monkeys. J Neurosurg 60:151–157

207. Cole DJ, Matsumura JS, Drummond JC, Schell RM (1992) Focal cerebral ischemia in rats: effects of induced hypertension, during reperfusion, on CBF. J Cereb Blood Flow Metab 12:64–69

208. Fischberg GM, Lozano E, Rajamani K, Ameriso S, Fisher MJ (2000) Stroke precipitated by moderate blood pressure reduction. J Emerg Med 19:339–346

209. Kassell NF, Peerless SJ, Durward QJ, Beck DW, Drake CG, Adams HP (1982) Treatment of ischemic deficits from vasospasm with intravascular volume expansion and induced arterial hypertension. Neurosurgery 11:337–343

210. Rordorf G, Cramer SC, Efird JT, Schwamm LH, Buonanno F, Koroshetz WJ (1997) Pharmacological elevation of blood pressure in acute stroke. Clinical effects and safety. Stroke 28:2133–2138

211. Rordorf G, Koroshetz WJ, Ezzeddine MA, Segal AZ, Buonanno FS (2001) A pilot study of drug-induced hypertension for treatment of acute stroke. Neurology 56:1210–1213

212. Hillis AE, Ulatowski JA, Barker PB, Torbey M, Ziai W, Beauchamp NJ, Oh S, Wityk RJ (2003) A pilot randomized trial of induced blood pressure elevation: effects on function and focal perfusion in acute and subacute stroke. Cerebrovasc Dis 16:236–246

213. Hillis AE, Wityk RJ, Beauchamp NJ, Ulatowski JA, Jacobs MA, Barker PB (2004) Perfusion-weighted MRI as a marker of response to treatment in acute and subacute stroke. Neuroradiology 46:31–39

214. Hillis AE, Barker PB, Beauchamp NJ, Winters BD, Mirski M, Wityk RJ (2001) Restoring blood pressure reperfused Wernicke's area and improved language. Neurology 56:670–672

215. Lo EH, Dalkara T, Moskowitz MA (2003) Mechanisms, challenges and opportunities in stroke. Nat Rev Neurosci 4:399–415

216. Yin W, Badr AE, Mychaskiw G, Zhang JH (2002) Down regulation of cox-2 is involved in hyperbaric oxygen treatment in a rat transient focal cerebral ischemia model. Brain Res 926:165–171

217. Yin D, Zhou C, Kusaka I, Calvert JW, Parent AD, Nanda A, Zhang JH (2003) Inhibition of apoptosis by hyperbaric oxygen in a rat focal cerebral ischemic model. J Cereb Blood Flow Metab 23:855–864

218. Wada K, Miyazawa T, Nomura N, Tsuzuki N, Nawashiro H, Shima K (2001) Preferential conditions for and possible mechanisms of induction of ischemic tolerance by repeated hyperbaric oxygenation in gerbil hippocampus. Neurosurgery 49:160–166; discussion 166–167

219. Menzel M, Doppenberg EM, Zauner A, Soukup J, Reinert MM, Bullock R (1999) Increased inspired oxygen concentration as a factor in improved brain tissue oxygenation and tissue lactate levels after severe human head injury. J Neurosurg 91:1–10

220. Rockswold SB, Rockswold GL, Vargo JM, Erickson CA, Sutton RL, Bergman TA, Biros MH (2001) Effects of hyperbaric oxygenation therapy on cerebral metabolism and intracranial pressure in severely brain injured patients. J Neurosurg 94:403–411

221. Zhang JH, Singhal AB, Toole JF (2003) Oxygen therapy in ischemic stroke. Stroke 34:E152–E153, author reply E153–E155

222. Badr AE, Yin W, Mychaskiw G, Zhang JH (2001) Effect of hyperbaric oxygen on striatal metabolites: a microdialysis study in awake freely moving rats after MCA occlusion. Brain Res 916:85–90

223. Ingvar HD, Lassen NA (1965) Treatment of focal cerebral ischemia with hyperbaric oxygen. Acta Neurol Scand 41:92–95

224. Badr AE, Yin W, Mychaskiw G, Zhang JH (2001) Dual effect of HBO on cerebral infarction in MCAO rats. Am J Physiol 280:R766–R770

225. Burt JT, Kapp JP, Smith RR (1987) Hyperbaric oxygen and cerebral infarction in the gerbil. Surg Neurol 28:265–268

226. Lou M, Eschenfelder CC, Herdegen T, Brecht S, Deuschl G (2004) Therapeutic window for use of hyperbaric oxygenation in focal transient ischemia in rats. Stroke 35:578–583

227. Veltkamp R, Warner DS, Domoki F, Brinkhous AD, Toole JF, Busija DW (2000) Hyperbaric oxygen decreases infarct size and behavioral deficit after transient focal cerebral ischemia in rats. Brain Res 853:68–73

228. Sunami K, Takeda Y, Hashimoto M, Hirakawa M (2000) Hyperbaric oxygen reduces infarct volume in rats by increasing oxygen supply to the ischemic periphery. Crit Care Med 28:2831–2836

229. Schabitz WR, Schade H, Heiland S, Kollmar R, Bardutzky J, Henninger N, Muller H, Carl U, Toyokuni S, Sommer C, Schwab S (2004 Neuroprotection by hyperbaric oxygenation after experimental focal cerebral ischemia monitored by MR-imaging. Stroke

230. Roos JA, Jackson-Friedman C, Lyden P (1998) Effects of hyperbaric oxygen on neurologic outcome for cerebral ischemia in rats. Acad Emerg Med 5:18–24

231. Kawamura S, Yasui N, Shirasawa M, Fukasawa H (1990) Therapeutic effects of hyperbaric oxygenation on acute focal cerebral ischemia in rats. Surg Neurol 34:101–106

232. Weinstein PR, Anderson GG, Telles DA (1987) Results of hyperbaric oxygen therapy during temporary middle cerebral artery occlusion in unanesthetized cats. Neurosurgery 20:518–524

233. Anderson DC, Bottini AG, Jagiella WM, Westphal B, Ford S, Rockswold GL, Loewenson RB (1991) A pilot study of hyperbaric oxygen in the treatment of human stroke. Stroke 22:1137–1142

234. Nighoghossian N, Trouillas P, Adeleine P, Salord F (1995) Hyperbaric oxygen in the treatment of acute ischemic stroke. A double-blind pilot study. Stroke 26:1369–1372

235. Rusyniak DE, Kirk MA, May JD, Kao LW, Brizendine EJ, Welch JL, Cordell WH, Alonso RJ (2003) Hyperbaric oxygen therapy in acute ischemic stroke: results of the hyperbaric oxygen in acute ischemic stroke trial pilot study. Stroke 34:571–574

236. Flynn EP, Auer RN (2002) Eubaric hyperoxemia and experimental cerebral infarction. Ann Neurol 52:566–572

237. Singhal AB, Wang X, Sumii T, Mori T, Lo EH (2002) Effects of normobaric hyperoxia in a rat model of focal cerebral ischemia-reperfusion. J Cereb Blood Flow Metab 22:861–868

238. Singhal AB, Dijkhuizen RM, Rosen BR, Lo EH (2002) Normobaric hyperoxia reduces MRI diffusion abnormalities and infarct size in experimental stroke. Neurology 58:945–952

239. Singhal AB, Benner T, Roccatagliata L, Schaefer PW, Koroshetz WJ, Buonanno FS, Lo EH, Gonzalez RG, Sorensen AG (2004) Normobaric oxygen therapy in hyperacute human stroke: attenuation of DWI abnormalities and improved NIHSS scores (abstract). Stroke 35:293

240. Singhal AB, Ratai E, Benner T, Koroshetz WJ, Roccatagliata L, Lopez C, Schaefer P, Lo EH, Gonzalez RG, Sorensen AG (2004) Normobaric hyperoxia in hyperacute stroke: serial NIHSS scores, diffusion-perfusion MRI and MR-spectroscopy (abstract). Neurology 62:464

241. Liu S, Shi H, Liu W, Furuichi T, Timmins GS, Liu KJ (2004) Interstitial pO_2 in ischemic penumbra and core are differentially affected following transient focal cerebral ischemia in rats. J Cereb Blood Flow Metab 24:343–349

242. Watson BD, Busto R, Goldberg WJ, Santiso M, Yoshida S, Ginsberg MD (1984) Lipid peroxidation in vivo induced by reversible global ischemia in rat brain. J Neurochem 42:268–274

243. Mickel HS, Vaishnav YN, Kempski O, von Lubitz D, Weiss JF, Feuerstein G (1987) Breathing 100% oxygen after global brain ischemia in mongolian gerbils results in increased lipid peroxidation and increased mortality. Stroke 18:426–430

244. Dubinsky JM, Kristal BS, Elizondo-Fournier M (1995) An obligate role for oxygen in the early stages of glutamate-induced, delayed neuronal death. J Neurosci 15:7071–7078

245. PROGRESS Collaborative Group (2001) Randomised trial of a perindopril-based blood-pressure-lowering regimen among 6,105 individuals with previous stroke or transient ischaemic attack. Lancet 358:1033–1041

246. Chapman N, Huxley R, Anderson C, Bousser MG, Chalmers J, Colman S, Davis S, Donnan G, MacMahon S, Neal B, Warlow C, Woodward M (2004) Effects of a perindopril-based blood pressure-lowering regimen on the risk of recurrent stroke according to stroke subtype and medical history: the progress trial. Stroke 35:116–121

247. Heart Protection Study Collaborative Group (2002) MRC/BHF heart protection study of cholesterol lowering with simvastatin in 20,536 high-risk individuals: a randomised placebo-controlled trial. Lancet 360:7–22

248. Hope Study and Micro-Hope Substudy Group (2000) Effects of ramipril on cardiovascular and microvascular outcomes in people with diabetes mellitus: results of the Hope study and micro-Hope substudy. Heart outcomes prevention evaluation study investigators. Lancet 355: 253–259

249. Laufs U, La Fata V, Plutzky J, Liao JK (1998) Upregulation of endothelial nitric oxide synthase by HMG CoA reductase inhibitors. Circulation 97:1129–1135

250. Yamada M, Huang Z, Dalkara T, Endres M, Laufs U, Waeber C, Huang PL, Liao JK, Moskowitz MA (2000) Endothelial nitric oxide synthase-dependent cerebral blood flow augmentation by L-arginine after chronic statin treatment. J Cereb Blood Flow Metab 20:709–717

251. Endres M, Laufs U, Huang Z, Nakamura T, Huang P, Moskowitz MA, Liao JK (1998) Stroke protection by 3-hydroxy-3-methylglutaryl (HMG)-CoA reductase inhibitors mediated by endothelial nitric oxide synthase. Proc Natl Acad Sci USA 95:8880–8885

Causes of Ischemic Stroke

W.J. Koroshetz, R.G. González

2.1 Introduction

Ischemic stroke occurs due to a multitude of underlying pathologic processes. The brain is such an exquisite reporting system that infarcts below the size that cause clinical signs in other organ systems can cause major disability if they affect brain. About 85 % of all strokes are due to ischemia, and in the majority of ischemic stroke the mechanism responsible is understood (Fig. 2.1). An illustration of the causes of the majority of ischemic strokes is shown in Fig. 2.2, including atherosclerotic, cerebrovascular, cardiogenic, and lacunar (penetrating vessel) mechanisms. However, in about 30 % of cases, the underlying causes are not known and these are termed cryptogenic strokes. This chapter reviews the pathways that lead to ischemic stroke.

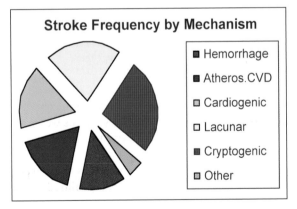

Stroke Frequency by Mechanism

- Hemorrhage
- Atheros. CVD
- Cardiogenic
- Lacunar
- Cryptogenic
- Other

Figure 2.1

Stroke frequency by mechanism. (*CVD* Cardiovascular disease)

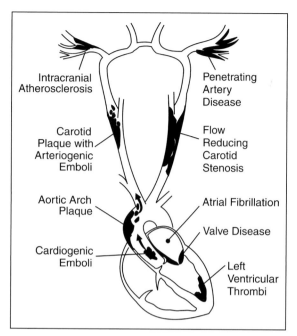

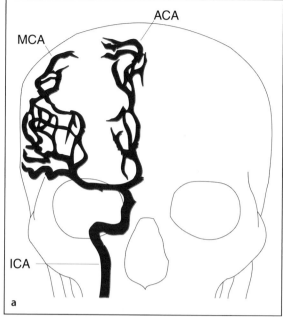

Figure 2.2

The most frequent sites of arterial and cardiac abnormalities causing ischemic stroke. Adapted from Albers GW, Amarenco P, Easton JD, Sacco RL, Teal P (2004) Antithrombotic and thrombolytic therapy for ischemic stroke: the Seventh ACCP Conference on Antithrombotic and Thrombolytic Therapy. Chest 126 (Suppl 3): 483S–512S

2.2 Key Concept: Core and Penumbra

Before embarking on a discussion of the causes of ischemic stroke, it is useful to consider the concepts of infarct core and penumbra. These terms were initially given specific scientific definitions. As applied in the clinic, their definitions have become operational, with the core generally defined as that part of the ischemic region that is irreversibly injured, while the penumbra is the area of brain that is underperfused and is in danger of infarcting. These are useful concepts for several reasons. If they can be identified in the acute ischemic stroke patient they provide prognostic information, and may help guide the

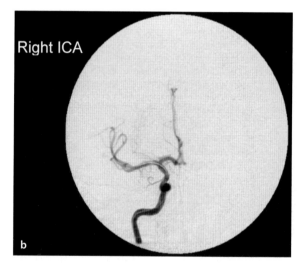

Figure 2.3 a, b

a Internal carotid artery feeds the middle cerebral artery (*MCA*) and anterior cerebral artery (*ACA*). b Right internal carotid artery (*ICA*)

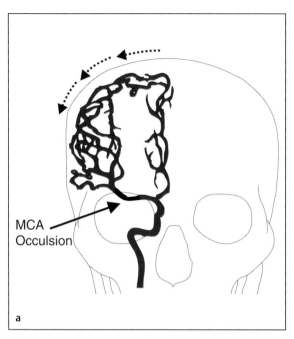

a

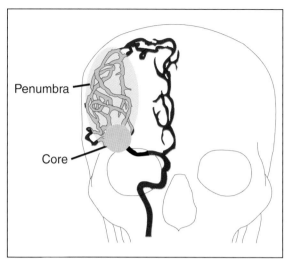

Figure 2.5

Core and penumbra after MCA occlusion.

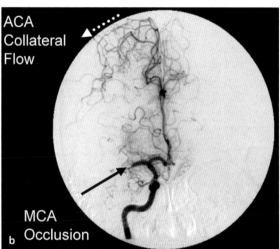

Figure 2.4 a, b

a ACA collateral flow after MCA occlusion. b ACA collateral flow

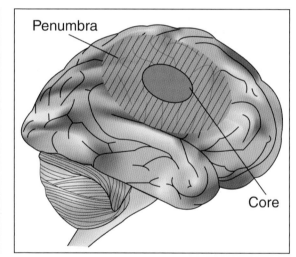

Figure 2.6

Penumbra/core

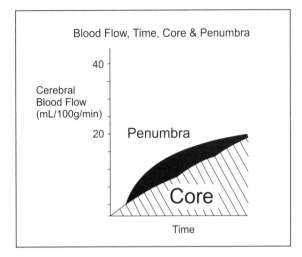

Blood Flow, Time, Core & Penumbra

Cerebral Blood Flow (mL/100g/min)

40

20

Penumbra

Core

Time

Figure 2.7

Blood flow, time, core and penumbra

patient's management. Importantly, it is now clear that neuroimaging can provide excellent estimates of the core and the penumbra in individual patients.

To illustrate the core/penumbra concept, let us consider the hypothetical case of an embolus to the main stem portion (M1) of the middle cerebral artery (MCA). The MCA along with the anterior cerebral artery (ACA) arise from the internal carotid artery (ICA) at the base of the frontal lobe (Fig. 2.3). When an embolus lodges in the M1 segment of the MCA, the MCA territory of the brain becomes underperfused (Fig. 2.4). However, in many cases the collateral circulation from the ACA and posterior cerebral artery can compensate to some degree. The amount of collateral flow determines the size of the core and the penumbra (Figs. 2.5, 2.6). However, it is critical to understand that both the core and penumbra are dynamic entities that depend on the complex physiology that is playing out in the acutely ischemic brain. If the occlusion is not removed, the core size usually increases, while the salvageable penumbra decreases with time (Fig. 2.7). The rate of change in the size of the core and the penumbra depends on the blood flow provided by the collaterals.

2.3 Risk Factors

In many respects stroke is a preventable disorder. Prevention is the target of a variety of programs to reduce risk factors for stroke. The greatest stroke risk occurs in those with previous transient ischemic attack or previous stroke (Table 2.1). For these patients risk factor reduction is essential and risk may be associated with specific cardiovascular, cerebrovascular or hematologic disorders. Secondary vascular risk has been shown to decrease with treatment of hypertension and hyperlipidemia and the institution of antiplatelet drug treatment. Globally, hypertension is the most significant risk factor for stroke, both ischemic and hemorrhagic. Elevation in blood pressure plays a large role in the development of vascular disease, including coronary heart disease, ventricular failure, atherosclerosis of the aorta and cerebrovascular arteries, as well as small vessel occlusion. Diabetes mellitus ranks highly as a stroke risk factor. Unless it is quelled, the current epidemic of obesity is expected to fuel greater stroke risk in the near future. Hyperlipidemia, tobacco abuse, cocaine and narcotic abuse, and lack of physical exercise also contribute to population stroke risk. There is an increased incidence of stroke during seemingly nonspecific febrile illnesses.

Table 2.1. Major risk factors for acute stroke

| Previous transient ischemic attack or previous stroke |
| Hypertension |
| Atherosclerotic cardiovascular and cerebrovascular disease |
| Diabetes mellitus |
| Obesity |
| Hyperlipidemia |
| Tobacco, cocaine and narcotic abuse |
| Hematologic abnormalities |
| Febrile illness |

Table 2.2. Primary lesions of the cerebrovascular system that cause ischemic stroke

Carotid stenosis
Intracranial atherosclerosis
Aortic atherosclerosis
Risk factors for atherosclerosis
Extracerebral artery dissection

2.4 Primary Lesions of the Cerebrovascular System

2.4.1 Carotid Stenosis

Many stroke patients have atherosclerosis, indicating a link between cardiac and cerebrovascular disease (see Table 2.2). But it is difficult for clinicians to predict the likelihood of stroke using signs and symptoms of heart disease. For instance, carotid bruits are more reliably predictive of ischemic heart disease than of stroke.

2.4.2 Plaque

A carotid plaque's variable composition may affect the associated stroke risk. Plaque is often echodense and calcified, and can be formed by the homogenous deposition of cholesterol. Plaque is dangerous not only because of its stenotic effects – plaque may rupture or dissect at the atherosclerotic wall, showering debris into the bloodstream, leading to multiple embolic cerebral infarcts downstream of the plaque. The ruptured, ulcerated plaque can also be a source of thrombus formation in that the anticoagulant properties of the endothelial surface are locally disrupted. Using transcranial Doppler, a number of groups have shown increased frequency of microembolic signals in the ipsilateral MCA in the days after symptom onset in patients with carotid stenosis.

Inflammation in the plaque wall has been postulated to influence thrombus formation in myocardial infarction (MI) as well as stroke. Recent studies have focused on the possibility that infection in the plaque contributes to thrombus formation and subsequent stroke or MI. *Chlamydia* particles have been recently discovered in carotid and coronary plaques.

2.4.3 Atherosclerosis Leading to Stroke: Two Pathways

An atherosclerotic lesion at the origin of the ICA can lead to stroke. The first pathway is a result of progressive narrowing of the ICA until the sluggish blood flow promotes the formation of a thrombus at the residual lumen, which results in complete occlusion. The acute occlusion may be symptomless if excellent collateral circulation exists along the circle of Willis and between leptomeningeal vessels; alternatively it may cause a large hemispheric stroke if collaterals are poor. The second pathway, termed "artery to artery" embolism, is a common pathway for MCA distribution stroke in patients with severe extracranial internal carotid stenosis. Commonly, this occurs at the time of ICA occlusion.

2.4.4 Collateral Pathways in the Event of Carotid Stenosis or Occlusion

In the pathway shown above (Fig. 2.4), leptomeningeal collateral blood sources traveling over the surface of the brain bring blood from the distal ACA branches into the distal MCA branches. This type of leptomeningeal collateral flow can also come from the posterior cerebral artery (PCA) branches to fill the distal MCA. Flow from the vertebrobasilar system can fill the distal ICA and its branches through the posterior communicating artery (PCoA). The potential for collateral flow in the case of carotid occlusion depends on the vascular anatomy of these alternative pathways. When collateral flow is not sufficient, ischemia occurs in the border zone (sometimes called "watershed") regions between the ACA/MCA or MCA/PCA.

2.4.5 Transient Neurological Deficits

Reoccurring transient neurological deficits also occur commonly in patients with MCA or intracranial carotid stenosis. These deficits generally last for less than 3 min and include transient monocular blindness as well as transient hemispheric neurologic deficits. Their pathologic basis is unknown, though in some cases of transient monocular blindness there is evidence of low flow (the "box car" appearance of red cell clumps separated by clear space) in the retinal arterioles. The retina may also contain highly refractile cholesterol emboli called Hollenhorst plaques. In many instances of severe carotid stenosis or occlusion, the intracranial collateral flow is sufficient to perfuse the brain and prevent ischemia.

2.4.6 Intracranial Atherosclerosis

Atherosclerosis can also occur intracranially to cause focal or multifocal stenosis in the siphon portion of the ICA, the MCA stem, the branch points of the major MCA branches, the ACA, A1 and A2 branches, the P1 and P2 segment of the PCA, the distal vertebral artery, the vertebral artery origin, the vertebrobasilar junction, and the basilar artery. Microatherosclerotic plaques can occur as described above in the proximal portion of the penetrator arteries arising from the major vessels at the base of the brain. They are not seen in the leptomeningeal vessels over the cortex.

Atherosclerosis in the intracranial portion of the carotid and in the MCA causes multiple strokes in the same vascular territory. It may also cause "slow stroke" syndrome, in which there is progressive worsening of focal cortical ischemic symptoms over days or weeks. In addition, the penetrator arteries flowing to the deep white matter and striatum originate from the MCA stem (M1) and may be occluded in patients with severe MCA stenosis. Atherosclerosis in the intracranial portion of the ICA and the MCA is more common in African Americans and Asian Americans for unknown reasons.

Additional common sites for atherosclerotic occlusion include the origin of the vertebral artery, the distal vertebral and vertebrobasilar junction, the mid-basilar artery, and the proximal PCA. Unlike ICA disease, severe atherosclerotic stenosis in the distal intracranial vertebral and basilar arteries can cause stroke via thrombotic occlusion of local branches as well as artery-to-artery embolus to the top of the basilar artery or the PCA(s). Low flow in the basilar artery can lead to thrombus formation with occlu-

sion of one brainstem penetrator vessel after another. Basilar thrombosis is not rare and is fatal because brainstem function is completely dependent on this vascular supply.

Low flow to the basilar artery can also be caused by vertebral disease. Sometimes one vertebral artery is small and terminates as the posterior inferior cerebellar artery, never making the connection to the basilar artery. Other times, one vertebral artery is occluded. In these two circumstances, flow-limiting disease in the dominant or remaining vertebral artery may then produce basilar ischemia. Thrombus at the site of vertebral artery stenosis can also dislodge and cause embolic stroke in the distal basilar artery or PCA territory.

In patients with left subclavian artery occlusion, the left vertebral artery commonly originates distal to the occlusion. This can result in the subclavian steal syndrome, in which blood flows in a retrograde direction down the vertebral artery to supply the arm. This anatomic condition is most frequently asymptomatic, but can result in low flow in the basilar artery during arm exercise.

In some patients with longstanding hypertension there is a dramatic dilatation of the intracranial vessels called "dolichoectasia." Basilar artery dolichoectasia can cause compression of the brainstem or cranial nerves. Thrombus can also form in these very dilated vessels leading to basilar-branch thrombotic occlusion or distal embolic stroke.

A recent trial of aspirin versus warfarin in patients with intracranial atherosclerosis did not demonstrate any difference in terms of efficacy, but bleeding complications were more common in the warfarin group.

2.4.7 Aortic Atherosclerosis

Atherosclerotic disease of the aorta is also likely to increase stroke risk. Transesophageal echocardiographic images can show plaque or thrombus on the aortic wall with dramatic flapping of a thrombus within the aortic lumen. Aortic atherosclerosis is a major cause of stroke during coronary artery bypass grafting; when the aortic cross clamp is released, atherosclerotic debris fills the aorta. Atherosclerotic emboli also occur as complications after coronary and aortic angiography due to vessel wall trauma from the catheter.

So-called cholesterol emboli disease can cause multiple strokes as well as joint pain, livedo reticularis skin rash, reduced renal function, and seizures. These cholesterol embolic strokes may not be amenable to thrombolysis.

Type I aortic dissection is one of the most difficult vascular lesions to manage in the presence of major stroke. The patient may present with chest pain and asymmetric pulses. Stroke may occur in the distribution of any major cerebral arteries because the dissection can involve both carotid and vertebral origins. Since rupture into the chest or extension of dissection into the pericardium or coronary origins is fatal, thrombolysis or anticoagulation cannot be used.

2.4.8 Risk Factors for Atherosclerosis

Hypercholesterolemia, family history of atherosclerotic disease, diabetes, homocysteinemia, elevated apolipoprotein a, hypertension, and smoking are all risk factors for generalized atherosclerosis. Inflammatory markers in the plaque and the systemic circulation are currently under study for their role in triggering symptoms in patients with atherosclerosis.

2.4.9 Extra-cerebral Artery Dissection

Extra-cerebral artery dissection is commonly responsible for stroke in young persons, including children. In adults, dissections tear the intima, and blood enters the wall of the vessel between the intima and the media. This blood causes the vessel wall to balloon outward, and compresses the lumen. If stroke results from this condition, it is most often caused by embolus; a thrombus forms at the tear site and is swept up the vessel into the brain. Dissection may also cause complete occlusion of the vessel and impair cerebral perfusion.

The outwardly distended vessel wall may also compress nearby structures. In carotid dissection at the base of the skull, compression palsies of cranial nerves IX, X, XI, and XII are sometimes seen. Carotid dissection can also interrupt the sympathetic nerve fibers that surround the carotid, causing a Horner's syndrome ptosis and miosis. The dissection site can be high up in the neck, often extending to the point where the ICA becomes ensheathed in the dura at the entry site into the petrous bone. Dissection also occurs in association with redundant looping of the carotid artery. Vertebral artery dissection commonly occurs where the vessel passes over the C2 lateral process to enter the dura.

Symptoms. Patients with carotid or vertebral dissection commonly present with pain. In extracranial carotid dissection the pain is localized to the region above the brow in front of the ear, or over the affected carotid. In vertebral dissection the pain is usually in the C2 distribution, ipsilateral posterior neck, and occipital regions.

Extracranial cerebral artery dissection occurs with massive trauma as well as minor neck injuries. It also occurs with seemingly trivial incidents, such as a strong cough or sneeze, chiropractic manipulation, hyperextension of the neck during hair washing, etc. In some cases, it appears to occur without known precipitants. Disorders of collagen such as fibromuscular dysplasia, Marfan's syndrome, and type IV Ehlers–Danlos syndrome are also associated with dissection.

Arterial dissection can result in the formation of a pseudo-aneurysm. Rupture of dissected vertebral arteries into the subarachnoid space is more common in children. Rupture of dissected carotid artery pseudo-aneurysms into the neck or nasal sinuses is generally rare. Dissection can occur intracranially and, on rare occasions, can spread intracranially from a primary extracranial origin.

2.5 Primary Cardiac Abnormalities

2.5.1 Atrial Fibrillation

Atrial fibrillation (AF) is a major risk factor for debilitating stroke due to embolism. The Framingham Stroke Study estimated that 14% of strokes occurred because of AF. The prevalence of AF is high and increases with age, peaking at 8.8% among people over the age of 80 years. The risk of stroke in patients with

AF also increases with age: as many as 5% of patients over 65 with AF suffer embolic stroke.

These emboli often originate as a mural thrombus, usually harbored by the fibrillating atrium, and more specifically the atrial appendage, because of its potential for regions of stagnant blood flow. Anticoagulation with warfarin has been shown to decrease stroke risk in elderly patients with AF or younger patients with concomitant heart disease, reducing the risk of thrombus formation.

In the evaluation of the patient with AF who experiences a stroke, it is important to determine whether the prothrombin time is elevated. The risk of warfarin-associated major hemorrhage, mostly intracranial, is approximately 0.5% per year. A hemorrhagic stroke, however, can still occur with a well-controlled prothrombin time.

2.5.2 Myocardial Infarction

Myocardial infarction (MI) commonly causes intraventricular thrombus to form on the damaged surface of the endocardium. Acute anterior wall infarction with aneurysm formation is especially associated with thrombus formation and stroke. Poor left ventricular function and ventricular aneurysm is also associated with increased risk of embolic stroke.

2.5.3 Valvular Heart Disease

Atrial fibrillation with mitral valve disease has long been considered a stroke risk factor. Mechanical prosthetic valves are prime sites for thrombus formation; therefore, patients with these valves require anticoagulation. Bacterial endocarditis can cause stroke as well as intracerebral mycotic aneurysms. Inflammatory defects in the vessel wall, when associated with systemic thrombolysis and anticoagulation, rupture with subsequent lobar hemorrhage, and precipitate stroke.

Nonbacterial, or "marantic," endocarditis is also associated with multiple embolic strokes. This condition is most common in patients with mucinous carcinoma and may be associated with a low-grade disseminated intravascular coagulation. A nonbacterial endocarditis, called Libman–Sacks endocarditis, oc-

curs in patients with systemic lupus erythematosus (SLE).

The role of mitral valve prolapse in stroke remains controversial. Strands of filamentous material attached to the mitral valve seen by echocardiography have recently been reported as a risk factor for embolic stroke.

2.5.4 Patent Foramen Ovale

Patent foramen ovale (PFO) occurs in approximately 27% of the population. Though the left-sided pressures are usually higher that those on the right, the flow of venous blood toward the foramen ovale can direct some blood to the left side of the heart. Increases in right-sided pressures, which can occur with pulmonary embolism or the Valsalva maneuver, increase blood flow from right to left atrium. PFO has been detected with increased incidence (up to 40%) in young persons with stroke. It is thought that venous clots in the leg or pelvic veins loosen and travel to the right atrium, and then cross to the left side of the heart causing embolic stroke. This conclusion is supported when stroke occurs in the context of deep vein thrombosis (DVT) or pulmonary embolus (PE) in a patient with PFO. Echocardiography has shown these paradoxical emboli crossing the foramen ovale. The diagnosis of PFO can be made by echocardiography when bubble contrast is seen to cross to the left side of the heart after intravenous injection, or bubble contrast is seen on transcranial Doppler examination of the intracranial vessels. Without concurrent DVT or PE it is never clear whether the PFO was causal. In the recent Warfarin Aspirin Reinfaction Study no difference in recurrent stroke risk was attributable to the presence of PFO; nor was there a difference in recurrent stroke in patients treated with aspirin compared to warfarin.

2.5.5 Cardiac Masses

Atrial myxoma is a rare atrial tumor that causes multiple emboli of either thrombus or myxomatous tissue. When the myxomatous emboli occur from the left atrium, they may cause the formation of multiple distal cerebral aneurysms with risk of hemorrhage.

Fibroelastoma is a frond-like growth in the heart that is also associated with a high stroke risk.

2.6 Embolic Stroke

2.6.1 The Local Vascular Lesion

The occlusion of an intracerebral vessel causes local changes in the affected vessel and its tributaries. There is also a vascular change in the microcirculation supplied by these vessels. As an embolus travels toward the brain, it is forced into progressively narrower vessels before it lodges in a vessel too small for it to pass. The initial shape of emboli and their course are not well known. Because the major vessels of the Circle of Willis have lumen diameters of only 1–2 mm, dangerous clots need not be very large. Some clots that have a string shape and curl, like those from a deep vein, become temporarily stuck at turns in the vessel, eventually becoming compacted into a plug when they finally lodge. The vessel is often distended. Symptoms localized to basilar branches sometimes occur in the moments before a top of the basilar ischemic syndrome occurs. Called the "basilar scrape," this is thought to result from temporary ischemia caused by the embolus as it travels up the vertebral and basilar vessels to the bifurcation at the top of the basilar artery. Emboli lodge at branch points, such as the T-like bifurcation of the basilar into two posterior cerebral arteries, and the T-like bifurcation of the carotid into the ACA and MCA. The fork of the MCA stem into the two or three divisions of the MCA is another common lodging site for emboli. Small branches coming off the large vessel at these sites will be occluded. There are a number of thin penetrator vessels that supply the midbrain and the overlying thalamus that are occluded in the top of the basilar embolus. The lumen of the anterior choroidal artery is in the distal carotid. Coming off the middle cerebral stem are penetrators to the striatum and internal capsule. Ischemia in these vascular territories that have little collateral flow channels can quickly lead to infarction as compared to ischemia in the cerebral cortex, which can receive blood flow via leptomeningeal collaterals.

2.6.2 Microvascular Changes in Ischemic Brain

In contrast to the situation in occluded small vessels, the vascular tree distal to an occlusion in a main cerebral vessel will not be occluded by the clot. In order to keep blood flow at normal levels, the distal vascular tree undergoes maximal vasodilatation. This vasodilatation is in part regulated by the action of nitric oxide on the vascular wall. Ischemic vasodilatation will attract collateral flow to the cortex from other vascular channels through leptomeningeal vessels. In the fully dilated bed, the cerebral blood flow will be driven by the blood pressure. As blood flow falls in the microvessels there is potential for microvascular thrombus formation. The endothelial surface of the microvascular circulation normally has an anticoagulant coating. Under ischemic conditions, it becomes activated to express white blood cell adhesion molecules. White blood cells attach to the vessel wall and may mediate microvascular injury and microthrombosis. In such a case, despite the recanalization of the main feeder vessel, there is "no reflow" of blood to the tissue. This loss of accessibility of the microvasculature to the blood pool and decreased cerebral blood volume are closely linked to infarction. In animal studies, stroke size is decreased if white blood cell counts are reduced or drugs are given to block white cell adhesion. Free radical production by the white blood cells is considered an important mediator of vessel-wall injury in stroke.

Damage to the vessel wall is manifested as hemorrhage into the infarct. Hemorrhagic conversion of embolic stroke is very common when examined by magnetic resonance imaging (MRI) sequences sensitive to magnetic susceptibility of the iron. In hemorrhagic conversion there are multiple small hemorrhages in the infarct that may not be apparent on CT scan or may be seen as a hazy or stippled increase in signal intensity. Large hemorrhages can also occur in the infarcted tissue. The latter are more common in large strokes that include the deep white matter and basal ganglia. As opposed to hemorrhagic conversion, which is usually not accompanied by clinical change, the large hematoma in the infarcted zone is often associated with worsened neurologic deficit. These hematomas frequently exert considerable mass effect on adjacent brain tissue and can increase intracranial pressure (ICP) and distort midbrain and diencephalic structures. Since these hemorrhages more commonly occur in the larger strokes, they often compound the mass effect due to ischemic edema. Hematoma formation is the major risk of thrombolytic therapy. The use of drugs that impair hemostasis (anticoagulants) may increase the probability of bleeding into a vascular territory with an injured vascular wall. Hemorrhage occurs when the blood flow and blood pressure are restored in a previously ischemic zone. The injured vascular wall is incompetent to withstand the hydrostatic pressure and the return of oxygen and white blood cells may also intensify the reperfusion injury at the vascular wall.

The vascular wall also regulates the flow of large molecules from the vascular space to the intercellular space (the so-called blood–brain barrier). In ischemia, there is net movement of water into the brain tissue. This is the basis of the increased T2 signal on MRI and the low density on CT in the first few days after stroke. At variable times after stroke, contrast imaging studies show that large molecules also cross into the brain tissue. The net water movement into brain, ischemic edema, can lead to secondary brain injury as a result of increased ICP and the distortion of surrounding tissues by the edematous mass effect. Mass effect, causing clinical worsening and classical herniation syndromes, is not uncommon in patients with large MCA strokes.

2.6.3 MCA Embolus

An embolus to the MCA is common and can cause a catastrophic stroke. It is also amenable to rapid therapy. For these reasons, special emphasis is placed here on this stroke subtype. As discussed above, carotid stenosis and occlusion cause stroke by artery-to-artery embolus into the MCA territory or by causing a low-flow state. This gives rise to the clinical syndrome of MCA stroke. Distinguishing features of carotid stenosis include the common occurrence of multiple stereotypic spells of transient ipsilateral hemispheric or monocular dysfunction. In addition, in carotid stenosis multiple emboli may occur over a short period of time. In some cases of embolus to the

MCA from a severely stenotic carotid, the embolus may be less well tolerated and the stroke more severe due to the lower perfusion pressure above the carotid lesion. Embolus from the carotid to the MCA can also occur from the stump of a completely occluded carotid. If the occlusion is hyperacute, then it is often possible to dissolve the fresh clot in the extracerebral carotid with urokinase and advance the catheter to treat the intracerebral clot. This can be followed by angioplasty of the carotid stenosis. However, if the carotid occlusion is more chronic, the organized clot extends up from the occlusion in the neck intracranially and may prevent passage of the catheter. This will preclude intra-arterial thrombolysis of the MCA clot.

2.6.4 Borderzone Versus Embolic Infarctions

Carotid stenosis can also cause low-flow stroke when the collateral flow from the anterior communicating artery (ACoA), PCoA, and retrograde through the ophthalmic artery is insufficient to perfuse the ipsilateral hemisphere. Low flow causes symptoms and infarction in the distal cortical watershed territory between the distal branches of the ACA, MCA, and PCA. The actual boundaries between these territories may shift due to increased flow through the ACA or PCA to supply the MCA. The classic presentation is called the "man in the barrel syndrome." The watershed ischemia causes dysfunction in the regions for motor control of the proximal arm and leg. There may be an aphasia known as "transcortical aphasia" due to disconnection of the laterally placed language areas and medial cortex. In transcortical aphasia, repetition is relatively preserved. In transcortical motor aphasia there is hesitant speech but preserved comprehension. In transcortical sensory aphasia, comprehension is more severely impaired than speech. Cortical watershed stroke is seen on imaging as a thin strip of infarction that runs from the posterior confluence of the MCA, ACA, and PCA branches in the posterior parietal cortex extending forward on the upper lateral surface of the cerebrum. On axial scans there is a small region of stroke on each of the upper cuts; only by mentally stacking the images does the examiner appreciate that the lesions are contiguous and form an anterior to posterior strip of stroke. The strip overlies the motor areas for control of the proximal leg and arm. A cortical watershed infarction is not entirely specific for low flow, because it can also be caused by showers of microemboli that lodge in the region of neutral hydrostatic pressure.

In addition to the cortical watershed, there is also an internal watershed formed by the junction of the penetrator arteries from the MCA and the leptomeningeal cortical vessels that enter the cortex and extend into the white matter. This watershed again forms a strip that lies in the white matter just above and lateral to the lateral ventricle. Instead of a strip of contiguous stroke the internal watershed region usually undergoes multiple discrete circular or oval shaped strokes that line up in an anterior to posterior strip. Internal watershed infarction may be more specific for low-flow stroke.

2.7 Lacunar Strokes

Penetrator vessels come off the basilar artery, the middle cerebral stem, and the PCA at right angles to the parent vessel. Small-vessel occlusive disease is almost entirely related to hypertension and is characterized pathologically by lipohyalinosis and fibrinoid necrosis of small 80- to 800-μm penetrator vessels. Occlusion of these penetrators causes small infarcts, termed lacunars, in their respective vascular territories, most commonly in the caudate, putamen, external capsule, internal capsule, corona radiata, pontine tegmentum, and thalamus. Hypertensive hemorrhage occurs in these same regions and is due to the same hypertensive changes in the penetrator vessels. The deficits caused by these small strokes are a function of their location. Because the penetrator vessels supply deep white matter tracts as they converge in the internal capsule or brainstem, the consequence of lacunar stroke is often related to disconnection of neural circuits.

Lacunar strokes are especially common in patients who have diabetes in addition to hypertension. Lacunar strokes can cause immediate motor and sensory deficits, though many patients recover considerable function in the weeks or months following lacunar-

stroke onset. In the National Institute of Neurological Disorders and Stroke Recombinant Tissue Plasminogen Activator Stroke Study (NINDS rt-PA Study), 50% of patients returned to a normal functional level within 3 months without rt-PA treatment. In the group receiving rt-PA, the probability of good recovery increased to 70%.

A number of clinical syndromes commonly occur due to lacunar strokes (see Table 2.3). However, the clinical symptoms may not be specific for the chronic occlusive disease of the small penetrator vessels described above. Of special importance is the infarct in a penetrator territory caused by disease of the parent vessel. In some cases, the penetrator stroke is only one, sometimes the first, of many regions to undergo infarction due to major vessel occlusion. In basilar artery occlusive disease, ischemia in the distribution of a single penetrator may occur as the "opening shot." On succeeding days, the origin of multiple penetrators becomes occluded due to the propagation of mural thrombus in the vessel. In addition, atherosclerosis in the parent vessel may narrow the lumen at the origin of the penetrators.

Atherosclerosis may also occur in some of the larger penetrators. Large strokes, or giant lacunes, occur as a result of the occlusion of multiple penetrators with occlusive disease in the parent vessel. This is particularly common in the MCA territory where leptomeningeal collateral flow preserves the cortex, but absence of collateral flow to the penetrator territory results in infarction.

In some cases, showers of small emboli cause penetrator strokes as well as cortical strokes. Small emboli may also reach these vessels. Chronic meningitis due to tuberculosis or syphilis commonly causes stroke in the penetrator territory due to inflammation around the parent vessel at the base of the brain with occlusion of the thin penetrators exiting through the inflammatory reaction (Table 2.4 lists the causes of lacunar infarcts).

Table 2.3. Clinical lacunar syndrome and infarct location

Clinical syndrome	Location of lacunar stroke
Pure motor hemiparesis involving face, arm, and leg	Contralateral posterior limb internal capsule or overlying corona radiata
	Contralateral pontine tegmentum
Pure unilateral sensory loss involving face, arm, and leg	Contralateral thalamus
Hemiparesis with homolateral ataxia	Contralateral thalamocapsular region
	Upper third of the contralateral medial pons
Dysarthria, clumsy hand	Contralateral lower third of the medial pons
Hemisensory loss and homolateral hemiparesis	Genu of the internal capsule
Sensory loss around corner of mouth and homolateral weakness of hand	Thalamocapsular region

Table 2.4. Causes of lacunar infarcts. (*CSF* Cerebrospinal fluid, *CTA* CT angiography, *ESR* erythrocyte sedimentation rate, *MRA* magnetic resonance angiography, *MRI* magnetic resonance imaging, *RPR* rapid plasma reagent)

Vascular lesion underlying penetrator vessel stroke	Clue to diagnosis
Hyalinization and fibrinoid necrosis	History of hypertension, especially with diabetes. Small lesion <1 cm diameter in the distal territory of the penetrator. Often multiple, bilateral, and even symmetrically placed lesions
Atherosclerosis of the parent vessel occluding the lumen of the penetrator by athero or thrombus	Stenosis in the parent vessel on MRA, CTA, transcranial ultrasound or direct angiography
	Large infarct that extends to the origin of the penetrator from the parent vessel.
	Multiple strokes in the distribution of the same parent vessel
Atherosclerosis in the penetrator vessel	Large infarct in penetrator territory with normal parent vessel lumen on CTA/MRA/direct angiography
Chronic meningitis	Large infarct in the penetrator territory.
	Rapidly progressive stroke course, presence of fever, chronic headache, elevated ESR, abnormal RPR, inflammatory CSF
	Narrowing of the lumen with gadolinium enhancement of the parent vessel on MRI
Emboli to the penetrator	Evidence of other small emboli. No history of hypertension or atherosclerosis

2.8 Other Causes of Stroke

2.8.1 Inflammatory Conditions

Primary granulomatous angiitis of the central nervous system causes progressive ischemic brain injury. Blood vessels of various sizes are affected by inflammation and, on occasion, hemorrhage occurs in addition to stroke. Granulomatous angiitis can occur in the MCA ipsilateral to V1-distribution Herpes zoster or in the vertebral after C2-distribution Herpes zoster. The cerebrospinal fluid (CSF) often shows signs of inflammation. Diagnosis is commonly made after a biopsy of the leptomeningeal vessels demonstrates the granulomatous inflammation. When caught in its early stages, treatment with cyclophosphamide and/or steroids can reverse the process. Left untreated, the disease is usually fatal and causes severe diffuse or multifocal brain injury.

Systemic lupus erythematosus (SLE) has a variety of presentations in the nervous system. Stroke-like events can occur, along with seizures and encephalopathy due to a small vessel vasculopathy. A circulating factor that increases the partial thrombin time (PTT), so-called lupus anticoagulant or anticardiolipin antibody, is associated with arterial thrombosis. A nonbacterial endocarditis may be a cause of embolic stroke.

Temporal arteritis is a giant cell arteritis seen in older adults with an elevated erythrocyte sedimentation rate, an elevated fibrinogen level, and a thickened wall of the extracranial carotid branches. Temporal arteritis can cause headache, tenderness over the temporal artery, jaw claudication, and transient visual loss. It is sometimes associated with polymyalgia rheumatica. It occasionally affects the vertebral artery.

Takayasu's arteritis is a giant cell arteritis of the large vessels off the arch of the aorta. It can cause occlusive disease in the carotid and the vertebrals, leading to stroke. Polyarteritis nodosa has rarely been reported to affect intracranial vessels. Sickle cell disease causes extracranial carotid stenosis or occlusion.

The beta amyloid that is deposited in plaques of patients with Alzheimer's disease can also infiltrate the walls of the small blood vessels that supply the cortex. This *amyloid angiopathy* is a common cause of lobar hemorrhage in the elderly, most of whom do not have Alzheimer's disease. Some patients present with transient neurologic deficits prior to their hemorrhage. Small microinfarctions can occur in the cortex, in addition to multiple hemorrhages. Hemorrhage is found to occur in those patients who have a combination of amyloid deposition in the vessel wall and fibrinoid necrosis of the vessel wall. Amyloid angiopathy is considered a major risk factor for intracerebral hemorrhage in patients receiving thrombolytic drugs for MI or stroke.

Moya-moya disease is an unusual condition causing progressive stenosis and occlusion of the internal carotid and the vessels of the Circle of Willis. Recurrent stroke as well as occasional hemorrhage characterize the clinical syndrome. A proliferation of collateral vessels into the deep penetrator territory leads to an appearance of a "puff of smoke" on direct angiography.

2.8.2 Venous Sinus Thrombosis

Venous sinus thrombosis can cause focal neurologic deficits, often with seizures, headache, and other signs of raised intracranial pressure. Venous strokes are frequently hemorrhagic and located in the proximity of the occluded sinus– parasagittal in a sagittal sinus thrombosis, temporal lobe in a transverse sinus thrombosis, and thalamus in a straight sinus thrombosis. Venous sinus thrombosis is seen in patients with hypercoagulable state or as a consequence of infiltration of the major sinus by tumor or infection.

2.8.3 Vasospasm in the Setting of Subarachnoid Hemorrhage

Subarachnoid hemorrhage (SAH) is most commonly caused by rupture of an intracranial aneurysm. It can result in vasospasm that may cause ischemia and infarction. Vasospasm due to SAH is thought to occur in the majority of cases of SAH, but is symptomatic in about a third of this population. Permanent neurological injury may occur in 10% or more. Vasospasm peaks around 1 week after SAH, but it can be seen as early as 3 days or as late as 3 weeks after the initial event. The underlying mechanisms are not understood, but vasospasm is clearly related to the amount of blood in the subarachnoid space.

2.8.4 Migraine

Epidemiological studies have demonstrated that migraine is associated with ischemic stroke independent of other risk factors. The mechanism is unknown, but potential factors include vascular hyper-reactivity, and sensitivity to or increased amount of vasoactive substances.

2.8.5 Primary Hematologic Abnormalities

Clotting systems disorders that cause systemic bleeding are associated with increased risk of intracerebral hemorrhage. Coumadin use is perhaps the most common cause of intracerebral hemorrhage, followed by thrombocytopenia. Thrombotic thrombocytopenic purpura (TTP) is most commonly manifested as ischemic stroke and should be treated by emergency plasmapheresis, which can reverse the microvascular thrombosis. Hypercoagulable states, such as protein C or S deficiency and Factor V Leiden mutation, increase the risk of venous sinus thrombosis. Arterial and venous occlusions occur in anticardiolipin syndrome along with fetal wasting and livedo reticularis. A hypercoagulable state with venous sinus thrombosis commonly occurs in the post-partum period or in severely dehydrated patients (see Table 2.5).

Table 2.5. Other causes of stroke

Inflammatory conditions
  Primary granulomatous angiitis
  Systemic lupus erythematosus
  Temporal arteritis
  Takayasu's arteritis

Venous sinus thrombosis

Vasospasm in the setting of subarachnoid hemorrhage

Migraine

Primary hematologic abnormalities
  Thrombotic thrombocytopenic purpura
  Protein C or S deficiency
  Factor V Leiden mutation
  Anticardiolipin syndrome
  Fetal wasting
  Livedo reticularis
  Post-partum period
  Severe dehydration states

2.9 Conclusion

There are many causes of stroke. In the past, the specific etiology of a stroke often remained mysterious. In present day medicine, specialists can often identify the etiology in minutes by analyzing the patient's history, clinical evaluation, and imaging results. Identifying the cause of a stroke in each case is critical for treating a hyperacute stroke, minimizing its progression, and preventing its recurrence.

PART II
Imaging of Acute Ischemic Stroke

Unenhanced Computed Tomography

Erica C.S. Camargo, Guido González,
R. Gilberto González, Michael H. Lev

Contents

3.1 Introduction

The speed, widespread availability, low cost, and accuracy in detecting subarachnoid and intracranial hemorrhage have led conventional computed tomography (CT) scanning to become the first-line diagnostic test for the emergency evaluation of acute stroke [1–6]. Head CT scans can detect ischemic brain regions within 6 h of stroke onset (hyperacute). According to reports by Mohr and González, the introduction of such early detection is comparable to that of conventional T2-weighted magnetic resonance imaging (MRI) [7–12]. For example, based on 68 patients imaged within 4 h of stroke onset, Mohr et al. [11] concluded that CT was equivalent to MRI in its ability to detect the earliest signs of stroke (Table 3.1, Figs. 3.1–3.5).

Importantly, the identification of ischemic brain tissue by CT not only defines regions likely to infarct, but also may predict outcome and response to intravenous (i.v.) or intra-arterial (i.a.) thrombolytic therapy [13]. Most commonly, CT is used to exclude parenchymal hemorrhage and significant established infarction. Unenhanced CT findings can additionally, in some settings, help to predict hemorrhagic transformation of already necrotic tissue following arterial reperfusion.

Sensitivity values for the CT detection of stroke vary in the literature. These differences are largely caused by the variance in study design and focus, the vascular territory in question, and the generation of CT scanner used. Because control groups without stroke are not commonly included as subjects in published reports, the specificity of CT scanning in stroke detection is not well established [14].

Table 3.1. CT findings that are useful in the detection of acute ischemia ("early ischemic signs"; EIS)

1. Focal parenchymal hypodensity
   – Of the insular ribbon (Fig. 3.1)
   – Of the lenticular nuclei (Fig. 3.2 a)

2. Cortical swelling with sulcal effacement (Figs. 3.2 a, 3.3, 3.4)

3. Loss of gray-white matter differentiation (Figs. 3.1, 3.2 a, 3.3, 3.4)

4. Hyperdense MCA sign (Fig. 3.5)

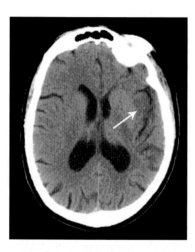

Figure 3.1

Brain CT image of a 56-year-old male, with acute onset of right hemiparesis and Broca's aphasia. Conventional noncontrast computed tomography (*NCCT*) demonstrates hypodensity of the left insular cortex, the so-called insular ribbon sign (*arrow*)

This chapter will review the role of conventional noncontrast CT (NCCT) scanning in the evaluation of hyperacute stroke patients, and will discuss data acquisition and image interpretation techniques, the physical basis of CT imaging findings, and the accuracy and clinical utility of CT scanning.

3.2 Technique

NCCT scanning of acute stroke patients presenting to the Massachusetts General Hospital is typically performed in the Emergency Department using a multidetector helical scanner. Precise imaging parameters will depend on the type (16-slice, 4-slice, etc.) and vendor of the CT scanner used; however, the overall goal of imaging is to maximize image quality – especially of the posterior fossa structures – while minimizing radiation dose, helical ("windmill") artifact, and image noise. To this end, a useful general principle is to use a helical pitch less than 1 (for maximal helical overlap, 0.5–0.66 is often optimal), a relatively slow table speed (5–8 mm/s), rapid gantry rotation (0.5–0.8 rotations/s, to better freeze motion), and the smallest possible focal spot setting. We present a sample head CT protocol, using the GE 4-slice LightSpeed Helical CT scanner, below (Table 3.2).

The following technique is routinely utilized: 140 kV, 170 mA (the maximal possible mA using small focal spot size), 5 mm slice thickness, 5 mm image spacing, 0.75 pitch, 0.8 s rotation time and 22 cm field of view. Image reconstruction is with both "head" and "bone" algorithms; use of other algorithms will degrade the quality of brain tissue visualization. Coverage is from the skull base to the vertex, using contiguous axial slices. The scans are sometimes obtained in a head-holder so as to optimize image registration between the noncontrast and contrast images for patients that undergo CT angiography (CTA) immediately following conventional CT. As already noted, the above scanning parameters were chosen as a tradeoff between maximizing reso-

Table 3.2. Technique for optimal NCCT image acquisition

Helical pitch <1 ("high-speed" helical techniques produce unacceptable reconstruction artifacts in the posterior fossa)
Slow table speed (5–8 mm/s)
Rapid gantry rotation (0.5–0.8 rotations/s)
Smallest possible focal spot setting

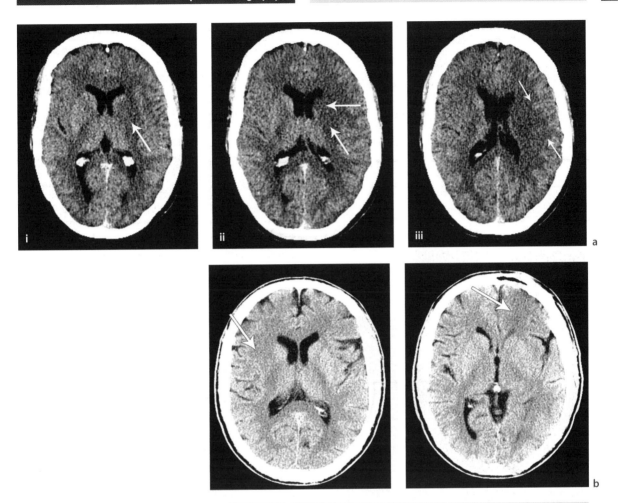

Figure 3.2 a, b

a Brain CT image of a 37-year-old white male, last seen normal at 10 p.m., found early next morning with right hemiplegia and severe aphasia. Axial noncontrast CT demonstrates early ischemic changes: i, ii hypodensity of the lenticular nucleus and caudate head (*arrows*), and iii cortical swelling with sulcal effacement (*arrows*). b Similar scan to a, showing right lenticular hypodensity (*left arrow*), but without stroke symptoms, which demonstrates the pitfall of patient's head tilt in the CT scanner gantry causing a "pseudolesion" due to right–left asymmetry within a given slice. This illustrates the importance of reviewing all contiguous CT slices, and awareness of possible imaging artifacts. Here, the patient is tilted, with asymmetry of the lateral ventricles and sylvian fissures. Additionally, the left frontal hypodensity (*right arrow*) is due to beam hardening artifact

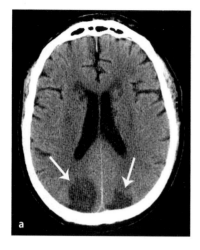

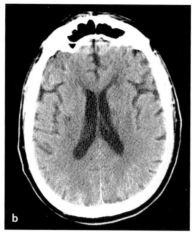

Figure 3.3 a, b

Patient found to be unrespon-sive following a coronary artery bypass graft (*CABG*) procedure. a NCCT obtained 36 h post-CABG demonstrates bilateral occipital hypodensities (*arrows*). b The "fogging effect" is noted on the NCCT obtained 18 days post-pro-cedure, with temporary resolu-tion of the parenchymal hypo-densities. On subsequent follow-up CT scans (not shown), cavita-tion occurred in the originally hypodense regions (see text)

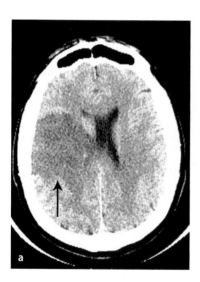

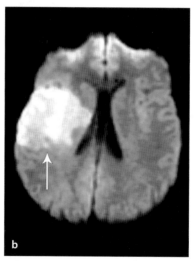

Figure 3.4 a, b

CT image of a 32-year-old right-handed male, found with left hemiparesis, dysarthria and left hemianopsia. a NCCT performed 12 h post-ictus shows extensive cortical and subcortical parenchymal hypodensity, with sulcal effacement and compression of the right lateral ventricle, covering an area greater than one-third of the MCA territory (*left arrow*). Such findings within the first 3–6 h of stroke onset would typically preclude thrombolytic therapy. b Correlative diffu-sion-weighted MRI (*MRI-DWI*), performed 1 h before the NCCT, demonstrates restricted diffusion in the same region (*right arrow*)

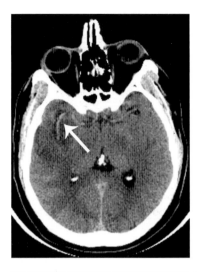

Figure 3.5

Figure 3.5

CT image of a 32-year-old right-handed male with left hemiparesis, dysarthria and left hemianopsia. NCCT performed 12 h post-ictus shows a hyperdense vessel sign of the right middle cerebral artery (*MCA*) ("*HMCAS*") (*arrow*)

Table 3.3. Hounsfield Scale

Negative	Zero	Positive
Air(<–1000 HU)	Water	Bone, metal (>1000 HU)
Fat (–30 to –70 HU)		Punctate calcifications (30–500 HU)
		Blood (60–100 HU)
		Gray matter (30–35 HU)
		White matter (20–25 HU)
		Muscle (20–40 HU)

A 1% increase in net tissue water → 2.5 HU decrease on NCCT

3.3 Physical Basis of Imaging Findings

CT scans measure x-ray beam attenuation through a region of interest, attenuation being directly proportional to tissue density. For the purpose of image reconstruction, attenuation values are expressed as Hounsfield Units (HU), a linear density scale in which water has an arbitrary value of zero [15]. Thus, tissues denser than water – including brain parenchyma, muscles, blood, and bone, which have higher attenuation values – occupy the positive side of the Hounsfield scale, and are assigned a gray-scale brightness that is "lighter" than water. Conversely, low-density tissues – including fat and air – have negative Hounsfield values, and hence appear "darker" than water on head CT images. Typically, gray matter has an attenuation value of approximately 30–35 HU; and white matter, 20–25 HU [15] (Table 3.3).

The pathophysiology underlying the ischemic changes detected by CT is outlined in a prior review by Marks [4]. The finding of *early* (up to 6 h) parenchymal hypodensity has been hypothesized to be secondary to cytotoxic edema, caused by lactic acidosis and failure of cell membrane ion pumps due to an inadequate ATP supply [16]. This process may involve redistribution of tissue water from the extracellular to the intracellular space, but because there is little overall change in *net* tissue water, there is only minimal reduction in gray and white matter brain

lution and image contrast of the brain parenchyma (most notably in the posterior fossa), and minimizing both scan time and patient radiation dose. Again, we discourage the use of "high-speed" helical technique (pitch >1) for brain imaging, as the degree of helical reconstruction artifact through the posterior fossa may produce images of unacceptable diagnostic quality. A value of 170 mA is specifically chosen in order to take advantage of the small x-ray tube focal spot setting. It is noteworthy that, using this scan protocol, the resulting axial 5-mm-thick source images can be reformatted to 2.5-mm-thick slices in either the bone or soft tissue algorithm, should the need arise. With the newest generation scanners (16-slice or greater) reformatting to even thinner slices can be achieved – of great value for three-dimensional (3D) reconstructions in the sagittal or coronal imaging planes.

parenchymal Hounsfield attenuation. Alternatively, hypodensity due to vasogenic edema (beyond 3–6 h) is caused by loss of tight junction endothelial cell integrity and appears only if residual or resumed perfusion is present [16]. The HU attenuation of acutely ischemic brain parenchyma is directly proportional to the degree of edema; for every 1 % increase in tissue water content, x-ray attenuation decreases by 3–5 %, which corresponds to a drop of approximately 2.5 HU on CT imaging [4, 17, 18]. This has also been observed in a recent rat model of acute middle cerebral artery (MCA) occlusion [19].

Such small changes in HU can be difficult to detect by eye, especially given the inherent noise in CT scanning – hence the need for optimal "window width" and "center level" review settings, discussed in the following section. In this regard, the superiority of diffusion-weighted imaging (DWI) in revealing cytotoxic edema in very early stages of infarction remains unrivaled. The "restriction" of apparent diffusion coefficient (ADC) values during the early stages of cerebral ischemia reflects decreased Brownian motion of water molecules in both the intra- and extracellular spaces. In the subacute period, between 7 and 10 days after stroke onset, the appearance of vasogenic edema leads initially to a recovery of ADC values, and afterwards to their increase. In acute stroke, a correlation between this ADC restriction and the decrease in CT attenuation has been observed; however, the time courses of these processes are different, suggesting a differing underlying physiology. Whereas the reduction in ADC is nearly complete within 90 min of stroke onset, CT attenuation continues to linearly decrease over several hours [20]. Interestingly, ADC values tend to be lower in regions with early NCCT hypodensity than in those without, supporting the observation that hypodense regions on CT are likely to be irreversibly infarcted, despite early recanalization [21].

Of note, an interesting phenomenon that sometimes occurs in the subacute phase of stoke is the "CT fogging effect," in which irreversibly infarcted regions "disappear" on unenhanced CT performed on older generation scanners, 2–6 weeks after stroke onset (Fig. 3.3). With "fogging," the acute-phase CT low attenuation – due to edema – is thought to re-solve, to be replaced by higher attenuation infiltration of macrophages and neo-capillarity within the infarcted tissue bed. The infarct "reappears" in the late phase, as tissue cavitation occurs [22].

3.4 Optimal Image Review

3.4.1 Window-Width (W) and Center-Level (L) CT Review Settings

Because the reductions in Hounsfield attenuation accompanying early stroke are small – indeed, often barely perceptible to the human eye – the precise window and level settings (measured in HU) used for CT image review are potentially important variables in the detection of subtle ischemic hypodensity. These settings are known to influence lesion conspicuity and diagnostic accuracy in diseases other than stroke. For example, in the CTA evaluation of severe carotid artery stenosis, optimal window and level viewing parameters are required for precise luminal diameter measurement [23, 24]. In abdominal CT, the routine use of narrow "liver windows" has been advocated in order to improve soft tissue contrast within the liver, thereby increasing the conspicuity of subtle lesions [25]. A study from our group has shown that the CT detection of acutely ischemic brain parenchyma is facilitated by soft copy review using narrow, nonstandard window and level settings, in order to accentuate the small attenuation difference between normal and ischemic gray and white matter (Fig. 3.6) [26].

Specifically, NCCT images from stroke patients were first reviewed using standard settings of approximately 80 HU W and 20 HU L (virtual hard copy), and then using nonstandard, variable soft copy, narrow window and level settings, initially centered at approximately 8 HU W and 32 HU L. Using the standard viewing parameters, the sensitivity and specificity for stroke detection were 57 % and 100 %, respectively. Sensitivity for stroke detection increased to 71 % when images were reviewed using the nonstandard, narrow window and level settings, with no loss of specificity ($P=0.03$). Moreover, the use of interactive, soft copy window and level settings did not significantly increase the time required for

Figure 3.6 a, b

a CT image of a 79-year-old female, 5 h post onset of left-sided hemiplegia. i, iii Images are displayed using standard noncontrast CT review settings (window width of 75 HU and center level of 20 HU). ii, iv Images are displayed using narrow, nonstandard review settings (window width of 16 HU and center level of 31 HU). Although early ischemic changes (insular ribbon sign and hypoattenuation of the lentiform nucleus) are subtly present on the standard setting images, these become more conspicuous with the nonstandard review settings (*arrows*). b Another example of the importance of nonstandard window and level review settings. An 18-year-old male, evaluated in the Emergency Department after a construction accident. i Standard NCCT review settings fail to accurately distinguish subtle right convexity subdural hematoma from bone. ii Nonstandard review settings (center level = 80 HU, window width = 200 HU), with which hemorrhage and bone are assigned different gray scale values, facilitate the detection of the subtle right frontal hematoma (*arrows*)

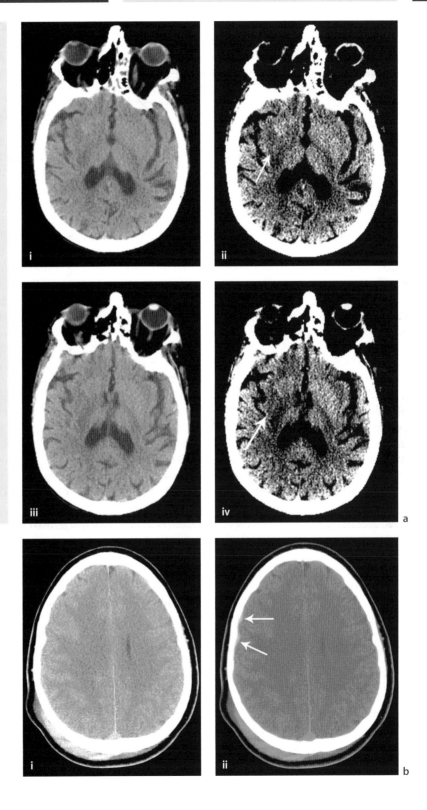

Table 3.4. Stroke detection with soft copy NCCT review. (*L* = Center-level CT review setting, *W* = window-width CT review setting)

	Standard settings (80 HU W, 20 HU L)	Narrow, non-standard settings (8 HU W, 32 HU L)
Sensitivity	57%	71%
Specificity	100%	100%

p = 0.03

scan interpretation over that needed using standard settings (Table 3.4).

3.4.2 Density Difference Analysis (DDA)

The idea of exploiting the subtle difference in density between normal and acutely edematous brain tissue in order to improve stroke detection is not new. A 1997 report described an automated post-processing method for the CT detection of MCA territory infarcts using histographic analysis of density values [14]. Attenuation values for each CT slice were recorded in both hemispheres, and a density-difference diagram was calculated by subtraction of the left hemisphere histogram from that of the right. Using DDA, the detection rate for infarcts increased from 61% to 96%. All normal studies were correctly interpreted, and in no case was a correct diagnosis on the unprocessed CT images revised using DDA [14]. Unlike the use of narrow soft-copy window and level-review settings however, DDA requires specialized post-processing equipment and additional interpretation time.

3.5 CT Early Ischemic Changes: Detection and Prognostic Value

3.5.1 Early Generation CT Scanners

Estimates of hyperacute stroke detection rates for NCCT vary. Early generation CT scanners often failed to detect stroke during the first 48 h after stroke onset [27]. In contrast to this, a 1989 study of 36 patients

with MCA infarction reported that 70% of CT examinations obtained within 4 h of stroke onset showed focal decreased attenuation consistent with tissue ischemia [28].

3.5.2 Early CT Findings in Hyperacute Stroke

NCCT findings within the first 3–6 h of stroke onset – when present – are typically subtle, and are mainly the result of tissue edema caused by early infarction, as previously described. The "classic" early ischemic changes (EIC) of stroke CT imaging are: (1) loss of gray–white matter differentiation in cortical gyri, basal ganglia or insula (the so-called insular ribbon sign); (2) loss of cortical sulci or narrowing of the sylvian fissure; (3) compression of the ventricular system and basal cisterns; and (4) hyperdensity in a Circle of Willis vessel due to the presence of occlusive thrombus, most notably in the middle cerebral artery (proximal MCA, also known as "hyperdense MCA sign," HMCAS, Fig. 3.5) [29]. The more recently described "MCA-dot sign" is indicative of thrombus in the more distal MCA sylvian branches (M2 or M3), and can frequently be seen without HMCAS. Normal attenuation values within the MCA are approximately 40 HU, whereas in the setting of thromboembolism, these values are increased to about 80 HU. An HU ratio >1.2 between the affected and contralateral, unaffected artery, in the setting of acute stroke symptoms, is considered suspicious of thrombus. The differential diagnosis of HMCAS includes calcified atherosclerosis, and high hematocrit levels [30].

Of the features listed above, parenchymal hypodensity is the most important. EIC have been reported in hyperacute, acute, and subacute stroke. In hyperacute stroke (0–3 h of stroke onset), EIC have been shown in up to 31–53% of cases [12, 31]. Tomura [7] reported a 92% rate of lentiform nucleus obscuration within 6 h of MCA stroke [7]. In another series of 53 patients studied within 5 h of angiographically proven MCA occlusion prior to i.v. thrombolysis, early CT showed hypodensity in 81%, brain swelling in 38%, and a hyperdense MCA in 47% [13]. Despite these different results with respect to the detection of EIC according to the stroke timeframe, it has been reported that there does not seem to be increased de-

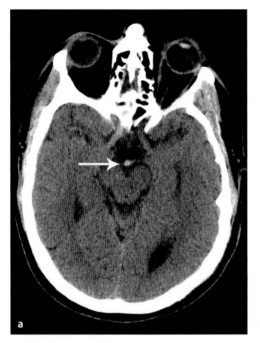
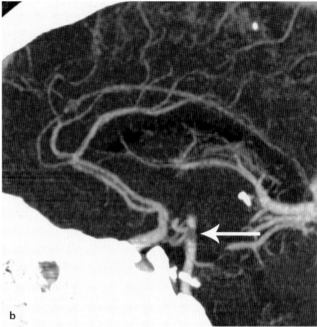

Figure 3.7 a, b

Image of a 44-year-old right-handed male, 5.5 h post onset of slurred speech, drowsiness, and left hemiparesis. The patient was immediately intubated in the Emergency Department. **a** NCCT shows dense vessel sign at the top of the basilar artery (*left arrow*). **b** CT angiography confirms the presence of a clot in the distal basilar artery (*right arrow*)

tection of EIC on NCCT within the 4–6 h post-stroke period as compared to the first 2–3 h post-stroke [11]. Early hypodensities have a high (87%) positive predictive value for stroke as seen on follow-up neuroimaging exams [13, 31].

Cortical swelling and sulcal effacement have not been clinically useful indicators of acute infarction. One series found no swelling in the first 3 h post-ictus; another found swelling in only 23% of patients imaged within 3 h [7, 8].

HMCAS, first described by Pressman in 1987, is a specific but insensitive indicator of acute MCA stroke; estimates of its incidence range from 1% to 50% [4, 29]. The presence of HMCAS depends on two factors: section thickness and delay between stroke onset and CT scanning [30]. Hyperdense attenuation of other arteries, such as the basilar, may also indicate the presence of thrombus; however, in our experi-

ence, this can frequently be seen with "normal" NCCT scans due to beam hardening of the posterior fossa, and therefore caution is advised in interpreting this finding (Fig. 3.7). Despite this, EIC in posterior circulation stroke has been reported: in one study of 40 patients with known acute basilar thrombosis, parenchymal signs of ischemia were seen in 27%, and a hyperdense basilar artery was present in 70%. A major criticism of these results is that CT evaluation was retrospective and unblinded, as all patients underwent i.a. thrombolysis [32].

3.5.3 Prognostic/Clinical Significance of EIC

The early CT findings listed above not only facilitate stroke detection, but can also help to predict prognosis and the response to thrombolytic therapy [10, 13, 33–35]. For example, in a study that revealed HMCAS in 18 of 55 (33%) patients presenting within 90 min of stroke onset, HMCAS was predictive of poor outcome after i.v. thrombolysis; a National Institutes of Health Stroke Scale (NIHSS) score of greater than 10 was an even better predictor of poor outcome [36]. Another group reported that early low attenuation in more than 50% of the MCA territory is predictive of up to 85% mortality, with poor outcome in survivors [13].

In the large i.v. thrombolysis trials, such as The European Cooperative Acute Stroke Study (ECASS) I, National Institute of Neurological Disorders and Stroke (NINDS) Study, and ECASS II, much attention was paid to the presence of EIC and their correlation with clinical outcome, in the hope of determining accurate prognostic indicators. The conclusions of these analyses – many of which were performed post-hoc – have been controversial, in part due to heterogeneous confounding variables such as varying reverse recombinant tissue plasminogen activator (rt-PA) doses, treatment times, stroke subtypes, and CT reader training.

ECASS I, a double-blind placebo-controlled trial of i.v. thrombolysis administered within 6 h of hemispheric stroke onset, was performed from 1992 to 1994, and involved 620 patients at 75 centers in 14 European countries [1, 37]. In this study, patients with initial CT findings of greater than one-third MCA territory hypodensity or sulcal effacement were shown to have an increased risk of fatal intraparenchymal hemorrhage after treatment (Fig. 3.4). Because of this, these findings are considered by some to be contraindications to thrombolytic therapy [10, 34, 35, 37, 38]. However, it is controversial whether this rule is applicable when only subtle early ischemic parenchymal changes are present (Table 3.5).

In the NINDS Study, which showed a benefit of i.v. thrombolysis administered within 3 h of stroke onset, there was a trend towards improved outcome despite the presence of early CT hypodensity [35]. In this trial, 624 patients were randomized to i.v. rt-PA versus placebo. Patients with hemorrhage on initial CT were excluded from the NINDS Study, a less strict entry criterion than was applied in the ECASS trial, in which patients with either early hemorrhage *or* significant parenchymal hypodensity on initial CT were excluded. In neither study was angiographic proof of

Table 3.5. NCCT predictors of poor stroke outcome

Hyperdense MCA sign on early NCCT
Early parenchymal hypoattenuation > 50% of the MCA territory
ASPECTS <7

a vascular occlusion amenable to thrombolytic treatment obtained prior to the administration of rt-PA. In NINDS, patients with hypodensity greater than one-third of the MCA territory had an odds-ratio of 2.9 for symptomatic hemorrhage, whereas patients with hypodensity less than one-third of the MCA territory had an odds-ratio of 1.5 [31]. In a different study of 1025 stroke patients treated with rt-PA, hypodensity greater than one-third of the MCA territory was also an independent risk factor for symptomatic hemorrhage [39].

Another controversy is that, in ECASS I, a positive effect of i.v. thrombolysis was revealed only after a careful *retrospective* review of the initial CT scans, with the application of strict, greater than one-third MCA territory hypodensity exclusion criteria [10, 35]. This difference from the NINDS trial may be partly related to the longer, 6-h treatment window applied to the ECASS patients. Furthermore, based on additional review of the ECASS data, it has been suggested that a subgroup of hyperacute stroke patients *without* demonstrable CT ischemia is also unlikely to benefit from i.v. thrombolysis. This is likely because, in patients with no or minimal ischemic change, the potential benefits of thrombolysis may be offset by the risk of hemorrhage [10].

3.6 ASPECTS

As already noted, regions of frank hypodensity on NCCT are likely to reflect severe and irreversible ischemic damage. Indeed, CT hypoattenuation seems to have a direct correspondence to critically hypoperfused tissue seen on positron emission tomography (PET) [21]. In an attempt to standardize the detection and reporting of the extent of ischemic hypodensity, the Alberta Stroke Program Early CT

Figure 3.8

Axial NCCT images showing the MCA territory regions as defined by ASPECTS. (*C* Caudate, *I* insular ribbon, *IC* internal capsule, *L* lenticular nucleus, *M1* anterior inferior frontal MCA cortex, *M2* inferior division, temporal lobe MCA cortex lateral to the insular ribbon, *M3* posterior temporal MCA cortex, *M4*, *M5* and *M6* are the corresponding anterior, lateral and posterior MCA cortices immediately rostral to M1, M2 and M3, respectively)

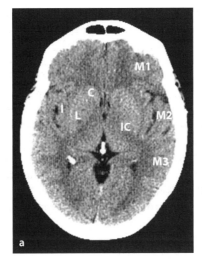

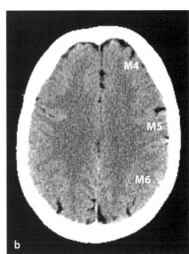

Score (ASPECTS) was proposed in 2000 [40]. With ASPECTS, the MCA territory is divided into ten regions of interest on two CT axial slices, including: caudate, insula, lenticular, internal capsule, and six other cortical regions ("M1"–"M6") (Fig. 3.8). The score is computed by subtracting, from 10, 1 point for each region containing an ischemic hypodensity. Hence, a completely normal MCA territory would receive a score of "10," and a completely infarcted MCA territory, a score of "0."

Although this method is reported to be more reliable and reproducible – with better inter- and intra-observer variability than the one-third MCA rule – this point is not without controversy [40–43]. In one study, Mak et al. [43] have suggested that the one-third MCA rule results in better interobserver agreement than ASPECTS in detecting clinically significant EIC, independent of prior knowledge of the clinical history. Further comparisons of these two methods for hypodensity quantification are warranted; however, it is clear that, at minimum, an important advantage to using ASPECTS is that it is easily taught to inexperienced observers, training them to carefully examine multiple regions for subtle hypodensity. This is especially important in the Emergency Department, where residents, fellows, and junior staff from Neurology, Emergency, and General Radiology Departments may be interpreting stroke CTs.

The correlation between ASPECTS and clinical outcomes in MCA stroke has also been examined. Within the first 3 h of MCA stroke onset, baseline ASPECTS values correlate inversely with the severity of NIHSS and with functional outcome; scores of 7 or less, indicating more extensive cerebral hypoattenuation in the MCA territory, are correlated with both poor functional outcome and symptomatic intracerebral hemorrhage [40].

3.6.1 Implications for Acute Stroke Triage

It is clear from the above that accurate, early identification of hypodense, ischemic brain parenchyma by CT has important clinical implications for acute stroke treatment. The advent of thrombolytic therapy makes the CT detection of hypodense brain tissue, as well as the better characterization of its predictive value for hemorrhage after treatment, exceedingly important. The ability of physicians to detect parenchymal hypodensity, however, is limited by potentially clinically relevant inter- and intra-observer variability [1, 9, 38, 44–46]. In the first ECASS trial, for example, almost half of the protocol violations were due to failure to recognize early NCCT signs of infarction [1, 37]. In discussing ECASS, one editorialist pointed out that, had the local, prospective readers been as capable of detecting subtle early signs of

Table 3.6. NCCT predictors of symptomatic intracranial hemorrhage post-thrombolysis for stroke

Parenchymal hypoattenuation >1/3 of the MCA territory
ASPECTS <7

ischemia as the panel of six expert neuroradiologists who later retrospectively reviewed the ECASS scans, the study results would have been dramatically improved [1] (Table 3.6).

In the ECASS II trial, in an attempt to control for confounding variables, lower doses of rt-PA were used than in the ECASS I trial, and patients with greater than one-third MCA territory hypodensities were excluded from the study; this resulted in very low hemorrhage rates in the rt-PA-treated patients [47]. In a more recent i.a. thrombolysis study, patients with a baseline ASPECTS >7 – implying less extensive MCA hypodensities on NCCT – had significantly more independent functional outcomes at 90 days than did patients with baseline ASPECTS ≤7 [48].

Despite its low sensitivity for stroke detection, HMCAS has been shown to have a high (91%) positive predictive value for neurological deterioration in MCA stroke [49]. In a series of 18 patients with proximal MCA occlusions suggested by HMCAS, 94% had poor final neurological outcomes [30]. In contrast, an isolated MCA-dot sign appears to be an indicator of less severe stroke at onset, with a more favorable long-term prognosis [50]. One study concluded that there was no difference in outcome between stroke patients with and without the MCA-dot sign [30].

HMCAS and MCA-dot sign were also reviewed with respect to outcomes after thrombolysis. In the ECASS I trial, HMCAS was associated with early cerebral edema, more severe neurological deficits, and poor clinical prognosis [10]. Nonetheless, patients with HMCAS treated with rt-PA, instead of placebo, remained more likely to have good neurological recovery [51]. In another study of 55 patients that received i.v. rt-PA within 90 min of stroke onset, HMCAS predicted poor outcome after i.v. thrombolysis, and this effect was even more pronounced in the subgroup of patients with HMCAS and NIHSS >10 [36]. Recently, a study comparing outcomes of pa-

tients treated with i.v. versus i.a. thrombolysis showed that, in i.a.-treated patients, outcomes were favorable regardless of the presence of HMCAS, whereas, in those treated with i.v. rt-PA, outcomes were less favorable when HMCAS was present [52]. Similarly, in posterior circulation strokes, EIC do not appear to be predictive of outcome in patients receiving i.a. thrombolysis [32].

Interestingly, although patients who present with a "top-of-carotid," "T" occlusion on NCCT or CTA commonly have larger final infarct volumes and poor clinical outcomes, additional EIC are not functional predictors of outcome following thrombolytic therapy [53].

3.6.2 Reading CT Scans

Some of the reported variability in CT scan interpretation is dependent on level of training. A study in *Journal of the American Medical Association* tested the ability of 103 emergency physicians, neurologists, and general radiologists to determine eligibility for thrombolytic therapy from a group of 54 acute head CTs [46]. Scan findings included intracerebral hemorrhage, acute infarction, intracerebral calcifications (impostor for hemorrhage), old cerebral infarction (impostor for acute infarction), and normal parenchyma. Of 569 CT readings by emergency physicians, 67% were correct; of 435 readings by neurologists, 83% were correct; and of 540 readings by radiologists, 83% were correct. Overall sensitivity for detecting hemorrhage was 82%; 17% of emergency physicians, 40% of neurologists, and 52% of radiologists achieved 100% sensitivity for identification of hemorrhage. The authors concluded that physicians in this study did not uniformly achieve a level of sensitivity for identification of intracerebral hemorrhage sufficient to permit safe selection of candidates for thrombolytic therapy.

Even brief periods of training, however, can improve inter-reader reliability in the early CT detection of stroke. At a 4-h training course for participants in the second ECASS trial, 532 readers were shown two different sets of ten CT scans before and after the course. After the completion of training, the average number of correct readings increased from

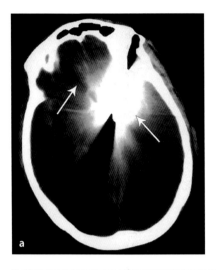
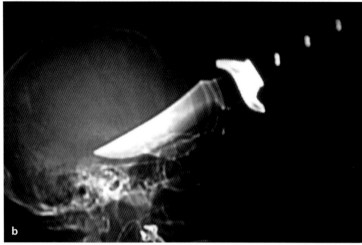

Figure 3.9 a, b

a NCCT with heavy streak artifact (*arrows*), due to the presence of a metallic foreign body (b)

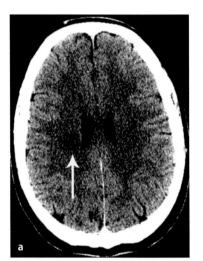
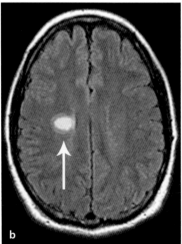
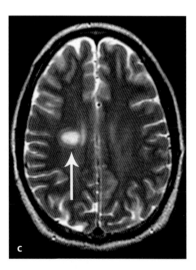

Figure 3.10 a–c

Example of one of the multiple differential diagnoses of NCCT hypodensity. Patient awoke with left hemiparesis. a NCCT shows hypodensity in the right corona-radiata (*arrow*). b Axial FLAIR and c axial T2-weighted MR images demonstrate corresponding high signal lesion in a horizontal peri-ventricular, or "dawson finger" distribution. The final diagnosis was multiple sclerosis

7.6 to 8.2 for the first set of cases, and from 6.3 to 7.2 for the second set of cases (*P*<0.001) [38].

The importance of having a relevant clinical history in the interpretation of subtle EIC findings – raising suspicion for stroke – should not be underestimated either. Mullins et al. [54] showed that availability of a clinical history indicating that early stroke is suspected significantly improves the sensitivity for detecting strokes on unenhanced CT (from approximately 38% to 52% in the cohort studied), without reducing specificity. In contradistinction, the availability of such a history did not significantly improve the sensitivity for detecting stroke using diffusion-weighted MR imaging (the findings of which are more conspicuous) [54].

We have found advantages to the use of both small and large image displays for CT analysis: with small size image display, an overall image review is facilitated, whereas the use of large size image display is useful for the analysis of specific structural details [55].

Finally, attention must be paid to avoiding interpretation pitfalls such as streak artifact (Fig. 3.9), patient tilt (Fig. 3.2b), and stroke mimics – such as multiple sclerosis – that can present with similar signs and symptoms (Fig. 3.10).

3.7 Conclusion

Despite ongoing technological advances in neuroimaging techniques and protocols for the assessment and treatment of patients with cerebrovascular diseases, NCCT remains the standard of care for acute stroke triage. Advantages of CT scanning in the assessment of acute stroke patients include convenience, accuracy, speed, and cost. At present, CT scanning is also the standard for the detection of acute subarachnoid and intraparenchymal hemorrhage, although newer MR susceptibility and fluid attenuated inversion recovery (FLAIR) techniques are challenging this claim [56–59]. The accuracy of CT scanning for stroke detection can be optimized by the use of an appropriate scanning technique, as well as interactive image review at a picture archival and communication system (PACS) workstation us-

ing narrow window and level settings. More importantly, CT scanning has prognostic value; for patients receiving thrombolytic treatment, it may help predict both responses to treatment and hemorrhage risk. Finally, as will be discussed in the following chapters, CT angiography (CTA) with or without CT perfusion (CTP) can be performed in the same imaging session as NCCT scanning without substantially delaying definitive thrombolytic treatment. This multimodal CT imaging provides data regarding both vascular patency and tissue perfusion, which has added value in the triage of acute stroke patients.

References

1. Russell E (1997) Diagnosis of hyperacute ischemic infarct with CT: key to improved clinical outcome after intravenous thrombolysis? Radiology 205:315–318
2. Del Zoppo GJ (1995) Acute stroke – on the threshold of a therapy. N Engl J Med 333:1632–1633
3. Powers WJ, Zivin J (1998) Magnetic resonance imaging in acute stroke: not ready for prime time (editorial). Neurology 50:842–843
4. Marks MP (1998) CT in ischemic stroke. Neuroimaging Clin North Am 8:515–523
5. Brant-Zawadzki M (1997) CT angiography in acute ischemic stroke: the right tool for the job? (Comment.) Am J Neuroradiol 18:1021–1023
6. Dillon WP (1998) CT techniques for detecting acute stroke and collateral circulation: in search of the Holy Grail (editorial, comment). Am J Neuroradiol 19:191–192
7. Tomura N, Uemura K, Inugami A, Fujita H et al (1988) Early CT findings in cerebral infarction: obscuration of the lentiform nucleus. Radiology 168:463–467
8. Truwit CL, Barkowich AJ, Gean-Marton A et al (1990) Loss of the insular ribbon: another early CT sign of acute middle cerebral artery infarction. Radiology 176:801–806
9. Von Kummer R, Holle R, Grzyska U, Hofmann E et al (1996) Interobserver agreement in assessing early CT signs of middle cerebral artery infarction. Am J Neuroradiol 17:1743–1748
10. Von Kummer R, Allen KL, Holle R et al (1997) Acute stroke: usefulness of early CT findings before thrombolytic therapy. Radiology 205:327–333
11. Mohr J, Biller J, Hilal S, Yuh W et al (1995) Magnetic resonance versus computed tomographic imaging in acute stroke. Stroke 26:807–812
12. Gonzalez RG, Schaefer PW, Buonanno F et al (1999) Diffusion-weighted MR imaging: diagnostic accuracy in patients imaged within 6 hours of stroke symptom onset. Radiology 210:155–162

13. Von Kummer R, Meyding-Lamade U, Forsting M et al (1994) Sensitivity and prognostic value of early CT in occlusion of the middle cerebral artery trunk. Am J Neuroradiol 15:9–15

14. Bendszus M, Urbach H, Meyer B, Schulthieb R, Solymosi L (1997) Improved CT diagnosis of acute middle cerebral artery territory infarcts with density-difference analysis. Neuroradiology 39:127–131

15. Lev MH, Gonzalez RG (2002) CT angiography and CT perfusion imaging. In: Toga AW, Mazziotta JC (eds) Brain mapping: the methods, 2nd edn. Academic Press, San Diego, Calif., pp 427–484

16. Bell BA, Symon L, Branston NM (1985) CBF and time thresholds for the formation of ischemic cerebral edema, and effect of reperfusion in baboons. J Neurosurg 62:31–41

17. Torack RM, Alcala H, Gado M et al (1976) Correlative assay of computerized cranial tomography CCT, water content and specific gravity in normal and pathological postmortem brain. J Neuropathol Exp Neurol 35:385–392

18. Unger E, Littlefield J, Gado M (1988) Water content and water structure in CT and MR signal changes: possible influence in detection of early stroke. Am J Neuroradiol 17:1743–1748

19. Dzialowski I, Weber J, Doerfler A, Forsting M, von Kummer R (2004) Brain tissue water uptake after middle cerebral artery occlusion assessed with CT. J Neuroimaging 14(1):42–48

20. Kucinski T, Vaterlein O, Glauche V, Fiehler J, Klotz E, Eckert B, Koch C, Rother J, Zeumer H (2002) Correlation of apparent diffusion coefficient and computed tomography density in acute ischemic stroke. Stroke 33(7):1786–1791

21. Grond M, von Kummer R, Sobesky J, Schmulling S, Rudolf J, Terstegge K et al (2000) Early x-ray hypoattenuation of brain parenchyma indicates extended critical hypoperfusion in acute stroke. Stroke 31(1):133–139

22. Lev MH, Ackerman RH (1999) In re: reversible ischemia determined by xenon-enhanced CT after 90 minutes of complete basilar artery occlusion. Am J Neuroradiol 20(10):2023–2024

23. Dix JA, Evans AJ, Kallmes DF, Sobel A, Phillips CD (1997) Accuracy and precision of CT angiography in a model of the carotid artery bifurcation. Am J Neuroradiol 18:409–415

24. Lev MH, Ackerman RH, Lustrin ES et al (1995) Two dimensional spiral CT angiography in carotid occlusive disease: measurement of residual lumen diameter with ultrasound correlation. Proceedings of the 33rd annual meeting of the American Society of Neuroradiology, Chicago, Ill.

25. Webb WR, Brant WE, Helms CA (eds) (1991) Introduction to CT of the abdomen and pelvis. In: Webb WR, Brant WE, Helms CA (eds) Fundamentals of body CT. Saunders, Philadelphia, Pa., p 137

26. Lev M, Farkas J, Gemmete J, Hossain S, Hunter G, Koroshetz W et al (1999) Acute stroke: improved nonenhanced CT detection- benefits of soft-copy interpretation by using variable window width and center level settings. Radiology 213:150–155

27. Wall SD, Brant-Zawadski M, Jeffrey RB, Barnes B (1982) High frequency CT findings within 24 hours after cerebral infarction. Am J Radiol 138:307–311

28. Bozzao L, Bastianello S, Fantozzi LM, Angeloni U, Argentino C, Fieschi C (1989) Correlation of angiographic and sequential CT findings in patients with evolving cerebral infarction. Am J Neuroradiol 10:1215–1222

29. Pressman BD, Tourje EJ, Thompson JR (1987) An early CT sign of ischemic infarction: increased density in a cerebral artery. Am J Neuroradiol 8:645–648

30. Somford DM, Nederkoorn PJ, Rutgers DR, Kappelle LJ, Mali WP, van der Grond J (2002) Proximal and distal hyperattenuating middle cerebral artery signs at CT: different prognostic implications. Radiology 223(3):667–671

31. Patel SC, Levine SR, Tilley BC, Grotta JC, Lu M, Frankel M et al (2001) Lack of clinical significance of early ischemic changes on computed tomography in acute stroke. J Am Med Assoc 286(22):2830–2838

32. Arnold M, Nedeltchev K, Schroth G, Baumgartner RW, Remonda L, Loher TJ et al (2004) Clinical and radiological predictors of recanalisation and outcome of 40 patients with acute basilar artery occlusion treated with intra-arterial thrombolysis. J Neurol Neurosurg Psychiatry 75(6):857–862

33. Tomsick TA, Brott T, Barsan W et al (1992) Thrombus localization with emergency cerebral computed tomography. Am J Neuroradiol 13:79–85

34. Adams HP, Brott TG, Furlan AJ et al (1996) Guidelines for thrombolytic therapy for acute stroke: a supplement to the guidelines for the management of patients with acute ischemic stroke. A statement for healthcare professionals from a Special Writing Group of the Stroke Council, American Heart Association. Circulation 94:1167–1174

35. The NINDS t-PA Stroke Study Group (1997) Intracerebral hemorrhage after intravenous t-PA therapy for ischemic stroke. Stroke 28:2109–2118

36. Tomsick T, Brott T, Barsan W, Broderick J et al (1996) Prognostic value of the hyperdense middle cerebral artery sign and stroke scale score before ultraearly thrombolytic therapy. Am J Neuroradiol 17:79–85

37. Hacke W, Kaste M, Fieschi C et al (1995) Intravenous thrombolysis with recombinant tissue plasminogen activator for acute hemispheric stroke: the European Cooperative Acute Stroke Study (ECASS). J Am Med Assoc 274:1017–1025

38. von Kummer R (1998) Effect of training in reading CT scans on patient selection for ECASS II. Neurology 51:S50–S52

39. Tanne D, Kasner SE, Demchuk AM, Koren-Morag N, Hanson S, Grond M et al (2002) Markers of increased risk of intracerebral hemorrhage after intravenous recombinant tissue plasminogen activator therapy for acute ischemic stroke in clinical practice: the Multicenter rt-PA Stroke Survey. Circulation 105(14):1679–1685

40. Barber PA, Demchuk AM, Zhang J, Buchan AM (2000) Validity and reliability of a quantitative computed tomography score in predicting outcome of hyperacute stroke before thrombolytic therapy. ASPECTS Study Group. Alberta Stroke Programme Early CT Score. Lancet 355(9216):1670–1674

41. Coutts SB, Demchuk AM, Barber PA, Hu WY, Simon JE, Buchan AM et al (2004) Interobserver variation of ASPECTS in real time. Stroke 35(5):103–105

42. Pexman JH, Barber PA, Hill MD, Sevick RJ, Demchuk AM, Hudon ME et al (2001) Use of the Alberta Stroke Program Early CT Score (ASPECTS) for assessing CT scans in patients with acute stroke. Am J Neuroradiol 22(8):1534–1542

43. Mak HK, Yau KK, Khong PL, Ching AS, Cheng PW, Au-Yeung PK et al (2003) Hypodensity of >1/3 middle cerebral artery territory versus Alberta Stroke Programme Early CT Score (ASPECTS): comparison of two methods of quantitative evaluation of early CT changes in hyperacute ischemic stroke in the community setting. Stroke 34(5):1194–1196

44. Tomsick T (1994) Sensitivity and prognostic value of early CT in occlusion of the middle cerebral artery trunk: a commentary. Am J Neuroradiol 15:16–18

45. Shinar D, Gross CR, Hier DB et al (1987) Interobserver reliability in the interpretation of computed tomographic scans of stroke patients. Arch Neurol 44:149–155

46. Schriger DL, Kalafut M, Starkman S, Krueger M, Saver JL (1998) Cranial computed tomography interpretation in acute stroke: physician accuracy in determining eligibility for thrombolytic therapy. J Am Med Assoc 279:1293–1297

47. Hacke W, Kaste M, Fieschi C, von Kummer R, Davalos A, Meier D et al (1998) Randomised double-blind placebo-controlled trial of thrombolytic therapy with intravenous alteplase in acute ischaemic stroke (ECASS II). Second European-Australasian Acute Stroke Study Investigators. Lancet 352(9136):1245–1251

48. Hill MD, Rowley HA, Adler F, Eliasziw M, Furlan A, Higashida RT et al (2003) Selection of acute ischemic stroke patients for intra-arterial thrombolysis with pro-urokinase by using ASPECTS. Stroke 34(8):1925–1931

49. Manno EM, Nichols DA, Fulgham JR, Wijdicks EF (2003) Computed tomographic determinants of neurologic deterioration in patients with large middle cerebral artery infarctions. Mayo Clin Proc 78(2):156–160

50. Leary MC, Kidwell CS, Villablanca JP, Starkman S, Jahan R, Duckwiler GR et al (2003) Validation of computed tomographic middle cerebral artery "dot" sign: an angiographic correlation study. Stroke 34(11):2636–2640

51. Manelfe C, Larrue V, von Kummer R, Bozzao L, Ringleb P, Bastianello S et al (1999) Association of hyperdense middle cerebral artery sign with clinical outcome in patients treated with tissue plasminogen activator. Stroke 30(4):769–772

52. Agarwal P, Kumar S, Hariharan S, Eshkar N, Verro P, Cohen B et al (2004) Hyperdense middle cerebral artery sign: can it be used to select intra-arterial versus intravenous thrombolysis in acute ischemic stroke? Cerebrovasc Dis 17(2–3):182–190

53. Kucinski T, Koch C, Eckert B, Becker V, Kromer H, Heesen C et al (2003) Collateral circulation is an independent radiological predictor of outcome after thrombolysis in acute ischaemic stroke. Neuroradiology 45(1):11–18

54. Mullins ME, Lev MH, Schellingerhout D, Koroshetz WJ, Gonzalez RG (2002) Influence of the availability of clinical history on the noncontrast CT detection of acute stroke. Am J Radiol 179(1):223–228

55. Seltzer SE, Judy PF, Feldman U, Scarff L, Jacobson FL (1998) Influence of CT image size and format on accuracy of lung nodule detection. Radiology 206(3):617–622

56. Singer MB, Atlas SW, Drayer BP (1998) Subarachnoid space disease: diagnosis with fluid-attenuated inversion-recovery MR imaging and comparison with gadolinium-enhanced spin-echo MR imaging- blinded reader study. Radiology 208:417–422

57. Atlas SW, Thulborn KR (1998) MR detection of hyperacute parenchymal hemorrhage of the brain. Am J Neuroradiol 19:1471–1507

58. Gilleland GT, Gammal T, Fisher W (1998) Hyperacute intraventricular hemorrhage revealed by gadolinium-enhanced MR imaging. Am J Radiol 170:787–789

59. Noguchi K, Ogawa T, Inugami A et al (1995) Acute subarachnoid hemorrhage: MR imaging with fluid attenuated inversion recovery MR imaging. Radiology 203:257–262

Stroke CT Angiography (CTA)

Shams Sheikh, R. Gilberto González,
Michael H. Lev

Contents

4.1 Introduction

Death or incapacitating disability can be prevented or diminished in some patients who present within 6 h of embolic stroke onset by thrombolytic therapy [1–14]. With the recent advent of the Desmotoplase in Acute Ischemic Stroke (DIAS) Trial results, this time window may soon be extended to as long as 9 h [15]. In the treatment of anterior circulation stroke, current guidelines support the use of intravenous (i.v.) recombinant tissue plasminogen activator (rt-PA) administered within 3 h of stroke [12, 13]. Intra-arterial (i.a.) thrombolysis, which has a longer treatment window, can be administered within 6 h of anterior circulation stroke ictus [9]. However, the risk of intracranial hemorrhage from these agents, as well as the probability of treatment failure, increases dramatically with time after stroke onset [6, 13, 16]. In the case of brainstem (posterior circulation) stroke, the treatment window for thrombolysis is greater than 6 h, not only because of the apparent increased resistance of the posterior circulation to hemorrhage, but also because of the uniformly poor outcome of untreated basilar artery strokes and the lack of alternative therapies [10].

Conventional, noncontrast head CT (NCCT) scanning is performed on all patients prior to treatment, in order to exclude hemorrhage or a large [greater than one-third middle cerebral artery (MCA) territory] infarction, both of which are contraindications to treatment [13, 16]. The role of unenhanced CT in the evaluation of acute stroke is fully discussed in the previous chapter. Although NCCT has some value in predicting patients most likely to be *harmed by* thrombolysis, it is of little value in predicting the patients – those with large vessel vascular occlusions – most likely to *benefit from* thrombolysis.

Because *NCCT and clinical exam alone are limited in their ability to detect large vessel thrombus, CT angiography (CTA) has been increasingly advocated as a first-line diagnostic test for patients presenting with signs and symptoms of acute stroke.* Advancements in scanner technology, novel contrast injection schemes that allow for uniform vascular and tissue enhancement, and the availability of rapid post-processing algorithms have all resulted in the clinically practical detection using CTA of both circle-of-Willis thrombus [17, 18] and parenchymal stroke [19–24].

Due to the narrow time window available for the initiation of thrombolytic treatment, speed is of the essence. The rationale in the workup for acute stroke is therefore to identify *as quickly as possible* those patients who may benefit from i.a. or i.v. thrombolysis or other available acute stroke therapies. Importantly, CTA *excludes* from treatment patients with occlusive stroke mimics [e.g., transient ischemic attack (TIA), complex migraine, seizure] *who will not benefit* from, and may be harmed by, such therapies.

The CTA protocol described in this chapter was designed to provide diagnostically useful information about both the vascular and parenchymal phases of brain enhancement. The administration of contrast serves two purposes: first, to visualize acute clot in the MCA, distal internal carotid artery (ICA), basilar artery, and other major circle of Willis vessels (Fig. 4.1); and second, to better delineate potentially salvageable, underperfused, ischemic areas of the brain that are at risk for full infarction if circulation is not restored. More specifically this includes those areas with a relative lack of contrast enhancement on CTA source images (CTA-SI), consistent with reduced blood volume. Indeed, simultaneous recording and subtraction, on a slice-by-slice basis, of the pre- from the post-contrast axial images results in *quantitative* maps of cerebral blood volume (CBV) [25]. The reasons for, and clinical significance of, this blood volume weighting of CTA-SIs is fully discussed in the next chapter on CT perfusion. Moreover, CTA-SI can also be of value in suggesting otherwise unsuspected regions of vascular occlusion. For example, CTA-SI

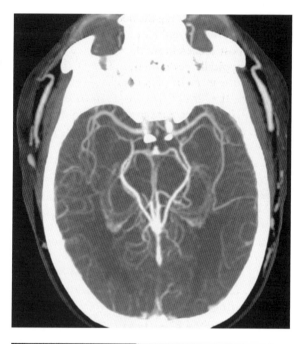

Figure 4.1

Axial maximal intensity projection (MIP) image obtained at the CT scanner console provides a rapid review of the major intracranial vessels for possible occlusion

"perfusion deficits" present in multiple vascular territories, visible on post- but not pre-contrast images, suggests cardiac emboli as the stroke source.

Helical CT is less expensive and more readily available at most hospital emergency departments compared to MRI; therefore, performing CTA can be a quick and natural extension of the NCCT exam, an exam that is already routinely obtained as part of the pre-thrombolysis workup at most institutions. The addition of CTA seldom adds more than 10 min of scanning and reconstruction time to that of the conventional CT examination. With the speed of the newer generation of multidetector row CT (MDCT) scanners, a complete "arch-to-vertex" CTA can be performed during the dynamic administration of a single bolus of contrast, allowing visualization of the great vessel origins, carotid bifurcations, and Circle of Willis – often obviating the need for further evaluation by MR angiography or ultrasound. Although complete post-processing of the entire neurovascular system is typically performed offline (during which time the patient can be prepared for thrombolysis, if necessary), the "critical" maximal intensity projection (MIP) reformatted images of the intracranial circulation can routinely be constructed directly at the CT console in under a minute.

This chapter will discuss the role of CTA in the diagnosis and triage of acute stroke patients. First, the general principles of helical CT scanning will be reviewed, including image acquisition and reconstruction techniques. The stroke CTA protocol will then be described, followed by specific issues regarding the accuracy and clinical utility of stroke CTA.

4.2 Background – General Principles of CTA

The development of helical CT in the early 1990s made possible the rapid acquisition of angiographic-type vascular images, with no greater risk of patient complications than that of routine i.v. contrast-enhanced CT scanning. With helical CT scanning, a slip-ring scanner design developed in the early 1990s, permits the x-ray tube and detectors to freely rotate around the gantry for a full 360°, allowing CT image data to be continuously and rapidly acquired as the scanner table moves uniformly through the gantry. This results in the creation of a three-dimensional helical "ribbon" of data that can be reconstructed at any arbitrary slice increment, and reformatted in any arbitrary plane (Fig. 4.2).

4.2.1 Advantages and Disadvantages of CTA

CTA has both advantages and disadvantages compared to other vascular imaging techniques [26–28]. Increasingly, as scanner speed and spatial resolution continue to improve – for a relatively constant total radiation dose – with the ongoing development of more advanced 16-, 32-, and 64-slice multidetector row CT scanners, these disadvantages are becoming less restrictive, especially with regard to total iodinated contrast dose.

4.2.1.1 Potential Advantages

Speed. The entire length of the ICA can be scanned in under 60 s (the extracranial ICA alone in less than 30 s), minimizing image misregistration from motion and breathing artifacts, and often reducing contrast requirements.

Accuracy. CTA provides truly anatomic, non-flow-dependent data with regard to length of stenoses, residual lumen diameters and areas, and calcifications; flow-dependent techniques such as MR angiography (MRA) and ultrasound (US) are not able to provide these data. Figure 4.3 illustrates the accuracy of CTA as compared to contrast-enhanced MRA.

Low Risk. CTA has a lower rate of patient discomfort, is less expensive, and has considerably lower risk of stroke and other vascular complications compared to conventional catheter arteriography. It is also advantageous in situations when MR is contraindicated or cannot be performed. CTA is typically more readily available than MR, especially in emergency settings. CTA, unlike MRA, lends itself to the imaging of acutely ill patients, as there are no restrictions on the type and quantity of associated support equipment, such as intravenous pumps, ventilators, or monitoring hardware. Because CT scan acquisition is more rapid than that of MRA, CTA is less prone to motion artifact. When CTA is combined with CT perfusion (CTP) for the evaluation of acute stroke, quantitative perfusion data can also be obtained, which is not typically possible with MR perfusion imaging.

4.2.1.2 Potential Disadvantages

Limited Field-of-view and Spatial Resolution. With slower, older generation, single slice helical scanners, CTA is limited in its ability to optimally evaluate tandem or multiple lesions of diverse vessels. This is usually due to restrictions imposed by either x-ray tube heating or the contrast bolus dose. Also, for a given set of imaging parameters (mAs, kV, slice thickness, etc.), single-slice CTA has slightly decreased in-plane resolution compared to conventional axial CT imaging. With the newer, faster, multidetector row scanners, these limitations do not typically exist.

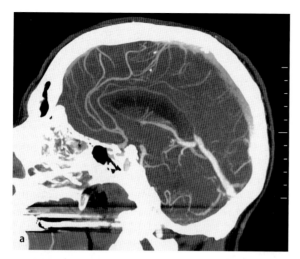

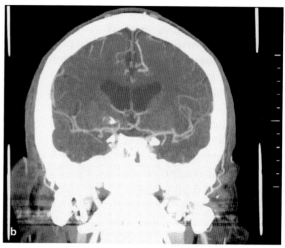

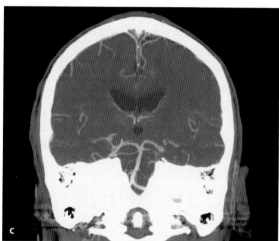

Figure 4.2

Sagittal and coronal MIP images, output from the CT scanner console, in the plane selected by the user. The slice thickness is adjusted to target the vessels of interest and "remove" overlying vessels that would obscure evaluation. **a** Sagittal MIP image shows the course of the anterior cerebral artery with variant additional vessels arising from the anterior communicating artery. **b** Coronal MIP image shows the ICA and MCA bifurcations bilaterally. **c** Second coronal MIP image adjusted to view the basilar artery in its entirety

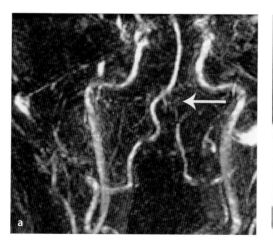

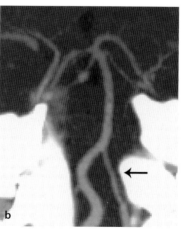

Figure 4.3

a Contrast-enhanced MRA: there is apparent nonfilling of the left vertebral artery (*arrow*). **b** Curved reformat from CTA of the vertebrobasilar junction now demonstrates patent vertebral arteries (*arrow*)

Long Post-processing. CTA reconstructions may require long post-processing times. Although axial, coronal, and sagittal MIP images of the circle of Willis can typically be obtained at the CT console by technologists in under a minute, more complex reconstructions, such as curved reformats of the entire length of the carotid or vertebral arteries, can take considerably longer.

Physiological Data. Unlike MRA and US, CTA is limited in its ability to provide physiological data, such as flow velocity or direction.

Accuracy of Reconstructions. Dense, circumferential calcifications can cause beam hardening and degrade the accuracy of vascular reconstructions. Optimal methods for measuring small (<1–1.5 mm) vascular stenosis are under investigation.

Iodinated Contrast Risk. The risks of routine i.v. contrast administration accompany CTA, including the possibility of allergic or idiosyncratic reactions or glomerular injury. Compared with US and MRA, which do not require i.v. contrast, CTA can be inconvenient for routine follow-up studies. Some hospitals commonly use US and MRA for noninvasive vascular screening and follow-up of carotid occlusive disease. In the nonemergency setting, CTA can be reserved for use as a problem-solving tool when the results of US and MRA are inconsistent, or when tandem lesions are present, such as in Fig. 4.4, and can often obviate the need for conventional catheter arteriography.

4.2.2 CTA Scanning Technique: Pearls and Pitfalls

The rapid acquisition of the large digital dataset required for CTA places great demands on CT imaging hardware and software. Because CT image noise is inversely proportional to x-ray photon flux through a given axial slice, optimal helical scanning requires a high x-ray tube heat load capacity.

Certain user-defined imaging parameters are unique to helical CT scanning. "Pitch" refers to the ratio between table increment per gantry rotation and x-ray beam collimation [29].

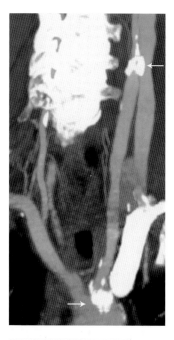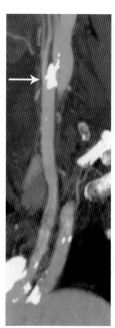

Figure 4.4

Tandem lesion, with stenosis at the origin of the left common carotid artery (LCCA) and origin of the left internal carotid artery (LICA)

Depending on the precise vendor and generation of scanner (single-slice, 4-slice, 8-slice, 16-slice, etc.), tube-heating constraints may limit the total deposited tube current [in milliampere-seconds (mAs)]. For a given tube current (in mAs) and voltage (in kV), increasing the pitch, by increasing the table increment per gantry rotation, will allow greater coverage; however, there will be fewer photons per slice, resulting in quantum mottle. When the table travel per rotation is equal to the beam collimation, there is a one-to-one ratio between the column of transmitted x-rays and the detector width; the pitch is "1," and image quality is improved [30]. When the table travel per rotation is less than the beam collimation, pitch is less than 1, and there is "overlap" of photon flux through the imaged tissue bed, resulting in even greater image quality. Figure 4.5 illustrates the advantage of overlapping the acquisition of helical data. Hence, in all our neuroimaging protocols at Massachusetts General

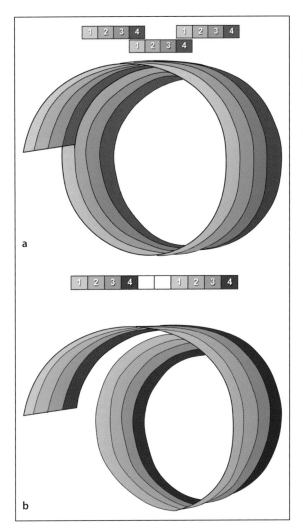

Figure 4.5

"Ribbons" of helical data as acquired from helical CT. a When the pitch is less than 1, such as in a four-channel system, and the table translation equals three channels, then the ribbon acquired from the first channel of the second rotation will overlap the ribbon of the fourth channel of the first rotation. b When the pitch is greater than 1, more longitudinal area can be covered; however, the helical data ribbons do not overlap, so each ribbon must receive a sufficiently high x-ray dose to obtain a diagnostic image, and the advantages of overlapping data cannot be used

Table 4.1. Optimization of posterior fossa image quality and minimization of "windmill artifact"

Minimal pitch (0.5–0.6)
Slow table speed (5–7 mm/gantry rotation)
Maximal gantry rotation rate (0.4–0.5 s/rotation)
Thinnest possible acquisition matrix; thick reformats for image review

Hospital (MGH), optimal visualization of posterior fossa structures is achieved using a pitch <1. In order to both optimize posterior fossa image quality and minimize helical "windmill artifact," we therefore typically employ a pitch of 0.5–0.6, along with a relatively slow table speed of 5–7 mm/rotation, with the newest generation of multidetector row scanners. Additionally, in an attempt to reduce motion artifact, our protocols typically call for the most rapid achievable gantry rotation rate. This can be as fast as 0.5 s per rotation on the newer 16-slice scanners. Moreover, spatial resolution in the z-direction is optimized by the acquisition of minimally thin slices, although image noise and quantum mottle are reduced by the review of thicker reformatted images (Table 4.1). Finally, we routinely choose our tube current (in mAs) setting to be no higher than that which will permit the use of the small – rather than the large – focal spot size.

By maximizing longitudinal coverage and image quality, the overall time to complete imaging increases. This demands an increased amount of iodinated contrast media, so as to adequately opacify the arterial tree being imaged, while minimizing arterial dilution and wash out, as well as venous opacification. Ideally, the overall dose of contrast agent should also be minimized so as to lessen the risk of contrast-induced nephropathy (CIN), as well as allergic reaction. Variations on the theme of contrast administration include injection strategies such as a saline bolus chaser and multiphasic injection, which are explained below. For a given pitch, an increased table speed permits greater z-direction coverage of the arterial tree during peak, uniform contrast enhancement, whereas a slower table speed, although providing greater image quality, may result in imaging portions of the vascular system with less than optimal enhancement, and more venous opacification.

4.2.2.1 Single-slice Protocols

In order to achieve optimal arterial image contrast and resolution, single-slice CTA protocols must therefore be tailored to the region being studied, the clinical question being asked, and the heat load capability of the scanner being used. In general, values for slice acquisition, thickness, scan field of view (FOV), and pitch should be as small as possible such that the entire region of interest can be covered in a single scan. Of note, for both single and multislice scanners, the diameter of the body part being scanned should never exceed the scan FOV, or beam-hardening artifact from outside the FOV will result. Conversely, tube current should be as large as possible, within tube heating constraints, so as to maximize photon flux and therefore minimize quantum mottle (image graininess). The image reconstruction interval should also be minimized in order to reduce the step or "zipper" artifact. For example, optimal characterization of a known, focal, carotid bifurcation stenosis can be achieved using the following single-slice CT parameters: 1 mm collimation, pitch of 1, 0.5 mm reconstruction interval, 12 cm FOV, 140 kV, and 250 mA, scanned narrowly around the level of maximal stenosis. Screening of the *entire* carotid artery, however, requires 3 mm collimation, a pitch >1, and typically a reduced tube current and voltage, to permit greater z-direction coverage [27, 28, 31].

4.2.2.2 Multi-slice Protocols

With multidetector row CT (MDCT), the choice of optimal scan parameters becomes more complex. Armed with newer x-ray tubes capable of higher heat capacity, as well as novel detector designs, multislice scanners can comfortably image entire vascular territories without the aforementioned constraints. The more rapid MDCT affords imaging of the arterial phase during more uniform contrast enhancement, more closely mimicking a catheter arteriogram [32]. Early MDCT scanners, circa 1994, had a detector ar-

ray of four rows along the z-axis, with four data channels to record the x-ray attenuation. Newer MDCT scanners employ 16 or more detector rows with varying combinations of individual detector widths, data channels, maximal z-direction coverage, and minimal slice thickness. Some vendors build detector arrays with narrower central rows than outer rows – so-called adaptive array detectors [33]. At the time of writing, 64-slice scanners will soon be commercially available, which will be capable of up to 4 cm of z-direction coverage and 0.6-mm-thick slices per gantry rotation. Such scanners will be ideally suited to coronary artery imaging. Overall, when compared with single-slice scanners, multislice scanners allow for reduced contrast dose, shorter scan duration, and thinner slices.

4.2.3 Radiation Dose Considerations

Interestingly, as the number of detector rows and channels increases in the evolution of MDCT scanners, allowing more coverage and better resolution, overall radiation dose to the patient has not significantly increased for a given level of image quality. At most institutions, the radiation dose for a typical head CT remains in the range of 0.06–0.12 Gy or 6–12 rad. To put this in context, the limits for occupational exposure to radiation (as set by the Nuclear Radiology Commission), for negligible likelihood of harmful effect, is no greater than 50 milli-sievert (mSv) per year (or 5 rem/year) [34]. In comparison, environmental exposure to radiation, such as from radon and cosmic x-rays, is approximately 3.5 mSv/year, and that of a single chest radiograph is roughly 0.05–0.1 mSv [35, 36]. It is noteworthy that these limits exist for occupational exposure, but not for patients, as it is assumed that patient exposure is diagnostically required.

To compare exposure between different CT protocols, one can use the absorbed dose, usually reported as the CT dose index (CTDI) in mGy. This concept was introduced by Jucius and Kambic to predict the multiple slice average dose at the center of a set of axial scans [37]. The product of the $CTDI_{vol}$ and the z-axis coverage for the particular scan then yields the "dose-length product" (DLP), where $CTDI_{vol}$ is the

Table 4.2. Strategies to reduce radiation dose

	Advantages	Disadvantages
Lower tube current (mAs)	Decreased radiation dose	Noisier image
Thinner slices with low tube current (mAs)	Decreased radiation dose Can reformat to any desired thickness	Source images are too grainy
Automated tube modulation	Decreased radiation dose	Complexity of scan setup

average dose in the standard head CT dosimetry phantom [38, 39].

With regard to MDCT radiation exposure, several factors must be weighed. There is up to a 4.5% loss of efficiency versus single-detector row scanners due to absorption of radiation in the z-axis by septa between the detector rows [33]. However, with MDCT, more of the x-ray beam is utilized per rotation due to the increased number of detector rows, with less of a penumbra [33]. Subsequently, these effects balance, and the dose efficiency of MDCT has been shown to be comparable to that of single-slice helical CT [33].

A related issue is the so-called cone beam effect, which to date has been a rate-limiting step in the development of larger (32-, 64-slice) detector arrays. This refers to the fact that the further a given detector row is from the center of the x-ray beam, the more angled the beam is through that detector, introducing nonlinearities to the image reconstruction algorithm.

There are several strategies to reduce radiation exposure in MDCT. Reducing photon flux is the primary means; however, decreasing tube current (mAs) results in increased image noise, as there are fewer x-rays per slice interrogated. This "quantum mottle" therefore becomes exaggerated with thinner slices. As already noted, the noise associated with thin slices can be compensated for by review of thicker slab reformatted images. Indeed, it has been shown that increasing depth from 4 to 8 cm requires doubling the tube current (mAs) to maintain the same amount of noise [38, 39]. Again, to lower the tube current (mAs) and maintain diagnostic image quality with MDCT, thinner slices with decreased tube current (mAs) can be acquired and reconstructed at thicker, less noisy slice intervals. Table speed and pitch can

also be increased, thereby decreasing exposure, so long as image quality is not degraded [40].

Lowering kilovoltage peak (kVp) is another strategy to reduce radiation exposure. The kVp setting reflects both photon number and photon energy. With higher kVp values, although fewer photons are absorbed (due to less interaction with biological tissue, which typically has a relatively low "k-edge"), each photon has higher energy. Hence, calculation of actual *absorbed* radiation dose becomes complex for low kVp scanning, in which tube current (mAs) is often increased to maintain image quality. Typical kVp for head CT scanning is 140 or 120 kVp [41]. A notable exception to this is CTP, which employs 80 kVp, so as to take advantage of the low k-edge of iodine, in order to increase conspicuity of the relatively small amounts of contrast reaching the brain parenchyma (see Chapter 5).

Specific advances in MDCT have been directed towards lowering radiation dose. Among these, automatic tube current modulation is more important for body than for head imaging. With this technique, the tube current is adjusted according to body diameter on the scout image, so as to maintain the same total amount of noise in the image (proportional to photon flux) for any given slice (Table 4.2) [42].

4.3 CTA Protocol for Acute Stroke

4.3.1 General Considerations

A successful CTA protocol requires balancing multiple *scanning, contrast administration, reformatting, and reconstruction parameters, in order to obtain diagnostically useful images* of the enhanced vascular tree. Reformatting here refers to the immediate post-process-

Table 4.3. General principles of single-slice CT and multidetector row CT (*MDCT*)

Single Slice CT	MDCT
Standard contrast dose	Reduced contrast dose
Longer imaging time	Shorter imaging time
Thicker slices	Thinner slices

ing of the raw image data into various slice thicknesses, FOVs, and "kernel" formats (such as "bone" or "brain" algorithms). Reconstruction refers to the creation of summary 2D and 3D projections for image review and interpretation (such as maximum intensity projection, "MIP," or volume rendering, "VR").

Ideally, there should be no venous enhancement; although, except for specific indications - such as cavernous sinus aneurysm and arterial venous malformation (AVM) assessment – this is seldom clinically limiting. *z*-direction coverage, in plane and longitudinal resolution, and signal-to-noise ratio should be maximized, while minimizing radiation dose, total amount of contrast administered, and acquisition slice thickness. Our routine stroke CTA protocol for 8-, 16-, 64-, and sometimes even 4-slice MDCT scanners covers from the great vessel origins at the aortic arch, to the cranial vertex. A typical 4-slice protocol might cover only the neck and Circle-of-Willis vessels, and a typical single-slice protocol might be restricted to the Circle of Willis only.

MDCT is preferred over single-detector row helical scanners, as there is improved heat load capacity of the x-ray tube, which results in more freedom in selecting the specific imaging parameters. The coverage area can be imaged more quickly with MDCT; there are more options in selecting pitch, table speed, and intrinsic slice thickness to obtain a desirable image quality. With continued scanner evolution, *the interaction between these variables is increasingly complex and nonintuitive; however, in our experience – for brain imaging – certain general principles have emerged, as enumerated in Table 4.3.* Although increasing pitch or table speed can lead to lowered image quality, this can be overcome by increasing tube current (mAs). With decreasing pitch, and hence

more overlap of the helical dataset, raw images benefit from increased density of the x-ray attenuation data, resulting in less noise.

After reformatting, MDCT data are displayed as both axial images (usually with a slice thickness that is a multiple of the acquisition slice thickness) and reconstructed images (discussed below). With MDCT, the interslice gap can be arbitrarily selected, so the subsequent 2D and 3D reconstructed images will not be subject to "zipper" or "stair step" artifact.

4.3.2 Contrast Considerations

Optimal CTA imaging is dependent on the concentration of intravascular iodine, which in turn is dependent on both choice of contrast and injection strategy. Nonionic CT contrast agents have been shown to be safe in an animal model of MCA stroke, without significant neuronal toxicity, even to already ischemic neurons [43, 44]. There are several forms of nonionic contrast, with varying concentrations of iodine. The relationship between concentration and enhancement is demonstrated graphically in Fig. 4.6 [45, 46].

Some patients are at higher risk for CIN, most notably those who are diabetic, who have pre-existing renal dysfunction, or who have a combination of the two. Nephrotoxicity from contrast media is dose dependent [47, 48]. Recently, Aspelin et al. [49] demonstrated the benefit of using iodixanol, an iso-osmolar agent, in patients with diabetes and borderline renal function, although this agent has both increased expense, and increased viscosity at room temperature, compared to other low osmolar (but not iso-osmolar) agents [49, 50]. In their randomized prospective multi-center study, diabetic patients with renal impairment undergoing angiography had a 3% incidence of CIN. To counter the increased viscosity of iodixanol, one can pre-warm the contrast media. It is noteworthy, however, that some studies have suggested that other low-osmolar agents, with lower cost and viscosity, may have similarly good safety profiles with regard to CIN.

For those patients who are allergic to iodinated contrast media, premedication with anti-histamines and steroids can blunt the anaphylactic response.

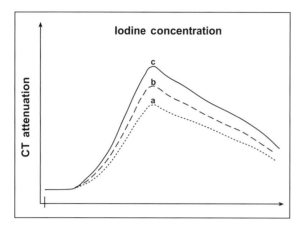

Figure 4.6

When iodine concentration is increased, there is a pro-portionally greater peak enhancement, shown with iodine concentration greatest in *c* and least in *a*

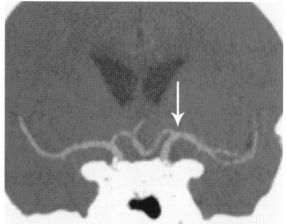

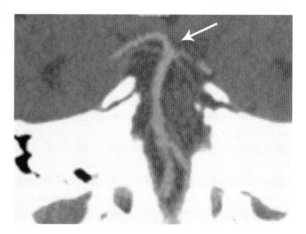

Figure 4.7

Gadolinium-enhanced CTA can be used in an urgent situation. Here, the top of the internal carotid arteries is clearly seen, as is the top of the basilar artery

Although a full discussion of the management of iodinated contrast allergy is beyond the scope of this text, it is noteworthy that, in the setting of an acute stroke, there is insufficient time to complete a course of steroid administration, which requires many hours. For such patients, gadolinium may be used as an alternative CT contrast agent for the evaluation of acute stroke [51]. Importantly, some researchers have suggested that – at the doses required for CTA – any potential advantage of gadolinium over iodinated contrast, for use in patients with high risk of CIN, is negated. Figure 4.7 demonstrates the clinical utility of gadolinium for emergent evaluation of the Circle of Willis by CTA.

Yet another strategy to decrease total contrast load is the use of a so-called bolus chaser – saline rapidly injected immediately following the contrast bolus. This has the advantage of clearing the "dead space" of contrast in the i.v. tubing and brachiocephalic/sub-clavian veins that does not typically contribute to im-aging (thereby also reducing streak artifact at the thoracic inlet). Bolus chasing, which requires the use of a dual-head CT power injector, has been shown to be effective in maintaining peak maximum enhance-ment, with a reduced total contrast dose [52–54]. The addition of a chaser results in a similar initial rate of enhancement, and can additionally contribute to a longer overall duration of enhancement [55], shown graphically by Fig. 4.8. It is estimated that bolus chas-ing can reduce total contrast load by an average of 25% or more [56, 57].

4.3.2.1 Contrast Timing Strategies

Achieving adequate arterial opacification depends on the volume, rate, and duration of contrast administra-tion, graphically depicted in Fig. 4.9. Ideally, imag-

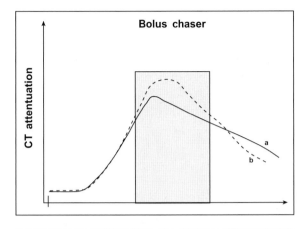

Figure 4.8

Use of a saline bolus chaser (*b, dashed line*) results in a greater maximum enhancement and a slower delay in wash out when compared to the standard bolus (*a, solid line*). The *rectangle* shows the ideal enhancement

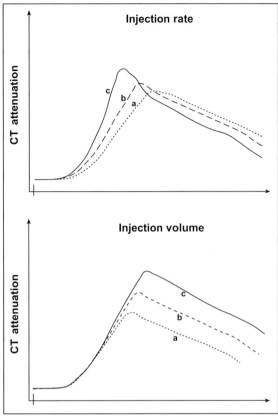

Figure 4.9

Increasing the injection rate (*c* has the fastest rate) or volume (*c* has the greatest volume) results in a greater maximum enhancement

ing should begin as the arterial tree enhances, and be completed prior to significant venous opacification – something not routinely achievable due to the relatively short mean transit time (2–4 s) of contrast through the capillary bed. This is not typically problematic unless the cavernous sinus is being evaluated, although, as noted earlier, the extremely rapid imaging achievable with the newest generation of 64-slice helical scanners lends new importance to various contrast-timing strategies (Table 4.4).

Indeed, with up to 16-slice scanners, our acute stroke protocol typically calls for a fixed 25-s prep delay between the onset of contrast administration and the onset of scanning, except for patients with atrial fibrillation (or other causes of significantly decreased cardiac output), who require a longer, 35- to 40-s delay.

Scanners equipped with a "bolus tracking" function can use a variable prep delay, in order to minimize venous enhancement; however, this adds complexity to scanning protocols, and is seldom clinically important unless scanning is very rapid. With bolus tracking, scanning starts once a preset Hounsfield opacification is reached in a vessel of interest. As already noted, venous opacification *does not* routinely interfere with diagnostic evaluation, with the pos-

sible exception of cavernous sinus evaluation. The inherent lag within the system, between the desired time to start imaging and the actual image acquisition, remains the main disadvantage with this technique. This can range from 5 to 15 s, as reported in several studies [58–60]. Modern scanners have a delay of as long as 4 s with the bolus tracking function.

As an alternative to bolus tracking, a "smartscan" type function can be used, in which a test bolus is administered to determine the scan delay [61]. A region of interest is selected, typically in the proximal ICA, and 10 ml of contrast is injected. This region is scanned continuously using the "low mAs/kVp"

Table 4.4. Strategies for contrast dose administration

	Advantages	Disadvantages
Higher iodine concentration	Better opacification	Higher contrast dose
Higher flow rate	Greater peak enhancement	Larger i.v. access Vascular injury
Higher injection volume	Greater peak enhancement	Higher iodine load
Iso-osmolar contrast	Less nephrotoxic	Costlier Increased viscosity
Gadolinium	Can be used in urgent situations, for patients with severe allergy	Vascular enhancement not as dense; risk of increased nephrotoxicity with large gadolinium doses
Saline chaser	Less contrast medium Decreased streak artifact at origin of great vessels Greater absolute difference in attenuation	Requires potentially expensive specialized dual head CT power injectors
Fixed delay	Simple, error free, straightforward for multiple technologists in large centers	Must lengthen delay for atrial fibrillation; may be inadequate for timing in very rapid newer (64-slice) scanners
Bolus tracking	Accounts for different patient physiology	More complex and time consuming for the technologist; scanning may not occur during peak or uniform contrast enhancement
Test bolus	Accounts for different patient physiology	More complex; requires 10–15 ml of additional contrast, not required for imaging
Multiphasic injection (Fleischmann)	Uniform plateau of enhancement Accounts for varying patient physiology	Requires test bolus Requires dual phase CT power injector
Multiphasic, with exponential decay (Bae)	Uniform plateau of enhancement	Requires multiple assumptions regarding patient factors that may not be known or justifiable Requires CT power injector capable of exponential decay mode

technique, and the prep delay is chosen as the time corresponding to 50% of maximal test vessel opacification. As with bolus tracking, however, a test bolus is seldom clinically necessary. Of the thousands of CTAs performed at MGH, scanning began too early with the use of a 25-s delay for only a handful of patients with low cardiac output secondary to atrial fibrillation. Figure 4.10 demonstrates the limited utility of a scan when the delay is not chosen correctly. Both mathematical and animal models have demonstrated that, when there is reduced cardiac output, intravenous injection will result in a delayed intra-

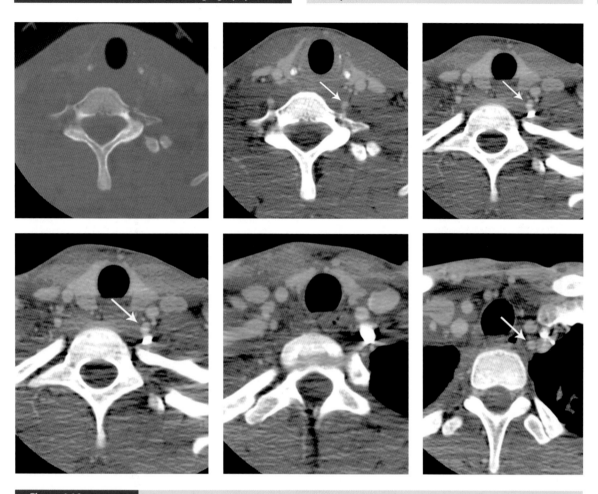

Figure 4.10

Limited evaluation of the vertebral artery due to streak artifact and poor choice of scan delay. In this example, there is a left C7 transverse process fracture through the foramen transversarium. Fortunately, the ipsilateral vertebral artery, although poorly opacified, does not enter the foramen at this level. There is poor visualization of the vertebral artery as the majority of the contrast is venous. Furthermore, sequentially caudad levels demonstrate streak artifact from dense contrast injected in the ipsilateral arm in the left subclavian vein, which obscures evaluation of the origin of the vertebral artery

arterial arrival time, and a greater peak arterial enhancement [62]. In patients with reduced cardiac output, therefore, once again, a 35- to 40-s prep delay is typically employed. Increasing the degree of arterial opacification can be accomplished simply by utilizing either a larger injection volume, or a faster injection rate. With a test bolus, the time density curve generally has a slightly different geometry from that of the main bolus, as shown in Fig. 4.11. This is likely due to injection of a smaller amount of contrast without a saline flush, which has different dilutional effects [55].

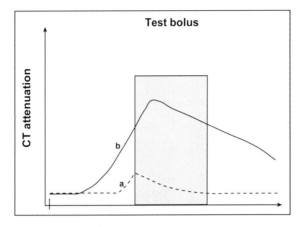

Test bolus

CT attenuation

b

a

Figure 4.11

Time density curve of a test bolus (*a*) as compared with the standard bolus (*b*). The *rectangle* demonstrates the ideal enhancement

As image acquisition takes a finite amount of time, usually longer than the time required for peak arterial enhancement, the resultant CTA image will include portions of the arterial tree that are not at peak enhancement. If the degree of arterial enhancement is not uniform, a thresholding-based reconstructed image may demonstrate a false occlusion [63, 64]. By using bolus-shaping strategies, so that arterial enhancement plateaus instead of peaks, more uniform vascular opacification is achieved and a more representative image of the vascular tree can be displayed. To determine the appropriate injection strategy, mathematical models of vascular enhancement have been developed. Bae et al. [62, 65] used a compartmental approach to model aortic enhancement. From this model, a multiphasic injection was proscribed by solving for the inverse of the model, the input function [66]. They found that an *exponentially decelerated injection method yields uniform vascular enhancement* [67].

Alternatively, Fleischmann and Hittmair [68] modeled aortic enhancement by treating the entire body as a "black box," where the input function was defined by the administration of a small contrast test bolus, and the output function was simply the resulting, measured time-attenuation curve. The "patient function" was the "black box," which substitutes for the multiple compartment model of Bae et al.'s approach. Using a discrete Fourier transform, the injection parameters that will result in a desired degree and duration of contrast enhancement in any given vessel can then be calculated. Unlike Bae et al.'s multi-compartmental model, no estimates or assumptions regarding patient weight, cardiac output, or other individual details needs to be included in the calculation. This tailored bolus can result in more uniform, optimal vascular enhancement, while simultaneously minimizing contrast requirements [69].

4.3.3 Post-processing: Image Reconstruction

4.3.3.1 Image Review

Appropriate image review is as important as optimal scanning technique for the correct interpretation of CTA studies. This applies to both image display parameters and three dimensional reconstruction techniques. With regard to soft copy image display, proper window and level settings are essential for optimizing parenchymal stroke detection. During image review of both NCCT and CTA images, windows and level settings should be chosen so as to exaggerate gray matter, white matter contrast, as discussed in Chapter 3 [70].

The CTA dataset is commonly reformatted into image slices twice that of the acquired scan width, however, with some degree of overlap. Even without overlap, this method may result in a prohibitive number of images for visual review. We therefore typically have two sets of axial reformatted images – one set with thick slices, for minimal quantum mottle, a minimal number of slices, and therefore optimal visual image review, and a second set with thin slices and maximal overlap, for use in 2D and 3D reconstruction. This second set minimizes certain reconstruction artifacts, such as the "zipper" effect.

By reconstructing the reformatted images into a composite view, with both thicker axial slices and optimally reconstructed images – including MIP, multiplanar volume reformat (MPR), curved reformat, shaded surface display (SSD), or VR – it is possible to evaluate the vessel in its entirety. This becomes important for lesions at branch points, such as aneurysms. While occlusions of large vessels may be obvious from sequential axial images, cutoff of a tortuous vessel, such as a distal M2 segment of the MCA, may not be entirely clear without a detailed and lengthy review of the source images.

Review of reconstructed 2D and 3D images assists review of the 2D axial source images by providing a composite image of the vessels. Once this review is complete, referral to the axial source images can be made for further evaluation, such as the degree of stenosis. Confirming the presence of a small aneurysm or venous sinus thrombosis may be better accomplished on the thin axial source images as well. Finally, vascular dissection can be directly visualized on the axial source images.

Both 2D and 3D reconstructions are time intensive. At our institution, there are dedicated 3D technologists who use stand-alone workstations to output the reconstructed images. Of note, however, *many scanners have easy-to-use reconstruction software that can be applied directly at the CT console by the technologist,* with only minimal interruption of patient throughput. Specifically, our technologists routinely reconstruct axial, coronal, and sagittal MIP views through the brain on *all* or our head CTAs. *These are done using 3-cm-thick slabs with 0.5 cm of overlap, take only approximately 30 s per imaging plane to reconstruct, and contribute greatly to a quick overview of the anterior cerebral artery (ACA, sagittal plane), MCA (axial and coronal plane), posterior cerebral artery (PCA, axial plane), and vertebral-basilar (coronal plane) anatomy, as shown in Figs. 4.1 and 4.2.*

One potential pitfall of *all* of these rendering techniques is the obscuration of internal blood vessel lumens by immediately adjacent calcified structures. This is most problematic for the characterization of cavernous sinus aneurysms, and for the measurement of residual lumen diameters in the presence of heavy circumferential calcifications, especially in cases of severe carotid bifurcation occlusive disease [28, 71]. A pitfall unique to SSD, which makes it unsuitable for CT venographic reconstructions, is its elimination of image pixels by thresholding. This feature

makes it possible to falsely create the appearance of a vascular stenosis if bone adjacent to a vessel is over-thresholded. In what follows, the various reconstruction methods are discussed in more detail:

4.3.3.2 Maximum Intensity Projection

As with MRA, a projected 2D image can be constructed by displaying only pixels with the maximum, or highest, CT attenuation along a given ray. One of the earliest descriptions of creating MIP images for CTA was by Napel [72]. As noted above, MIP images can be quickly and easily reconstructed at the scanner console, and are thereby readily available and convenient for review. These images can be constructed with a user-defined thickness. Furthermore, they are less sensitive than axial source images and SSD images to varying window and level settings. At Stanford, they have suggested that MIP is superior to SSD for renal artery stenosis evaluation [73]. Other

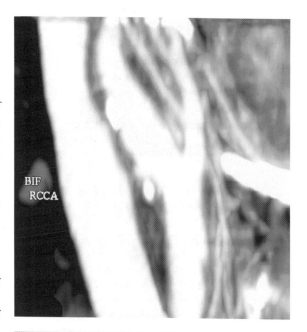

Figure 4.12

MIP image of normal carotid bifurcation; atherosclerosis may obscure the underlying enhancing lumen. (BIF Bifurcation, RCCA right common carotid artery)

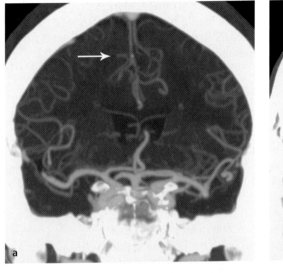
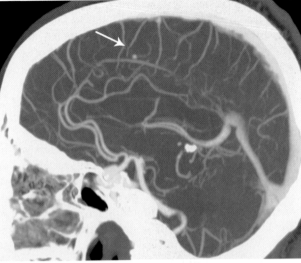

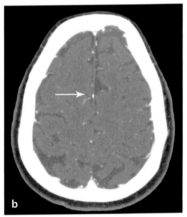
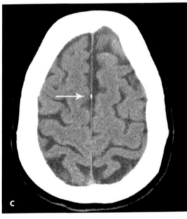

Figure 4.13

a Coronal and sagittal MIP images demonstrate an apparent aneurysm of the callosomarginal artery (*arrows*). b Axial contrast-enhanced source image confirms the presence of a density in the location shown on the MIP images (*arrow*). c Comparison with noncontrast image at the same location demonstrates calcification of the falx, there is no aneurysm (*arrow*)

groups have suggested similar results for carotid artery stenosis.

As this technique relies on detecting the highest pixel on a given ray, it is sensitive to overlap from adjacent bony and opacified venous structures, as shown in Figs. 4.12 and 4.13. Currently attempts are being made to subtract the underlying bony structures, but to date these have been limited by multiple technical factors, not least of which is subtle patient motion resulting in inaccurate representation of the composite image.

4.3.3.3 Multiplanar Volume Reformat

Instead of taking the highest attenuation in a pixel along a given ray, an MPR image is formed by the *mean* CT attenuation. It not routinely used by our group for image review, as the vascular images are more commonly confounded by overlap from adjacent bone or opacified venous structures. The slab can be reconstructed at an arbitrary slab thickness, as in an MIP; here the vertebrobasilar system is shown in Fig. 4.14. Unlike SSD and VR techniques, 2D MPR reconstructions do not obscure partially occlusive thrombus.

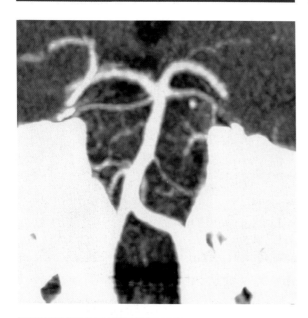

Figure 4.14

MPR image of vertebrobasilar system

4.3.3.4 Curved Reformat

To quickly delineate and review the entire course of a long, tortuous vessel, such as the carotid or vertebral arteries, a curved reformatted image is helpful. Here, the vessel is traced along its course, with the user selecting the pixels to display on consecutive axial images. The resultant reconstructed image is displayed in a 2D format. The process of creating curved reformatted (CR) images is the most time intensive of any of the rendering techniques discussed here. It is

also subject to interpretative error, analogous to that of a conventional angiogram; hence, two orthogonal views are required to accurately screen for vascular stenosis (which may be elliptical, rather than spherical in nature), as shown in Fig. 4.15. CR is especially useful for quickly screening for dissection, of both the cervical internal carotid artery and the vertebral artery at the skull base, provided these reconstructions are included with the reconstructed image set, demonstrated in Fig. 4.16.

4.3.3.5 Shaded Surface Display

This is a thresholding technique to display all pixels with attenuation values greater than a user-specified Hounsfield threshold. Bone, opacified vessels, and calcification will be captured with a threshold of 80–100 HU; however, most parenchymal structures will be excluded [74]. SSD is not as useful in acute stroke evaluation, as only pixels on the surface are displayed. This limits evaluation for partially occlusive thrombus. It has been most successfully used for surgical planning, such as for paraclinoid aneurysms.

4.3.3.6 Volume Rendering

With VR, unlike with SSD, nonsurface pixels are included in the dataset [75]. This is advantageous, in that, using thresholding, layers of the vessel can be "peeled" away or made transparent, so as to demonstrate underlying structures, as shown in Fig. 4.17. To date, however, there have been no convincing studies demonstrating the efficacy of VR in evaluation for acute stroke. This is likely due to the intensive user interaction required to set user-defined parameters of opacity, window, and level to create diagnostically appropriate VR projections.

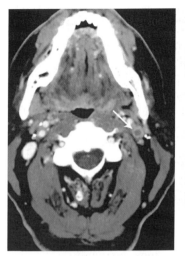
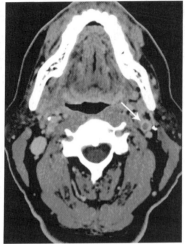
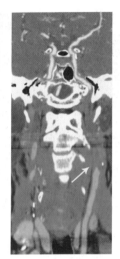
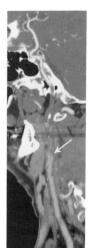

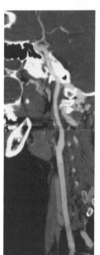
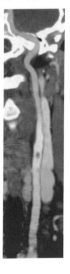

Figure 4.15

Occlusion of left internal carotid artery (*LICA*). Early and delayed axial images confirm the occlusion. Curved reformatted images of the LICA display the occlusion. Included are AP and lateral CR images of a normal LICA for comparison

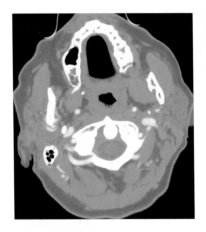 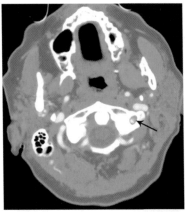 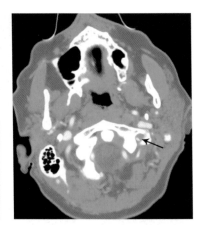

Figure 4.16

Left vertebral artery (*LVA*) dissection on both axial images and as shown on a curved reformatted image

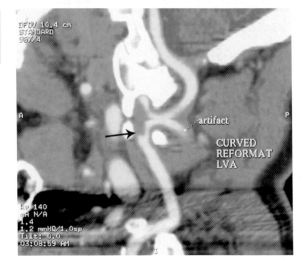

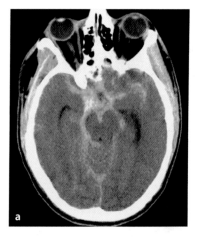
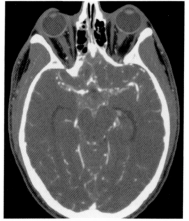
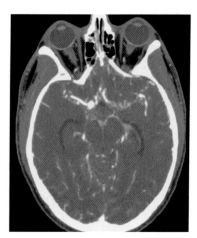

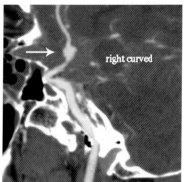
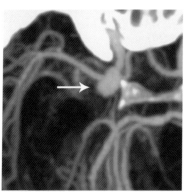

right curved

Figure 4.17

a Axial noncontrast and CTA source images with a subarachnoid hemorrhage (*SAH*) and the suggestion of an underlying top of carotid aneurysm. b Curved reformat, axial MIP, and volume rendered image confirm aneurysm at the top of the right carotid artery

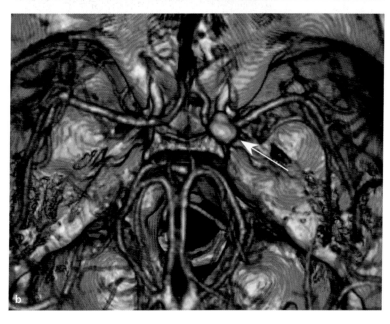

4.4 CTA Protocol for Acute Stroke

Multislice scanners allow flexibility in designing a rapid, efficient CTA protocol for acute stroke. The intracranial and extracranial vasculature can be imaged in less than 60 s. Even with the rapid scanning protocols designed for acute stroke, it remains necessary to tailor the acquisition, so that the images provide optimal visualization not only of an occlusive circle-of-Willis thrombus, but also of the possible *origin* or source of this thrombus. Because detection of an acute intracranial embolus is our first priority, the initial phase of our protocol is focused at the circle of Willis. By acquiring the intracranial CTA source images (also known as: "whole brain perfused blood volume images" – see Chapter 5) first, we simultaneously acquire the best possible CTA images of the circle of Willis. These images have the least venous contamination, as well as the most uniform arterial opacification, which is especially critical in the region of the cavernous sinus, Fig. 4.18.

Subsequently, CTA acquisition of the neck is performed, to evaluate for carotid stenosis as a possible source of emboli. In this "neck" phase of our protocol, it is not detrimental if venous opacification is present. Importantly, however, delayed scanning through the arch typically permits contrast that has pooled in the subclavian or brachiocephalic veins to be cleared prior to imaging, decreasing the resultant streak artifact from highly concentrated contrast in these vessels; subsequently, the origin of the great vessels can be more clearly evaluated. Figure 4.19 shows how streak at the origin by early scanning can result in misinterpretation.

After acquiring the CTA of the neck, single slab quantitative cine CT perfusion can additionally be performed, depending on the clinical need for these data in acute stroke triage. This is discussed at length in Chapter 5, along with specific scanning parameters. A sample stroke CTA protocol, optimized for the GE 16-slice scanner, is, however, provided for reference in Table 4.5. Using the aforementioned techniques for contrast reduction, including saline bolus chaser and bolus shaping, it is increasingly possible to obtain maximal uniform arterial enhancement –

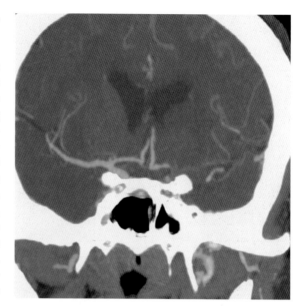

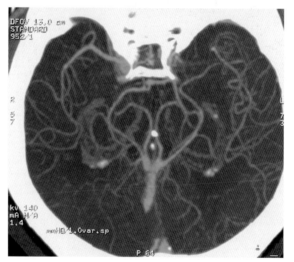

Figure 4.18

Occlusion at the top of the carotid, as best seen on coronal and axial MIP images

and hence diagnostic CTA images – without compromising the contrast dosage required for the addition of CT cine perfusion.

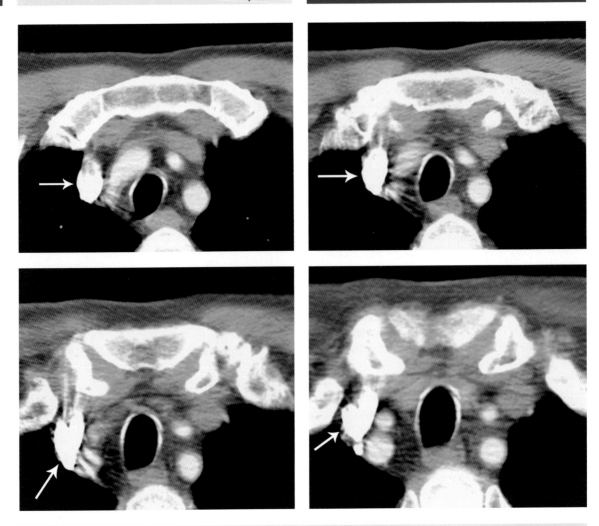

Figure 4.19

Dense contrast results in streak artifact in the right innominate vein and accounts for apparent nonopacification of the right common carotid artery (*RCCA*). On an axial image superior to the apparent obstruction, there is uniform enhancement

Table 4.5. Sample acute CTA/CTP protocol for GE 16-slice scanner. (*CTA* CT angiography, *CTP* CT perfusion, *FOV* field of view, *ICA* internal carotid artery, *NCCT* noncontrast CT)

	Contrast	Range	Slice thickness (mm)	Image spacing (mm)	Table feed (mm/s)	Pitch	Tube voltage (kV)	Tube current (mA)	Rota-tion time (s)	Scan FOV	Display FOV
NCCT	None	C1 to vertex	2.5	2.5	5.62	0.562	140	220	0.5	Head	22
CTA Head	4 ml/s for 40 ml, 25 s delay	C1 to vertex	2.5	2.5	5.62	0.562	140	200	0.5	Head	22
CTA Neck	0.8 ml/s for 30 ml	Arch to C1	2.5	2.5	5.62	0.562	140	250	0.5	Large	22
Cine CTP	7 ml/s for 40 ml, 5 s delay	Top of ICA	5	None, cine	None	N/A	80	200	1	Head	22

4.5 Accuracy and Clinical Utility of CTA in Acute Stroke

4.5.1 Optimal Image Review

As noted above, review of both "thick" reformatted axial source images and 2D/3D reconstructions is required for appropriate stroke CTA interpretation. Indeed, given the enormous number of thin slice axial sections required for 3D reconstruction, a systematic, practical approach to image review is required.

Initially, the axial 5-mm-thick noncontrast CT images are reviewed, primarily to exclude hemorrhage – an absolute contraindication to thrombolysis – but also to assess for parenchymal hypodensity (a strong relative contraindication to thrombolysis, if more than one-third of a vascular territory is involved). Care is taken to perform image review using narrow "window width" and "center level" display settings, so as to maximize the subtle difference between gray matter and white matter attenuation – thereby maximizing the detection of subtle, edematous, hypodense ischemic regions, as discussed at length in Chapter 3 [70].

Subsequently, the 2.5- to 3-mm-"thick" axial CTA source images are reviewed, typically at the scanner console. Large, proximal circle-of-Willis occlusions,

such as top-of-carotid T-lesions, are easily recognizable, even from the axial source images, and the "stroke team" can be immediately activated. Simultaneously, at most modern scanner consoles, the CTA dataset can be reformatted into "thin" (1.25 mm or less) slices, and quickly reconstructed into axial, coronal, and sagittal MIP images, facilitating more sensitive detection of secondary and tertiary branch occlusions. Even more detailed reconstructions, including curved reformats of the entire neurovascular system, from arch to vertex, can be created offline on a 3D workstation by a dedicated technologist.

4.5.2 Role of CTA in Acute Stroke

A major clinical role of CTA in acute stroke management remains the exclusion of unnecessary i.a. thrombolytic therapy in patients presenting with acute embolic stroke, but who *do not* have large vessel occlusions amenable to thrombolysis. Such occlusive stroke mimics include, but are not limited to, small vessel strokes (e.g., lacunar infarcts), TIAs, migraine headaches, seizures, and hypoglycemic events. CTA offers a convenient solution to the problem of efficiently diagnosing primary, secondary, and – increasingly – tertiary branch levels of intracranial vascular occlusion, *prior* to the initiation of thrombolytic therapy.

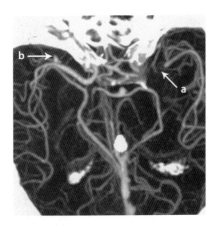
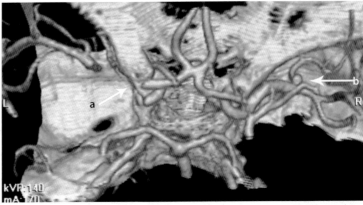

Figure 4.20

Incidental aneurysm found during evaluation for acute stroke. The collapsed MIP image shows cutoff of the left MCA stem (*arrow, a*) and right MCA aneurysm (*arrow, b*). Corresponding shaded surface display

When considering the possible need for thrombolysis, assessment of Circle-of-Willis anatomy, as well as of collateral flow distal to an occlusion, was demonstrated on CTA as early as in 1998 [25]. Indeed, Kucinski et al. [80] recently showed that collateral circulation is an independent predictor for outcome in acute ischemic stroke. Associated lesions in the setting of an acute intracranial vessel occlusion, such as aneurysms, which would preclude thrombolytic therapy, although rare, can also be demonstrated by CTA [21], as shown in Figs. 4.20 and 4.21.

CTA has been shown to be highly accurate in delineating the presence and extent of intracranial thrombus, Fig. 4.22. In a study of 44 consecutive intra-arterial thrombolysis candidates who underwent both CTA and the "gold standard" of catheter arteriography, CTA demonstrated a sensitivity and specificity of 98.4% and 98.1%, respectively, for the detection of proximal large vessel thrombus [76].

The degree and level of occlusion have been shown to be important factors in planning acute stroke therapy. In early studies, intravenous rt-PA for clot lysis was more likely to be effective in secondary and tertiary MCA branch occlusions than in larger, more proximal occlusions [6, 81]. In another study using CTA, there was little benefit from intravenous rt-PA

when there was poor collateralization, autolyzed thrombi, or proximal "top of carotid" saddle emboli [82]. In still other studies, "top of ICA" carotid terminus occlusion was demonstrated to be a better predictor of fatal outcome than an admission unenhanced CT showing greater than one-third MCA territory hypodensity [83, 84].

Moreover, the source images from the CTA dataset, assuming an approximate steady-state level of contrast enhancement during scan acquisition, are intrinsically blood volume weighted. Like DWI, these images can be used to determine tissue with a high likelihood of infarction in the absence of early, complete recanalization [77]. This topic is discussed more fully in Chapter 5.

Unlike unenhanced (or perhaps even enhanced) MRA, CTA is an anatomic imaging technique, and is therefore not highly likely to yield false-positive results for occlusion due to slow flow or artifact. Carotid sonography is also known to be inaccurate in distinguishing a true carotid occlusion from a hairline lumen. Indeed, accuracy for distinguishing hairline residual lumen from total occlusion of the internal carotid artery using single-slice helical CTA was found to be excellent, compared to a gold standard of catheter arteriography [78]. Accuracy rates were 95%

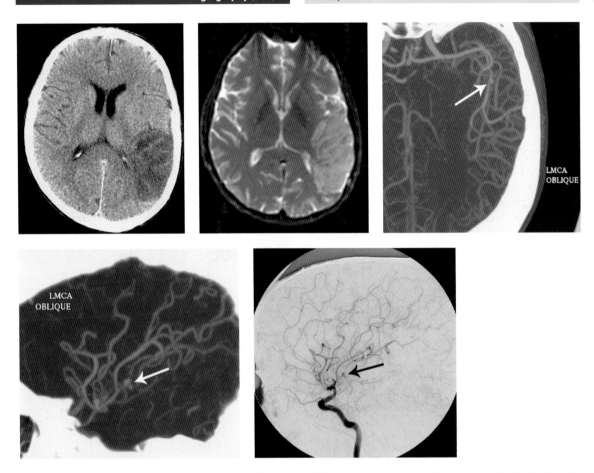

Figure 4.21

Acute stroke in a patient with endocarditis. The unenhanced and corresponding diffusion-weighted image (*DWI*) demonstrates acute infarct in the left parietal/temporal lobe. Evaluation with CTA MIP images clearly demonstrates a bilobed aneurysm (*arrow*), which is confirmed on the catheter cerebral angiogram

and 80% for two independent raters, with no statistically significant difference in accuracy between the two readers.

CTA has also been used to perform serial monitoring of patients with proven internal carotid artery occlusions. Surprisingly, spontaneous recanalization of an occluded internal carotid artery has been demonstrated [79]. In such cases, serial catheter angiography would have been prohibitive in terms of time, cost, and risk of complications.

Neck CTA can often elucidate the etiology of an intracranial occlusion. In older patients, carotid plaque can be accurately assessed by CTA. In a study of 82 patients, CTA was shown to be comparable to, and at times more accurate than, carotid sonography in determining the degree of stenosis [89]. Agreement in determination of vessel abnormality, plaque morphology, and ulceration between the two methodologies was reported to be 82%, 89%, and 96%, respectively. Moreover, 11 tandem lesions reported by

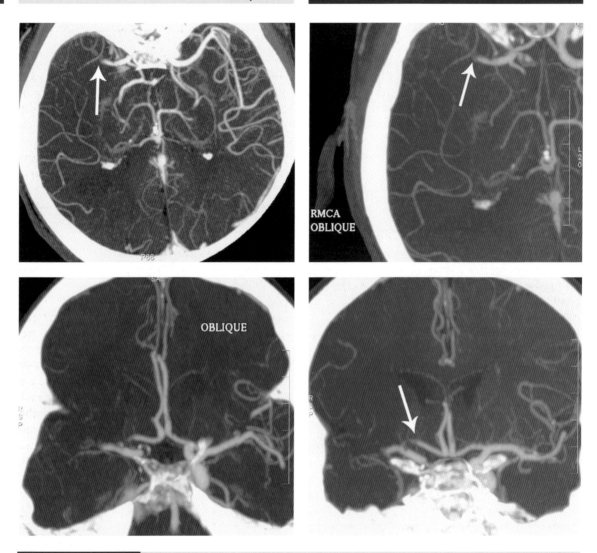

Figure 4.22

CT angiography (CTA) maximum intensity projection (*MIPs*) images with four different orientations demonstrate occlusion of the M1 segment of the right middle cerebral artery

CTA were not detected by sonography. When compared to a surgical gold standard, using North American Symptomatic Carotid Endarterectomy Trial (NASCET) criteria, degree of stenosis was correctly shown on CTA 89% of the time, as opposed to 83% with sonography. CTA did not overestimate stenosis.

CTA was superior to sonography in detecting plaque ulcerations and vessel abnormalities.

In younger patients, dissection of the carotid and/or vertebral arteries must be included in the differential diagnosis of acute stroke [85–87]. In 1999, Oelerich [88] reported satisfactory results with MRA in demonstrating craniocervical artery dissection. Although MR can demonstrate intramural hematoma, this is typically time-dependent, and, as noted previously, CTA is less prone to error from slow flow or other artifacts, and can provide a true anatomical image of the intravascular lumen. CTA can also provide information regarding the false lumen, flap, and extra-luminal structures – information not necessarily provided even by catheter arteriography.

4.6 Future Directions

As MDCT scanner technology advances, both acquisition speed and extent of z-direction coverage continue to improve. These advances should make possible the use of lower total contrast volumes and more rapid scanning, without loss of image quality or significantly increased radiation dose.

Increased coverage will not only be of benefit for cine CT perfusion studies, which are limited to the detector size of the given MDCT scanner (see Chapter 5), but it may also facilitate more complete neurovascular coverage than is currently obtainable, namely from the aortic arch to the vertex. Specifically, it may be possible to extend the neck portion of the CTA acquisition inferiorly to include the left atrium and left ventricle, so as to assess for endoluminal thrombus in stroke patients who present with atrial fibrillation as a possible embolic source. If successful, this technique has the potential to obviate the need for more invasive trans-esophageal echocardiography (TEE), which carries the rare but life-threatening risk of esophageal rupture [90]. CTA could therefore prove to be of greater value than TEE in acute stroke patients with atrial fibrillation [91].

Additionally, faster gantry rotation speeds may make possible "cine CTA fluoroscopy," with which difficult-to-detect lesions, such as cavernous sinus aneurysms or arterial venous malformations, could be visualized with greater temporal resolution during arterial, capillary, and venous phases of contrast enhancement. Dedicated studies could display a temporally parsed image, which would mirror the temporal resolution of the standard cerebral catheter arteriography.

4.7 Conclusion

CTA is a highly accurate tool for defining the level of intracranial vascular occlusion in patients presenting within 6 h of embolic stroke onset. CTA data will likely prove valuable in the rapid triage of such patients to appropriate therapy, including i.v. and i.a. thrombolytic treatment. For the evaluation of acute stroke patients, CTA is fast, simple, accurate, and convenient. Clinically relevant information regarding both vascular patency and parenchymal perfusion can be obtained during the first pass of a single contrast bolus in CTA.

Compared with single detector row CTA, there are fewer restrictions on designing a scanning protocol with the newer multislice CT scanners, especially those employing 16 channels or more – facilitating increased longitudinal coverage within a shorter scanning time. Complete imaging of the arterial tree – from arch to vertex – to evaluate for both acute occlusions and chronic stenoses – can be accomplished during peak arterial opacification. Contrast dose can be minimized with the use of a saline bolus and multiphasic injection. CTA not only compares favorably with catheter angiography for detection of acute large vessel occlusion, but can also provide information regarding collateral flow and lesion extent. By including neck CTA for acute stroke evaluation, embolic source and plaque burden at the origins of the internal carotid arteries can additionally be determined. Other stroke etiologies, such as dissection, can also be displayed. Finally, CTA of the neck affords an opportunity to plan catheter angiography, decreasing the time and contrast load required for i.a. thrombolysis, should it be required.

References

1. Adams HP, Brott TG, Ferlan AJ et al (1996) Guidelines for thrombolytic therapy for acute stroke: a supplement to the guidelines for the management of patients with acute ischemic stroke. Circulation 94:1167–1174
2. Alberts MJ (1998) tPA in acute ischemic stroke – United States experience and issues for the future. Neurology 51:S53–S55

3. Barr JD, Mathis JM, Wildenhain SL, Wechsler L, Jungreis CA, Horton JA (1994) Acute stroke intervention with intraarterial urokinase infusion. J Vasc Intervent Radiol 5:705–713

4. Caplan L, Mohr JP, Kistler P et al (1997) Should thrombolytic therapy be the first-line treatment for acute ischemic stroke? N Engl J Med 337:1309–1310

5. Chiu D, Krieger D, Villar-Cordova C et al (1998) Intravenous tissue plasminogen activator for acute ischemic stroke: feasibility, safety, and efficacy in the first year of clinical practice. Stroke 29:18–22

6. Del Zoppo GJ, Poeck K et al (1992) Recombinant tissue plasminogen activator in acute thrombotic stroke. Ann Neurol 32:78–86

7. Del Zoppo GJ, Pessin MS, Mori E, Hacke W (1991) Thrombolytic intervention in acute thrombotic and embolic stroke. Semin Neurol 11:368–384

8. Del Zoppo GJ (1995) Acute stroke – on the threshold of a therapy. N Engl J Med 333:1632–1633

9. Del Zoppo GJ, Higashida RT, Furlan AJ, Pessin MS, Rowley HA, Gent M (1998) PROACT: a phase II randomized trial of recombinant pro-urokinase by direct arterial delivery in acute middle cerebral artery stroke. PROACT Investigators. Prolyse in acute cerebral thromboembolism. Stroke 29: 4–11

10. Hacke W, Zeumer H, Ferbert A et al (1988) Intra-arterial thrombolytic therapy improves outcome in patients with acute vertebrobasilar occlusive disease. Stroke 19:1216–212

11. Hacke W, Kaste M, Fieschi C et al (1995) Intravenous thrombolysis with recombinant tissue plasminogen activator for acute hemispheric stroke: the European Cooperative Acute Stroke Study (ECASS). J Am Med Assoc 274:1017–1025

12. National Institute of Neurological Disorders for Stroke rt-PA Stroke Study (1995) Tissue plasminogen activator for acute ischemic stroke. N Engl J Med 333:1581–1587

13. NINDS Stroke Study Group (1997) Effect of rt-PA on ischemic lesion size by computed tomography. Preliminary results from the NINDS rt-PA Stroke Trial. Stroke 28: 2109–2118

14. Sussman BJ, Fitch TS (1958) Thrombolysis with fibrinolysis in cerebral arterial occlusion. J Am Med Assoc 167: 1705–1709

15. Hacke W, Albers G, Al-Rawi Y et al (2005) The DIAS Study Group. The Desmoteplase in Acute Ischemic Stroke Trial (DIAS) a phase II MRI-based 9-hour window acute stroke thrombolysis trial with intravenous desmoteplase. Stroke 36:66–73

16. Von Kummer R, Allen KL, Holle R et al (1997) Acute stroke: usefulness of early CT findings before thrombolytic therapy. Radiology 205:327–333

17. Lev MH, Nichols SJ (2000) Computed tomographic angiopgraphy and computed tomographic perfusion imaging of hyperacute stroke. Top Magn Reson Imaging 11: 273–287

18. Lev MH, Farkas J, Rodriguez VR et al (2001) CT angiography in the rapid triage of patients with hyperacute stroke to intraarterial thrombolysis: accuracy in the detection of large vessel thrombus. J Comput Assist Tomogr 25:520–528

19. Esteban JM, Cervera V (2004) Perfusion CT and angio CT in the assessment of acute stroke. Neuroradiology 46:705–715

20. Garg N, Eshkar N, Tanenbaum L et al (2004) Computed tomography angiographic correlates of early computed tomography signs in acute ischemic stroke. J Neuroimag 14:242–245

21. Chuang YM, Chao AC, Teng MM et al (2003) Use of CT angiography in patient selection for thrombolytic therapy. Am J Emerg Med 21:167–172

22. Cullen SP, Symons SP, Hunter G et al (2002) Dynamic contrast-enhanced computed tomography of acute ischemic stroke: CTA and CTP. Semin Roentgenol 37:192–205

23. Smith WS, Roberts HC, Chuang NA et al (2003) Safety and feasibility of a CT protocol for acute stroke: combined CT, CT angiography, and CT perfusion imaging in 53 consecutive patients. Am J Neuroradiol 24:688–690

24. Verro P, Tanenbaum LN, Borden NM, Sen S, Eshkar N (2002) CT angiography in acute ischemic stroke: preliminary results. Stroke 33:276–278

25. Hunter GJ, Hamberg LM, Ponzo JA et al (1998) Assessment of cerebral perfusion and arterial anatomy in hyperacute stroke with three-dimensional functional CT: early clinical results. Am J Neuroradiol 19:29–37

26. Schwartz RB (1995) Helical (spiral) CT in neuroradiologic diagnosis (review; 8 refs). Radiol Clin North Am 33:981–995

27. Lev MH, Ackerman RH, Lustrin ES et al (1995) Two dimensional spiral CT angiography in carotid occlusive disease: measurement of residual lumen diameter with ultrasound correlation. Proceedings of the 33rd Annual Meeting of the American Society of Neuroradiology, Chicago, Ill.

28. Lev MH, Ackerman RH, Lustrin ES, Brown JH (1995) A procedure for accurate spiral CT angiographic measurement of lumenal diameter. Proceedings of the 81st Scientific Assembly and Annual Meeting of the Radiological Society of North America, Chicago, Ill.

29. Silverman PM, Kalendar WA, Hazle JD (2001) Common terminology for single and multislice helical CT. Am J Radiol 176:1135–1136

30. Fox SH, Tanenbaum LN, Ackelsberg S (1998) Future directions in CT technology. Neuroimag Clin North Am 8:497–513

31. Kallmes DF, Evans AJ, Woodcock RJ et al (1996) Optimization of parameters for the detection of cerebral aneurysms: CT angiography of a model. Radiology 200:403–405

32. Napoli A, Fleischmann D, Chan FP et al (2004) Computed tomography angiography: state-of-the-art imaging using multidetector-row technology. J Comput Assist Tomogr 28:S32–S45

33. Rydberg J, Bukwalter KA, Caldemeyer KS et al (2000) Multisection CT: scanning techniques and clinical applications. Radiographics 20:1787–1806

34. NRC Committee on the Biological Effects of Ionizing Radiation BV (1990) In: Health effects of exposure to low levels of ionizing radiation. National Academy Press, Washington DC

35. Wall BF, Hart D (1997) Revised radiation doses for typical X-ray examinations. Report on a recent review of doses to patients from medical X-ray examinations in the UK by NRPB. National Radiological Protection Board. Br J Radiol 70:437–439

36. McCollough CH, Schueler BA (2000) Calculation of effective dose. Med Phys 27:828–837

37. Jucius RA, Kambic GX (1980) Measurements of computed tomography x-ray fields utilizing the partial volume effect. Med Phys 7:379–382

38. Kalendar WA, Wolf H, Suess C (1999) Dose reduction in CT by anatomically adapted tube current modulation. II. Phantom measurements. Med Phys 26:2248–2253

39. Kalendar WA, Prokop M (2001) 3D CT angiography. Crit Rev Diagn Imaging 42:1–28

40. Nickoloff EL, Alderson PO (2001) Radiation exposures to patients from CT: reality, public perception, and policy. Am J Roentgenol 177:285–287

41. Ertl-Wagner BB, Hoffmann RT, Bruning R (2004) Multidetector row CT angiography of the brain at various kilovoltage settings. Radiology 231:528–535

42. Kalra MK, Maher MM, Saini S (2004) Radiation exposure and projected risks with multidetector-row computed tomography scanning: clinical strategies and technologic developments for dose reduction. J Comput Assist Tomogr 28:S46–S49

43. Kendall BE, Pullicino P (1980) Intravascular contrast injection in ischaemic lesions. II. Effect on prognosis. Neuroradiology 19(5):241–243

44. Doerfler A et al (1998) Are iodinated contrast agents detrimental in acute cerebral ischemia? An experimental study in rats. Radiology 206(1):211–217

45. Han JK et al (2000) Factors influencing vascular and hepatic enhancement at CT: experimental study on injection protocol using a canine model. J Comput Assist Tomogr 24(3):400–406

46. Bluemke DA, Fishman EK, Anderson JH (1995) Effect of contrast concentration on abdominal enhancement in the rabbit: spiral computed tomography evaluation. Acad Radiol 2(3):226–231

47. Morcos SK, Thomsen HS, Webb JA (1999) Contrast-media-induced nephrotoxicity: a consensus report. Contrast Media Safety Committee, European Society of Urogenital Radiology (ESUR). Eur Radiol 9(8):1602–1613

48. Morcos SK (1998) Contrast media-induced nephrotoxicity–questions and answers. Br J Radiol 71(844):357–365

49. Aspelin P et al (2003) Nephrotoxic effects in high-risk patients undergoing angiography. N Engl J Med 348(6):491–499

50. Pugh ND (1996) Haemodynamic and rheological effects of contrast media: the role of viscosity and osmolality. Eur Radiol 6 [Suppl 2]:S13–S15

51. Henson JW et al (2004) Gadolinium-enhanced CT angiography of the circle of Willis and neck. Am J Neuroradiol 25(6):969–972

52. Schoellnast H et al (2003) Abdominal multidetector row computed tomography: reduction of cost and contrast material dose using saline flush. J Comput Assist Tomogr 27(6):847

53. Schoellnast H et al (2004) Aortoiliac enhancement during computed tomography angiography with reduced contrast material dose and saline solution flush: influence on magnitude and uniformity of the contrast column. Invest Radiol 39(1):20–26

54. Bader TR, Prokesch RW, Grabenwoger F (2000) Timing of the hepatic arterial phase during contrast-enhanced computed tomography of the liver: assessment of normal values in 25 volunteers. Invest Radiol 35(8):486–492

55. Cademartiri F et al (2002) Parameters affecting bolus geometry in CTA: a review. J Comput Assist Tomogr 26(4):598–607

56. Hopper KD et al (1997) Thoracic spiral CT: delivery of contrast material pushed with injectable saline solution in a power injector. Radiology 205(1):269–271

57. Haage P et al (2000) Reduction of contrast material dose and artifacts by a saline flush using a double power injector in helical CT of the thorax. Am J Roentgenol 174(4):1049

58. Kopka L et al (1995) Parenchymal liver enhancement with bolus-triggered helical CT: preliminary clinical results. Radiology 195(1):282–284

59. Paulson EK et al (1998) Helical liver CT with computer-assisted bolus-tracking technology: is it possible to predict which patients will not achieve a threshold of enhancement? Radiology 209(3):787–792

60. Shimizu T et al (2000) Helical CT of the liver with computer-assisted bolus-tracking technology: scan delay of arterial phase scanning and effect of flow rates. J Comput Assist Tomogr 24(2):219–223

61. Puskas Z, Schuierer G (1996) Determination of blood circulation time for optimizing contrast medium administration in CT angiography. Radiologe 36(9):750–757

62. Bae KT, Heiken JP, Brink JA (1998) Aortic and hepatic contrast medium enhancement at CT, part II. Effect of reduced cardiac output in a porcine model. Radiology 207(3):657–662

63. Rubin GD et al (1998) Measurement of the aorta and its branches with helical CT. Radiology 206(3):823–829

64. Rubin GD et al (1993) Three-dimensional spiral computed tomographic angiography: an alternative imaging modality for the abdominal aorta and its branches. J Vasc Surg 18(4):656–664; discussion 665

65. Bae KT, Heiken JP, Brink JA (1998) Aortic and hepatic contrast medium enhancement at CT, part I. Prediction with a computer model. Radiology 207(3):647–655

66. Bae KT, Tran HQ, Heiken JP (2000) Multiphasic injection method for uniform prolonged vascular enhancement at CT angiography: pharmacokinetic analysis and experimental porcine model. Radiology 216(3):872–880

67. Bae KT, Tran HQ, Heiken JP (2004) Uniform vascular contrast enhancement and reduced contrast medium volume achieved by using exponentially decelerated contrast material injection method. Radiology 231(3):732–736

68. Fleischmann D, Hittmair K (1999) Mathematical analysis of arterial enhancement and optimization of bolus geometry for CT angiography using the discrete Fourier transform. J Comput Assist Tomogr 23(3):474–484

69. Fleischmann D et al (2000) Improved uniformity of aortic enhancement with customized contrast medium injection protocols at CT angiography. Radiology 214(2):363–371

70. Lev MH, Farkas J, Gemmete JJ et al (1999) Acute stroke: improved nonenhanced CT detection – benefits of soft-copy interpretation by using variable window width and center level settings. Radiology 213:150–155

71. Dix JA, Evans AJ, Kallmes DF, Sobel A, Phillips CD (1997) Accuracy and precision of CT angiography in a model of the carotid artery bifurcation. Am J Neuroradiol 18:409–415

72. Napel S et al (1992) CT angiography with spiral CT and maximum intensity projection. Radiology 185(2):607–610

73. Rubin GD et al (1994) Spiral CT of renal artery stenosis: comparison of three-dimensional rendering techniques. Radiology 190(1):181–189

74. Vieco PT, Morin EE 3rd, Gross CE (1996) CT angiography in the examination of patients with aneurysm clips. Am J Neuroradiol 17(3):455–457

75. Kuszyk BS et al (1995) CT angiography with volume rendering: imaging findings. Am J Roentgenol 165(2):445–448

76. Lev MH et al (2001) CT angiography in the rapid triage of patients with hyperacute stroke to intraarterial thrombolysis: accuracy in the detection of large vessel thrombus. J Comput Assist Tomogr 25(4):520–528

77. Schramm P et al (2002) Comparison of CT and CT angiography source images with diffusion-weighted imaging in patients with acute stroke within 6 hours after onset. Stroke 33(10):2426–2432

78. Lev MH et al (2003) Total occlusion versus hairline residual lumen of the internal carotid arteries: accuracy of single section helical CT angiography. Am J Neuroradiol 24(6):1123–1129

79. Nguyen-Huynh MN, Lev MH, Rordorf G (2003) Spontaneous recanalization of internal carotid artery occlusion. Stroke 34(4):1032–1034

80. Kucinski T et al (2003) Collateral circulation is an independent radiological predictor of outcome after thrombolysis in acute ischaemic stroke. Neuroradiology 45(1):11–18

81. Wolpert SM et al (1993) Neuroradiologic evaluation of patients with acute stroke treated with recombinant tissue plasminogen activator. The rt-PA Acute Stroke Study Group. Am J Neuroradiol 14(1):3–13

82. Wildermuth S et al (1998) Role of CT angiography in patient selection for thrombolytic therapy in acute hemispheric stroke. Stroke 29(5):935–938

83. Kucinski T et al (1998) The predictive value of early CT and angiography for fatal hemispheric swelling in acute stroke. Am J Neuroradiol 19(5):839–846

84. Zivin JA (1998) Factors determining the therapeutic window for stroke. Neurology 50(3):599–603

85. Provenzale JM (1995) Dissection of the internal carotid and vertebral arteries: imaging features. Am J Roentgenol 165(5):1099–1104

86. Adams HP Jr. et al (1995) Ischemic stroke in young adults. Experience in 329 patients enrolled in the Iowa Registry of stroke in young adults. Arch Neurol 52(5):491–495

87. Bogousslavsky J, Regli F (1987) Ischemic stroke in adults younger than 30 years of age. Cause and prognosis. Arch Neurol 44(5):479–482

88. Oelerich M et al (1999) Craniocervical artery dissection: MR imaging and MR angiographic findings. Eur Radiol 9(7):1385–1391

89. Debernardi S et al (2004) CT angiography in the assessment of carotid atherosclerotic disease: results of more than two years' experience. Radiol Med (Torino) 108(1–2):116–127

90. Shapira MY et al (1999) Esophageal perforation after transesophageal echocardiogram. Echocardiography 16(2):151–154

91. Zaidat O et al (2002) The utility of ultrafast cardiac cycle gated and contrasted spiral computerized axial chest tomography in evaluation of patients with acute stroke and comparison with transesophageal echocardiography. Proceedings of the 27th International Stroke Conference. American Stroke Association, San Antonio, Tex.

CT Perfusion (CTP)

Sanjay K. Shetty, Michael H. Lev

5.1 Introduction

Acute stroke is a common cause of morbidity and mortality worldwide: it is the third leading cause of death in the United States (responsible for approximately 1 in 15 deaths in 2001) and affects approximately 700,000 individuals within the United States annually [1]. The ability to treat patients in the acute setting with thrombolytics has created a pressing need for improved detection and evaluation of acute stroke, with a premium placed on rapid acquisition and generation of data that are practically useful in the clinical setting. Recanalization methods for acute ischemic stroke remain limited to a restricted time window, since intravenous (i.v.) and intra-arterial (i.a.) thrombolysis carry hemorrhagic risk that increases with time post-ictus [2–4]. Clinical exam and unenhanced CT, the existing imaging standards for acute stroke, are limited in their ability to identify individuals likely to benefit from successful recanalization [3, 5–11].

Advanced imaging techniques extend traditional anatomic applications of imaging and offer additional insight into the pathophysiology of acute stroke, by providing information about the arterial-level cerebral vasculature, capillary-level hemodynamics, and the brain parenchyma. Our evolving understanding of acute stroke emphasizes knowledge of each of these levels to guide treatment decisions in the acute setting. As a modality, MR in particular has gained acceptance in the evaluation of acute stroke, in large part due to the rapidity and accuracy of diffusion-weighted imaging (DWI) in the detection of acute infarction when compared to traditional unenhanced CT [12, 13].

Table 5.1. The four key questions in the imaging evaluation of acute stroke and the roles of various CT techniques. (*CBF* Cerebral blood flow, *CTA* CT angiography, *CTP* CT perfusion, *CTA-SI* CTA source images)

Is there hemorrhage?
Unenhanced CT

Is there intravascular thrombus that can be targeted for thrombolysis?
CTA

Is there a "core" of critically ischemic irreversibly infarcted tissue?
CTP (CBV/CTA-SI)

Is there a "penumbra" of severely ischemic but potentially salvageable tissue?
CTP (CBF)

CT perfusion (CTP) expands the role of CT in the evaluation of acute stroke by providing insight into areas in which CT has traditionally suffered in comparison to MR – capillary-level hemodynamics and the brain parenchyma – and in doing so forms a natural complement to the strengths of CTA [14–17]. The imaging of acute stroke demands answers to four critical questions [10, 18, 19]:

- Is there hemorrhage?
- Is there intravascular thrombus that can be targeted for thrombolysis?
- Is there a "core" of critically ischemic irreversibly infarcted tissue?
- Is there a "penumbra" of severely ischemic but potentially salvageable tissue?

CTP attempts to address the latter two of these questions to better guide management in the acute setting. (Table 5.1).

CTP imaging techniques are relatively new compared to MR-based methods; their clinical applications are therefore less thoroughly reported in the literature [20–22]. Despite this, because the general principles underlying the computation of perfusion parameters such as cerebral blood flow (CBF), cerebral blood volume (CBV), and mean transit time (MTT) are the same for both MR and CT, the overall clinical applicability of perfusion imaging using both of these modalities is likely to be similar. In addition,

as will be discussed, first-pass CTP, unlike MR perfusion-weighted imaging (MR-PWI), readily provides high-resolution, quantitative data using commercially available software. In addition, CTA with CTP is fast [14], increasingly available [23], safe [24], and affordable [25]. It typically adds no more than 10 min to the time required to perform a standard unenhanced head CT, and does not hinder i.v. thrombolysis, which can be administered – with appropriate monitoring – directly at the CT scanner table immediately following completion of the unenhanced scan [8, 14, 16, 17, 20, 24, 26–49]. Like DWI and MR-PWI, CTA/CTP has the potential to serve as a surrogate marker of stroke severity, likely exceeding the NIH Stroke Scale (NIHSS) score or Alberta Stroke Program Early CT Score (ASPECTS) as a predictor of outcome [26, 50–57]. Because of these advantages, increasing evidence that advanced CT imaging can accurately characterize stroke physiology could have important implications for the management of stroke patients worldwide [32, 33, 58, 59].

5.2 CTP Technical Considerations

Acute Stroke Protocol. A protocol for the imaging of acute stroke should address the central questions necessary to triage patients appropriately (Table 5.1). The acute stroke protocol employed at our institution has three components: the unenhanced CT, an "arch-to-vertex" CTA, and dynamic first-pass cine CTP (Table 5.2). A similar CTA/CTP protocol, or its equivalent, could be applied using any commercially available multidetector row helical CT scanner with only minor variations that should not adversely alter image quality. The protocol is routinely completed within 10 min. Perhaps the most important aspect of patient preparation for CTP imaging may be to have an 18- or 20-gauge catheter already placed in an appropriately large vein *prior* to the patient's arrival in the CT suite. It is similarly useful for the power injector to be loaded prior to patient arrival. Total scanning time can be drastically reduced if such details are attended to before the examination. It is important to secure the head with tape or Velcro straps, as motion artifact can severely degrade CTA/CTP image quality.

Table 5.2. Sample acute stroke CT protocol employed at the authors' institution, incorporating CTA and CTP. The protocol is designed to answer the four basic questions necessary for stroke triage described in Table 5.1. The parameters are presented for illustrative purposes and have been optimized for the scanner currently employed in our Emergency Department (General Electric Healthcare Lightspeed-16). The parameters should be optimized for each scanner (*FOV* Field of view)

Series	Unenhanced	CTA head	CTA neck	Cine perfusion ×2
		Biphasic contrast injection: 4 ml/s for 40 ml, then 0.8 ml for 30 ml		7 ml/s for 40 ml for each CTP acquisition
		Delay: 25 s (35 s if poor cardiac output including atrial fibrillation)		Delay: 5 s; each is a 60-s cine acquisition
Range	C1 to vertex	C1 to vertex	Arch to C1	Two CTP slabs
Gantry angle	0	0	0	0
Algorithm	Standard	Standard	Standard	Standard
Slice thickness	5 mm	2.5 mm	2.5 mm	5 mm
Image spacing	5 mm	2.5 mm	2.5 mm	
Table feed	5.62 mm	5.62 mm	5.62 mm	N/A
Pitch	0.562	0.562	0.562	N/A
Mode	0.562:1	0.562:1	0.562:1	16*1.25 CINE 4i
kVp	140	140	140	80
mA	220	200	250	200
Rotation time	0.5 s	0.5 s	0.5 s	1 s
Scan FOV	Head	Head	Large	Head
Display FOV	22 cm	22 cm	22 cm	22 cm
Retrospective helical reconstructions		Thick 1.25 mm Interval 0.625 mm FOV 18 cm	Thick 1.25 mm Interval 1.0 mm FOV 18 mm	

The role of unenhanced CT in stroke triage, discussed in more detail in Chapter 3, is principally to exclude hemorrhage prior to thrombolytic treatment [60]. A large, greater than one-third middle cerebral artery (MCA) territory hypodensity at presentation is considered by most to be a contraindication to thrombolysis [61]. CT remains suboptimal in its ability to correctly subtype stroke, localize embolic clot, predict outcome, or assess hemorrhagic risk [3, 5–11]. Early ischemic signs of stroke are typically absent or subtle, and their interpretation is prone to significant inter- and intra-observer dependency [11, 56, 62–65].

The technical considerations and interpretation of the second portion of the acute stroke protocol, CTA, are discussed in detail in Chapter 4. Importantly, however, the source images from the CTA vascular acquisition (CTA-SI) also supply clinically relevant data concerning tissue-level perfusion. It has been theoretically modeled that the CTA-SI are weighted predominantly by blood volume rather than blood flow [22, 29, 66]. The potential utility of the CTA-SI series in the assessment of brain perfusion is discussed in detail below. This perfused blood volume technique requires the assumption of an approximately steady-state level of contrast during the period of image acquisition [29]. It is for this reason – in order to approach a steady-state – that our protocols call for a biphasic contrast injection that can achieve a better approximation of the steady-state [67, 68]. More complex methods of achieving uniform contrast concentration with smaller doses have been proposed that may eventually become standard, such as exponentially decelerated injection rates [69] and biphasic boluses constructed after analysis of test bolus kinetics [68, 70].

CTP Acquisition. The cine acquisition of CTP forms the final step in the acute stroke imaging evaluation. With dynamic, quantitative CTP, an additional contrast bolus is administered (at a rate of 4–7 ml/s) during continuous, cine imaging over a single brain region. Using the "standard" cine technique, imaging occurs for a total of 45–60 s, sufficient to track the "first pass" of the contrast bolus through the intracranial vasculature without recirculation effects. Our current scanner (General Electric Lightspeed 16) offers 2 cm of coverage per bolus (two 10-mm-thick or four 5-mm-thick slices) [28, 38, 46]; however, the coverage volume of each acquisition depends greatly on the manufacturer and generation of the CT scanner and continues to increase with enlarging detector arrays and improving technology. The maximum degree of vertical coverage could potentially be doubled with each bolus using a "toggle table" technique, in which the scanner table moves back and forth, switching between two different cine views, albeit at a reduced temporal resolution of data acquisition [42]. Our current protocol employs two boluses to acquire two slabs of CTP data at different levels, increasing overall coverage [48]. Importantly, at least one imaged slice in each acquisition must include a major intracranial artery for CTP map reconstruction. Because the previously acquired CTA data are available prior to CTP acquisition, one can target the tissue of interest through the selection of an appropriate imaging plane for the CTP acquisition, which is particularly important given the relatively restricted CTP coverage obtained even with two CTP acquisitions. It has been our experience that a scan plane positioned parallel and superior to the orbital roof can provide sufficient sampling of the middle (both superior and inferior divisions), anterior, and posterior cerebral artery territories to assess perfusion in cases of large vessel anterior circulation stroke, and, when positioned parallel and inferior, in cases of large vessel posterior circulation stroke [15, 71, 72]. An important consideration in the design of an acute stroke protocol is the total contrast dose; in the sample protocol presented here, the contrast used for the CTA has been restricted in order to allow two 40-ml boluses during the CTP acquisitions.

Considerable variability exists in the protocols used for CTP scanning, because CTP imaging has only recently gained acceptance as a clinical tool, and because construction of perfusion maps is dependent on the specific mathematical model used to analyze the dynamic, contrast-enhanced datasets. Algorithm-dependent differences in contrast injection rates exist; for example, models that assume "no venous outflow" necessitate extremely high injection rates (which in practice can be difficult to achieve) in order to achieve peak arterial enhancement before venous opacification occurs [30]. Considerably slower injection rates can be used with the deconvolution-based models [73]. However, regardless of injection rate, as with MR perfusion imaging, higher contrast concentrations are likely to produce maps with improved signal-to-noise ratios [74].

One accepted deconvolution CTP imaging protocol calls for scanning at 80 kV, rather than at a more conventional 120–140 kV (Table 5.2). Theoretically, given a constant tube current, this tube voltage setting would not only reduce the administered radiation dose to the patient but would also increase the conspicuity of i.v. contrast, due, in part, to the greater importance of the photoelectric effect for 80 kV photons, which are closer to the "k-edge" of iodine [46]. Images are acquired in cine mode at a rate of approximately one image per second. Improved temporal resolution is possible with some scanners, with acquisition rates as fast as one image per half second, however the resulting moderate improvement in tissue-density curve noise may not justify the increased radiation dose.

Table 5.3. Advantages and disadvantages of CTP relative to MR perfusion-weighted imaging (*PWI*)

Advantages

Availability and decreased cost of CT

Speed of acquisition

Ease of monitoring and intervention
in an unstable clinical setting

Can be performed in patients with pacemakers
or other contraindications to MR,
or in patients who cannot be screened for MR safety

Improved resolution

Quantitative perfusion information

Disadvantages

Limited scan coverage

Risks and complications of iodinated contrast

Ionizing radiation

More complex post-processing

5.3 Comparison with MR-PWI

5.3.1 Advantages

Quantitation and Resolution. While CTP and MR-PWI both attempt to evaluate the intricacies of capillary-level hemodynamics, the differences in technique create several important differences that should be considered (Table 5.3). While dynamic susceptibility contrast (DSC) MR-PWI techniques rely on the indirect T2* effect induced in adjacent tissues by high concentrations of intravenous gadolinium, CTP relies on direct visualization of the contrast material. The linear relationship between contrast concentration and attenuation in CT readily lends itself to quantitation, which is not possible with MR-PWI techniques. MR-PWI may also be more sensitive to "contamination" by large vascular structures and is also limited in some areas due to susceptibility effects from adjacent structures. In addition, CTP has greater spatial resolution than MR-PWI. These factors contribute to the possibility that visual evaluation of core/penumbra mismatch is more reliable with CTP than with MR-PWI [75, 76].

Availability and Safety. CT also benefits from the practical availability and relative ease of scanning, particularly when dealing with critically ill patients and the attendant monitors or ventilators. CT may also be the only option for a subgroup of patients with an absolute contraindication to MR scanning, such as a pacemaker, and is a safe option when the patient cannot be screened for MR safety.

5.3.2 Disadvantages

Limited Coverage. A major disadvantage of current CTP techniques is the relatively limited coverage; while MR-PWI is capable of delivering information about the whole brain, the coverage afforded by CTP depends greatly on the available CT technology. Our current protocol (using a GE Lightspeed 16 scanner) provides four slices (5 mm each) derived from a 2-cm-thick slab of tissue for each contrast bolus. Even with two CTP cine acquisitions, the overall coverage necessitates a tailored approach that acquires perfusion data in areas of interest. Importantly, however, the limited coverage offered by current CTP techniques may be less of a problem with further advances in multidetector CT technology.

Ionizing Radiation. CTA/CTP also requires ionizing radiation and iodinated contrast. The safety issues involved are no different from those of any patient group receiving contrast-enhanced head CT scanning, and are discussed at length in multiple papers [15, 77]. The CTP protocol, in particular, has been optimized to provide maximum perfusion signal with minimum dose [46]. Overall, each of the CTA and CTP components of our protocol delivers approximately the same low radiation dose to the head as a conventional CT.

Iodinated Contrast. Our current protocol employs two 40-ml boluses of iodinated contrast material for the CTP cine acquisitions, in addition to the contrast required for the CTA acquisition. This is a not insignificant dose of iodinated contrast, particularly in the relatively older population most at risk for stroke, and the dose may be of even higher concern if the patient subsequently requires additional contrast for endovascular intervention. However, nonionic iodinated contrast has been shown not to worsen stroke outcome [78–80]. In patients with preexisting renal dysfunction (abnormally elevated creatinine) or insulin-dependent diabetes, our protocol calls for nonionic, iso-osmolar contrast administration, minimizing the chance of nephrotoxicity [81].

Complex Post-Processing. Post-processing of CTA and CTP images is more labor intensive than that of MRA and MRP images, although with training and quality control, 3D reconstructions of CTA datasets, as well as quantitative CTP maps, can be constructed rapidly and reliably [82–84].

5.4 CTP: General Principles

Perfusion-weighted CT and MR techniques – as opposed to those of MR and CT *angiography* which detect bulk vessel flow – are sensitive to capillary, tissue-level blood flow [85]. This evaluation of capillary-level hemodynamics extends the traditional anatomic role of imaging to provide insight into the delivery of blood to brain parenchyma. The idea of contrast-enhanced CT perfusion imaging emerged as early as 1976, when a computerized subtraction technique was used to measure regional cerebral blood volume (rCBV) using the EMI scanner. Sodium iothalamate was administered intravenously to increase x-ray absorption in the intracranial circulation, permitting regional differences in CBV to be measured [86]. More recently, prior to the advent of helical CT scanning, "time to peak" analysis of cerebral perfusion was proposed as a means of evaluating stroke patients. Patients with a prolonged (greater than 8 s) time to peak parenchymal enhancement had poor clinical outcomes. This dynamic CT study took 10–15 min longer to perform than a conventional CT exam. Therefore, given the absence of faster scanning or an approved treatment for acute stroke, this method never gained clinical acceptance [87].

The generic term "cerebral perfusion" refers to tissue-level blood flow in the brain. This flow can be described using a variety of parameters, which primarily include CBF, CBV, and MTT (Table 5.4). Understanding the dynamic relationships between these parameters as cerebral perfusion pressure drops in the setting of acute stroke is crucial to the accurate interpretation of perfusion maps. Definitions of these parameters are as follows:

Table 5.4. Normal values for perfusion parameters in brain tissue (Adapted from [143])

	CBF (ml · 100 g^{-1} · min^{-1})	CBV (ml · 100 g^{-1})	MTT (s)
Gray matter	60	4	4
White matter	25	2	4.8

Cerebral blood volume (CBV) is defined as the total volume of blood in a given unit volume of the brain. This definition includes blood in the tissues, as well as blood in the large capacitance vessels such as arteries, arterioles, capillaries, venules, and veins. CBV has units of milliliters of blood per 100 g of brain tissue (ml · 100 g^{-1}).

Cerebral blood flow (CBF) is defined as the volume of blood moving through a given unit volume of brain per unit time. CBF has units of ml of blood per 100 g of brain tissue per minute (ml · 100 g^{-1} · min^{-1}).

Mean transit time (MTT) is defined as the *average* of the transit time of blood through a given brain region. The transit time of blood through the brain parenchyma varies depending on the distance traveled between arterial inflow and venous outflow. Mathematically, MTT is related to both CBV and CBF according to the central volume principle, which states that MTT=CBV/CBF [88, 89].

5.5 CTP Theory and Modeling

Although easy to define in theory, the perfusion parameters of CBV, CBF, and MTT can be difficult to quantify in practice. The *dynamic, first-pass* approach to CT perfusion measurement involves the dynamic i.v. administration of an intravascular contrast agent, which is tracked with serial imaging during its first-pass circulation through the brain tissue capillary bed. Depending on the assumptions regarding the arterial inflow and the venous outflow of the tracer, the perfusion parameters of CBV, CBF, and MTT can then be computed mathematically. Dynamic first-pass contrast-enhanced CTP models assume that the tracer (i.e., the contrast) used for perfusion measurement is *nondiffusible*, neither metabolized nor absorbed by the tissue bed through which it traverses. "Leakage" of contrast material outside of the intravascular space, which can occur in cases of blood–brain barrier (BBB) breakdown associated with tumor, infection, or inflammation, requires a different model to be used and therefore adds an additional layer of complexity to the calculations. Other means of assessing cerebral perfusion, including PET and xenon CT imaging for example, employ *diffusible tracer* models which generally involve fewer assumptions regarding steady-state CBF than do the *dynamic, first-pass* contrast-enhanced models used with MR and CT imaging. The two major types of mathematical models involved in performing these calculations are the deconvolution-based and nondeconvolution-based methods.

Nondeconvolution Techniques. Nondeconvolution-based perfusion methods rely on the application of the *Fick principle* to a given region of interest (ROI) within the brain parenchyma. This "conservation of flow" is expressed by the equation:

$$dC_t(t)/dt = CBF \cdot \left[C_a(t) - C_v(t) \right]$$

In the above formula, $C_t(t)$ is the tissue contrast concentration versus time curve (commonly referred to as the time density curve, TDC) measured within a given brain region. $C_a(t)$ is the TDC for the feeding artery (also known as the arterial input function, or AIF), and $C_v(t)$ is the TDC for the draining vein. In order to create "maps" of cerebral blood flow using cross-sectional imaging techniques, an independent TDC is obtained for each pixel. Because $C_t(t)$, $C_a(t)$, and $C_v(t)$ are known quantities, the equation can be solved, in principle, on a pixel-by-pixel basis, for CBF.

The ease of the mathematical solution to this differential equation, however, is highly dependent on the assumptions made regarding inflow and outflow to the region. One common model assumes no venous outflow, which simplifies the calculation at the cost of necessitating extremely high injection rates as described above.

CBV can be approximated as the area under the "fitted" (smoothed) tissue TDC, divided by the area under the fitted arterial TDC [66].

$$CBV = \int C_t(t) / \int C_a(t)$$

Note that when it is assumed that the contrast concentration in the arteries and capillaries is at a steady state, this equation forms the basis for the quantitative computation of CBV using the "whole brain perfused blood volume" method of Hunter and Hamberg [22, 29] described above. After soft tissue components have been removed by co-registration and subtraction of the pre-contrast scan, CBV then simply becomes a function of the density of tissue contrast, normalized by the density of arterial contrast.

Deconvolution Techniques. Direct calculation of CBF, applicable for even relatively slow injection rates, can be accomplished using deconvolution theory [73], which compensates for the inability to deliver a complete, instantaneous bolus of contrast into the artery supplying a given region of brain. In reality, a contrast bolus (particularly when administered in a peripheral vein) will undergo delay and dispersion before arriving in the cerebral vasculature; deconvolution attempts to correct for this reality, based on the following formula:

$$C_t(t) = CBF \cdot \left[C_a(t) \otimes R(t) \right]$$

Since the tissue and arterial TDCs [$C_t(t)$ and $C_a(t)$, respectively] can be determined directly from the CTP cine images, one can use deconvolution to solve for the product CBF·$R(t)$, the "scaled" residue function. CBF can then be obtained directly as proportional to the maximum *height* of this scaled residue function curve, whereas CBV is reflected as the *area* under the scaled residue function curve. Once CBF and CBV are known, MTT can be calculated using the central volume principle.

Mathematically, deconvolution of the arterial (AIF) and tissue curves can be accomplished using a variety of techniques, including the Fourier transform and the singular value decomposition methods. These methods vary in their sensitivity to such factors as: (1) the precise vascular anatomy of the underlying tissue bed being studied, and (2) the degree of delay, or dispersal, of the contrast bolus between the measured arterial and tissue TDCs [90]. In current clinical software, the singular value decomposition method, which is more sensitive to contrast dispersal factors than to specific local arterial anatomy, is the more commonly employed.

The creation of accurate, quantitative maps of CBV, CBF, and MTT using the deconvolution method has been validated in a number of studies [28, 37–39, 47, 90–93]. Specifically, validation has been accomplished by comparison with xenon [47, 94], PET [95], and MRP [96–98] in humans, as well as with microspheres in animals [28, 37, 38].

5.6 CTP Post-Processing

In urgent clinical cases, perfusion changes can often be observed immediately following scanning by direct visual inspection of the axial source images at the CT scanner console. Soft copy review at a workstation using "movie" or "cine" mode can reveal relative perfusion changes over time, although advanced post-processing is required to appreciate subtle changes, and to obtain quantification.

Axial source images acquired from a cine CT perfusion study are networked to a freestanding workstation for detailed analysis, including construction of CBF, CBV, and MTT maps. Prior to loading these data into the available software package, the source images should be visually inspected for motion artifact. Images showing significant misregistration with the remaining dataset can be deleted or corrected, depending on the sophistication of the existing software.

The computation of quantitative first-pass cine cerebral perfusion maps typically requires some combination of the following user inputs (Fig. 5.1):
- *Arterial input ROI*: A small ROI (typically 2×2 to 4×4 pixels in area) is placed over the central portion of a large intracranial artery, preferably an artery orthogonal to the imaging plane in order to minimize "dilutional" effects from volume averaging. An attempt should be made to select an arterial ROI with maximal peak contrast intensity.
- *Venous outflow ROI*: A small venous ROI with similar attributes is selected, most commonly at the superior sagittal sinus. With some software packages, selection of an appropriate venous ROI is critical in producing quantitatively accurate perfusion maps, while others are less sensitive to this selection [84].
- *Baseline*: The baseline is the "flat" portion of the arterial TDC, prior to the upward sloping of the curve caused by contrast enhancement. The baseline typically begins to rise after 4–6 s.
- *Post-enhancement cutoff*: This refers to the "tail" portion of the TDC, which may slope upwards towards a second peak value if recirculation effects are present. When such upward sloping at the "tail" of the TDC is noted, the data should be truncated to avoid including the recirculation of contrast. The perfusion analysis program will subsequently ignore data from slices beyond the cutoff.

Other user-defined inputs, such as "threshold" or "resolution" values, are dependent on the specific software package used for image reconstruction. It is worth noting that major variations in the input values described above may not only result in perfusion maps of differing image quality, but, potentially, in perfusion maps with variation in their quantitative values for CBF, CBV, and MTT. As previously noted, special care must often be taken in choosing an optimal venous outflow ROI, because that ROI value may be used to normalize the quantitative parameters.

Although the precise choice of CTP scanning level is dependent on both the clinical question being asked and other available imaging findings, an *essential caveat* in selecting a CTP slice is that the imaged

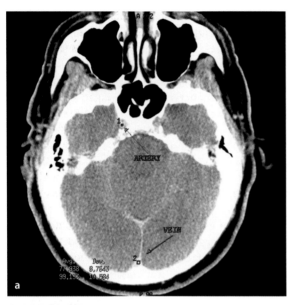

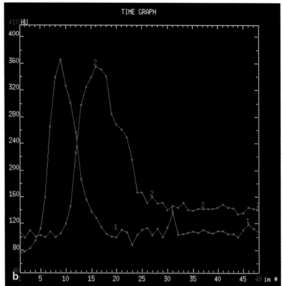

Figure 5.1 a, b

CT perfusion (*CTP*) post-processing. a Appropriate region of interest (*ROI*) placement on an artery (a major vessel running perpendicular to the plane of section to avoid volume averaging) and on a vein (the superior sagittal sinus, also running perpendicular to the plane of section and placed to avoid the inner table of the skull). b The time density curves (*TDC*) generated from this artery (*A*) and vein (*V*) show the arrival, peak, and passage of the contrast bolus over time. These TDCs serve as the arterial input function (*AIF*) and the venous output for the subsequent deconvolution step

level must contain a major intracranial artery. This is necessary in order to assure the availability of an AIF, to be used for the computation of perfusion maps using the deconvolution software.

In the construction of perfusion maps from either CT or MR datasets, voxels comprising the AIF can be selected in a semi-automated manner. In general, deconvolution is also less sensitive to variations in underlying vascular anatomy than are the nondeconvolution-based methods. This is because, for simplicity, the fundamental assumption of most nondeconvolution cerebral perfusion models is that a single feeding artery and a single draining vein support all blood flow to and from a given tissue bed, and that the precise arterial, venous, and tissue TDCs can be uniquely identified by imaging. This assumption is clearly an oversimplification. While MR-PWI maps (CBF and MTT) have been shown to have increased

accuracy with a bolus delay-corrected technique (BDC) [99], a delay correction is built into most available CTP processing software, so this is less of a concern in CTP.

Potential imaging *pitfalls* (Table 5.5) in the computation of CBF using the deconvolution method include both patient motion and partial volume averaging, which can cause the AIF to be underestimated. The effects of these pitfalls can be minimized by the use of image coregistration software to correct for patient motion, as well as by careful choice of ROIs for the AIF. In addition, comparison with the contralateral (normal) side to establish a percentage change from normal is a useful interpretive technique, since the reliability of quantitative data is in the range of 20–25% variation and the robustness of the quantitative data has not been established in large clinical trials.

Table 5.5. Pitfalls of CTP acquisition and post-processing

Failure to minimize or correct for motion during the cine CTP acquisition

Failure to continue cine CTP acquisition for at least 45–60 s to ensure return to baseline of venous enhancement

Failure to include a major intracranial artery in the CTP acquisition

Inappropriate arterial ROI selection, including use of an in-plane or obliquely oriented artery

Inappropriate venous ROI selection, including incorporation of the inner table of the skull into the ROI

Failure to truncate the time density curve to avoid incorporating recirculation of contrast into the CTP calculations

5.7 Clinical Applications of CTP

Indications (and potential indications) for advanced "functional" imaging of stroke in the first 12 h include the following: (1) exclusion of patients most likely to hemorrhage and inclusion of patients most likely to benefit from thrombolysis; (2) extension of the time window beyond 3 h for i.v. and 6 h for anterior circulation i.a. thrombolysis; (3) triage to other available therapies, such as hypertension or hyperoxia administration; (4) disposition decisions regarding neurological intensive care unit (NICU) admission or emergency department discharge; and (5) rational management of "wake up" strokes, for which precise time of onset is unknown [100]. The Desmoteplase in Acute Ischemic Stroke Trial (DIAS) suggests that the i.v. use of desmoteplase can be extended to a therapeutic window of 3–9 h post-ictus, with significantly improved reperfusion rates and clinical outcomes achieved in patients with a diffusion–perfusion mismatch on MR [101]. Indeed, based on this evidence and while awaiting information from other large trials such as EPITHET (Echoplanar Imaging Thrombolysis Evaluation Trial), some authors have cautiously proposed the use of either advanced MR or CT for extending the traditional therapeutic time window [18, 102], pointing to evidence of a relevant volume of salvageable tissue present in the 3- to 6-h time frame in >80% of stroke patients [101, 103, 104]. Methods that accurately distinguish salvageable from nonsalvageable brain tissue are being increasingly promoted as a means to select patients for thrombolysis beyond the 3-h window for i.v. therapy.

5.8 CTP Interpretation: Infarct Detection with CTA-SI

A number of groups have suggested that CTA source images, similar to DWI, can sensitively detect tissue destined to infarct despite successful recanalization [26, 36, 105]. Theoretical modeling indicates that CTA-SI, assuming an approximately steady state of contrast in the brain arteries and parenchyma during image acquisition, are weighted predominantly by blood volume, rather than blood flow, although this has yet to be validated empirically in a large series [22, 29, 66, 98]. An early report from our group indicated that CTA-SI typically defines minimal final infarct size and, hence, like DWI and CBV, can be used to identify "infarct core" in the acute setting [36] (Fig. 5.2). Co-registration and subtraction of the conventional, unenhanced CT brain images from the axial, post-contrast CTA source images should result in quantitative blood volume maps of the entire brain (Fig. 5.3) [15, 22, 29]. CTA-SI subtraction maps, obtained by co-registration and subtraction of the unenhanced head CT from the CTA source images, are particularly appealing for clinical use because – unlike quantitative first-pass CT perfusion maps – they provide whole brain coverage. Rapid, convenient co-registration/subtraction software is now commercially available on multiple platforms, allowing generation of these maps outside of the research arena [106, 107]. Subtraction maps, despite the improved conspicuity of blood volume lesions, may be limited by increased image noise [27]. A pilot study from our group of 20 consecutive patients with MCA stem occlusion who underwent i.a. thrombolysis following imaging demonstrated that CTA-SI and CTA-SI subtraction maps improve infarct conspicu-

Figure 5.2

An infarct in the left middle cerebral artery (*MCA*) distribution is more conspicuous on the CT angiography source image (*CTA-SI*) (*top right, arrows*) than the unenhanced CT (*top left*) performed in the acute setting. Subsequent diffusion-weighted image (*DWI, bottom left*) and unenhanced CT (*bottom right*) confirm the territory of infarction seen on CTA-SI

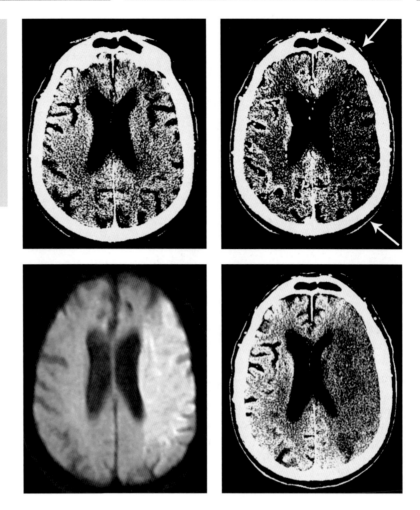

ity over that of unenhanced CT in patients with hyperacute stroke. True reduction in blood pool (as reflected by CTA-SI subtraction), rather than an increase in tissue edema (as reflected by unenhanced CT), may explain much of the improved infarct delineation in CTA-SI imaging. Concurrent review of unenhanced CT, CTA-SI, and CTA-SI subtraction images may be indicated for optimal CT assessment of hyperacute MCA stroke.

In another study, CTA-SI preceding DWI imaging was performed in 48 consecutive patients with clinically suspected stroke, presenting within 12 h of symptom onset (42 patients within 6 h) [26]. CTA-SI and DWI lesion volumes were independent predictors of final infarct volume, and overall sensitivity and specificity for parenchymal stroke detection were 76% and 90% for CTA-SI, and 100% and 100% for DWI, respectively. When cases with an initial DWI lesion volume <15 ml (small lacunar and distal infarctions) were excluded from analysis, CTA-SI sensitivity and specificity increased to 95% and 100%, respectively. Although DWI is more sensitive than CTA-SI for parenchymal stroke detection of small lesions (Fig. 5.4), both DWI and CTA-SI are highly accurate predictors of final infarct volume. DWI tends to underestimate final infarct size, whereas

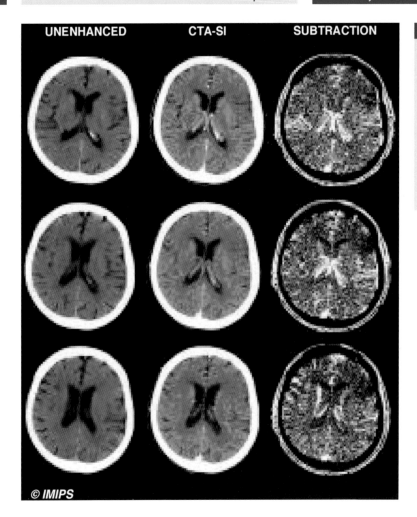

UNENHANCED   **CTA-SI**   **SUBTRACTION**

© IMIPS

Figure 5.3

Unenhanced, CTA-SI, and CTA-SI subtraction images demonstrate the value of the CTA-SI and CTA-SI subtraction images in improving conspicuity of acute stroke. The infarct is most obvious on the subtraction image, although the contrast-to-noise ratio is increased on these images as well. Figure courtesy Integrated Medical Image Processing Systems (*IMIPS*)

CTA-SI more closely approximates final infarct size, despite the bias towards DWI being obtained *after* the CTA-SI in this cohort of patients with unknown recanalization status.

Finally, it is noteworthy that, as with DWI, not every acute CTA-SI hypodense ischemic lesion is destined to infarct [108, 109]. In the presence of early complete recanalization, sometimes dramatic sparing of regions with reduced blood pool on CTA-SI can occur (Fig. 5.5). This suggests that, as with CBV, CBF, and DWI, time-dependent thresholds exist for distinguishing viable from nonviable CTA-SI (or CTA-SI subtraction) ischemia. Hunter et al. [110] studied the normalized blood volume on CTA-SI from 28 acute stroke patients at the *very* thin boundary between infarcted and spared tissue. They found that the probability of infarction in the core, inner boundary, and outer boundary were 0.99, 0.96, and 0.11 respectively, supporting the concept that CTA-SI thresholds predictive of tissue outcome exist [110].

Figure 5.4

A "false-negative" CTA-SI due to early imaging of a small infarct, retrospectively seen to be present on both the unenhanced CT and CTA-SI. It is noteworthy that the DWI lesion, although clearly more conspicuous, was imaged at a much later time point. *Top row*: unenhanced CT and CTA-SI at 3.5 h. *Bottom row*: DWI at 11 h and follow-up unenhanced CT at 33 h

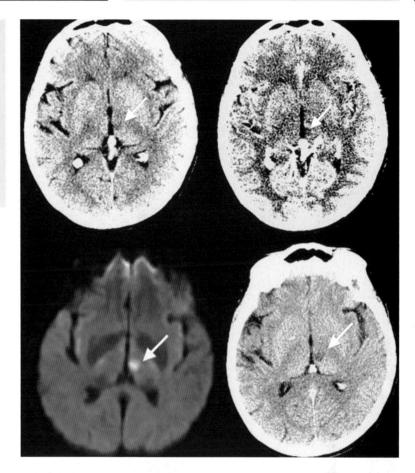

Figure 5.5

Reversal of CTA-SI abnormality. A patient with a right M1 thrombus who had complete recanalization after 90 min following intra-arterial (*i.a.*) thrombolysis. There is a large MCA territory blood pool deficit on the CTA-SI (*left, arrows*), but only a small deep gray lenticular hypodensity on the post-lysis unenhanced CT (*right*). Late follow-up showed lenticular infarct with minimal, patchy, incomplete infarction in other portions of the MCA territory. (Courtesy of Jeffrey Farkas, MD)

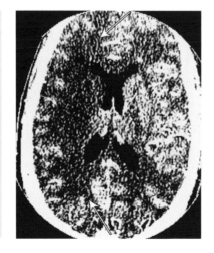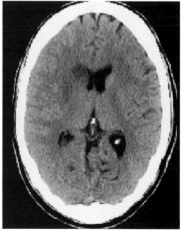

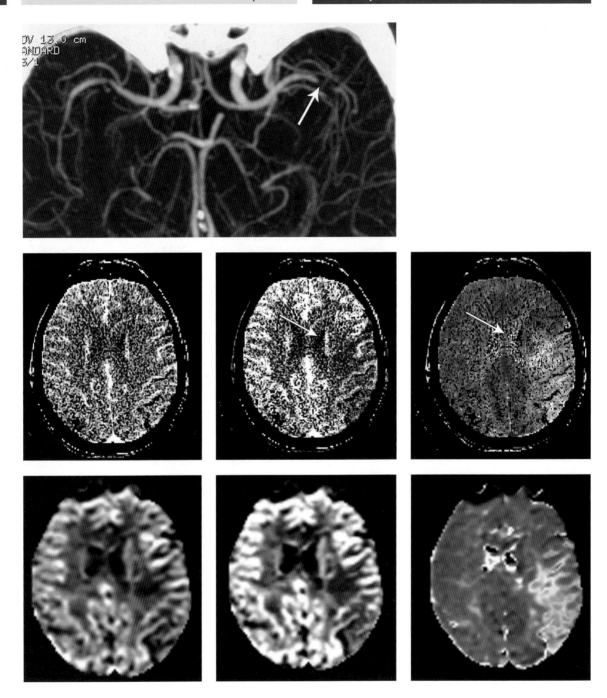

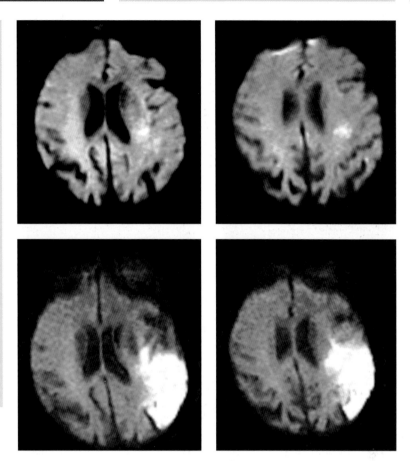

Figure 5.6 (continued)

A 65-year-old man, improving clinically at 5 h post-ictus, was monitored in the Neurology ICU based on his labile blood pressure, a fixed left M2 occlusion on CTA, and a significant core/penumbra mismatch on CTP/MRP. His 24-h follow-up DWI showed a small infarction. However, 24 h after cessation of hypertensive therapy there was infarct growth into the region of penumbra. From *top to bottom*: admission CTA, CTP [cerebral blood volume (*CBV*), cerebral blood flow (*CBF*) and mean transit time (*MTT*)] at 4.5 h, MR-PWI (*CBV/ CBF/MTT*) at 5.25 h, DWI at 24 h, and follow-up DWI at 48 h. The CTP and MR-PWI demonstrate a mismatch between the CBV (no abnormality) and the CBF/MTT penumbra (*arrows*). After cessation of hypertensive therapy, the DWI abnormality grows into the region predicted by the CBF/ MTT maps

5.9 CTP Interpretation: Ischemic Penumbra and Infarct Core

An important goal of advanced stroke imaging is to provide an assessment of ischemic tissue viability that transcends an arbitrary "clock-time" [111–113]. The original theory of penumbra stems from experimental studies in which two thresholds were characterized [114]. One threshold identified a CBF value below which there was cessation of cortical function, without an increase in extracellular potassium or reduction in pH. A second, lower threshold identified a CBF value below which there was disruption of cellular integrity. With the advent of advanced neuroimaging and modern stroke therapy, a more clinically relevant "operationally defined penumbra"

– that identifies hypoperfused but potentially salvageable tissue – has gained acceptance [111, 115–117].

Ischemic Penumbra. Cine single-slab CT perfusion imaging, which can provide quantitative maps of CBF, CBV, and MTT, has the potential to describe regions of "ischemic penumbra" – ischemic but still viable tissue. In the simplest terms, the "operationally defined penumbra" is the volume of tissue contained within the region of CBF–CBV mismatch on CTP maps, where the region of CBV abnormality represents the "core" of infarcted tissue and the CBF–CBV mismatch represents the surrounding region of tissue that is hypoperfused but salvageable (Figs. 5.6–5.8). The few papers that have investigated the role of CTP in acute stroke triage have typically

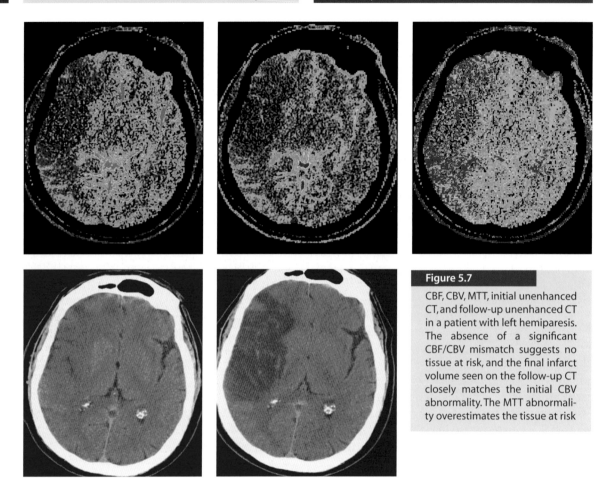

Figure 5.7

CBF, CBV, MTT, initial unenhanced CT, and follow-up unenhanced CT in a patient with left hemiparesis. The absence of a significant CBF/CBV mismatch suggests no tissue at risk, and the final infarct volume seen on the follow-up CT closely matches the initial CBV abnormality. The MTT abnormality overestimates the tissue at risk

assumed predefined threshold values for "core" and "penumbra" based on human and animal studies from the PET, MR, SPECT, or xenon literature, and determined the accuracy of these in predicting outcome [48]. By assuming cutoff values of ≥34% reduction from baseline CT-CBF for penumbra and ≤2.5 ml/100 g CT-CBV for core, Wintermark et al. [48] found good correlation between DWI and CT-CBV infarct core (r=0.698) and the MR-MTT and CT-CBF ischemic penumbra (r=0.946). Of note, the CT-CBV maps suffer from decreased signal-to-noise relative to CT-CBF maps, suggesting that the interpretation of CBV maps may benefit from a semiautomated thresholding approach to segmentation to more accurately gauge the size of infarct [76]. The interpreta-

tion of CTP in the setting of acute stroke is summarized in Table 5.6.

CT-CBF–CBV mismatch correlates significantly with lesion enlargement. Untreated or unsuccessfully treated patients with large CBF–CBV mismatch exhibit substantial lesion growth on follow-up, whereas those patients without significant mismatch – or those with early, complete recanalization – do not exhibit lesion progression of their admission CTA-SI lesion volume (Figs. 5.6–5.8). CTP-defined mismatch might therefore serve as a marker of salvageable tissue, and thus prove useful in patient triage for thrombolysis [118]. This result clearly has implications for the utility of a CTP-based model for predicting outcome in patients *without* robust recanalization. Sim-

Table 5.6. Summary of CTP interpretation

CBV, CBF match
No treatment regardless of lesion size

Large CBV, larger CBF
Possible treatment based on time post ictus, size
Consider no treatment if CBV >100 ml

Small CBV, larger CBF
Typically a good candidate for treatment
Consider no treatment if prolonged time-post-ictus

ilarly, in an earlier pilot study of CTP imaging, ultimate infarct size was most strongly correlated with CT-CBF lesion size in 14 embolic stroke patients *without* robust recanalization [119], again demonstrating the importance of this mismatch region as tissue at risk for infarction.

Several studies of MR-PWI suggest that CBF maps are superior to MTT maps for distinguishing viable from nonviable penumbra [120–122]. The reason for this relates to the fact that MTT maps display circulatory derangements that do not necessarily reflect ischemic change, including large vessel occlusions with compensatory collateralization (Fig. 5.9) and reperfusion hyperemia following revascularization (Fig. 5.10).

Refinements of the Traditional Penumbra Model. The "operationally defined penumbra," however, oversimplifies reality, as not all tissue contained within the operationally defined penumbra is destined to infarct. There is a region of "benign oligemia" contained within the region of the CBV–CBF mismatch that is not expected to infarct even in the absence of reperfusion. This refinement of the traditional model has important clinical implications, since treatment regimens that are based on an overestimated volume of tissue at risk will likely be too aggressive, exposing the patient to the risks and complications of treatment for tissue that would not likely have proceeded to infarct even without intervention. Few studies have reported specific CBF thresholds for distinguishing penumbra likely to infarct in the absence of early recanalization (nonviable penumbra) from penumbra likely to survive *despite* persistent vascular occlusion (viable penumbra) [120, 122]. Fewer

still have addressed this problem using CTP. Previous work from our group and others has: (1) detected a significant difference between the MR-CBF thresholds for penumbra likely to infarct and penumbra likely to remain viable [120, 122], and (2) also revealed a good correlation between MR and CT perfusion parameter values [58, 96–98, 123].

In a pilot study of CTP thresholds for infarction, we found that normalized, or relative CBF is the most robust parameter for distinguishing viable from nonviable penumbra. All regions with a less than 56% reduction in mean CBF survived whereas all regions with a greater than 68% reduction in mean CBF infarcted. In rough approximation, therefore, CT-CBF penumbra with less than one-half reduction from baseline values has a high probability of survival, whereas penumbra with a greater than two-thirds reduction from baseline values has a high probability of infarction. No region with a mean relative CBV less than 0.68, absolute CBF less than $12.7 \text{ ml} \cdot 100 \text{ g}^{-1} \cdot \text{min}^{-1}$, or absolute CBV less than $2.2 \text{ ml} \cdot 100 \text{ g}^{-1}$ survived. The latter compares well with the CBV threshold of $2.5 \text{ ml} \cdot 100 \text{ g}^{-1}$ selected by Wintermark et al. [48] to define "core." Because of differences in CBV and CBF between gray and white matter (Table 5.4), it is essential for the contralateral ROI used for normalization to have the same gray matter/white matter ratio as the ipsilateral ischemic region under study. Moreover, a number of studies suggest that, due to different cellular populations, gray and white matter may respond differently to ischemic injury.

There is little literature addressing perfusion thresholds in patients undergoing i.a. recanalization procedures [124]. Our results of mean relative CBF thresholds of 0.19 for core, 0.34 for nonviable penumbra, and 0.46 for viable penumbra are in general agreement with those of a SPECT study of patients with complete recanalization following i.a. thrombolysis. Pre-treatment SPECT showed CBF>55% of cerebellar flow in viable penumbra, even with treatment initiated 6 h after symptom onset [125]. Ischemic tissue with CBF >35% of cerebellar flow may remain salvageable if recanalization is achieved in under 5 h. Our results for mean relative CBF thresholds are also in agreement with SPECT and MR studies performed in patients who received other stroke therapies [120, 126–128].

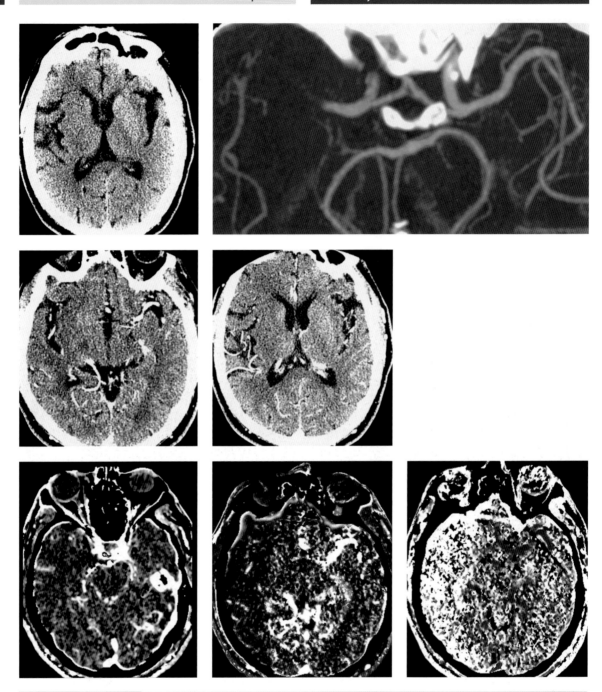

Figure 5.8

A 77-year-old bartender presenting with a left facial droop. Subtle changes of the insula and right lentiform nucleus were seen on initial unenhanced CT, and CTA revealed acute occlusion of the right M1 segment. The infarct is more conspicuous on CTA-SI, and CTP demonstrates an ischemic penumbra involving the entire right MCA territory, consistent with a large territory at risk for subsequent infarction. Successful i.a. thrombolysis at 3 h was performed. Follow-up DWI showed an infarct limited to the initial CTA-SI abnormality. *Top row*: initial unenhanced CT and CTA. *Second row*: CTA-SI. *Third row*: CTP (CBV/CBF/MTT).

Figure 5.8 (continued)

Fourth row: follow-up DWI at 36 h

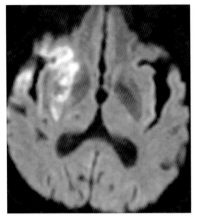

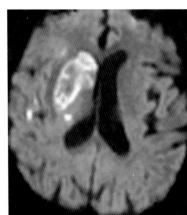

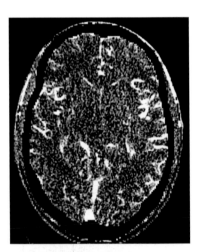

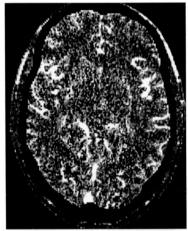

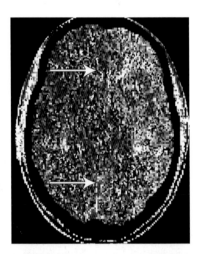

Figure 5.9

Perfusion abnormalities associated with a left internal carotid artery (*ICA*) dissection at the skull base. Despite the MTT abnormality that might have been mistaken for ischemic penumbra, follow-up unenhanced CT shows no evidence of infarction. The prolonged MTT was related to collateral flow necessitated by the ICA dissection. *Top row*: CBV, CBF, and MTT reveals prolonged MTT in the left hemisphere (*arrows*). *Bottom row*: curved reformat from a CTA shows the site of dissection (*arrow*)

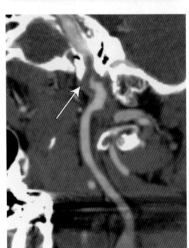

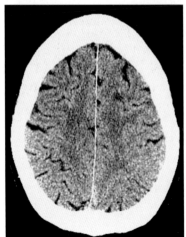

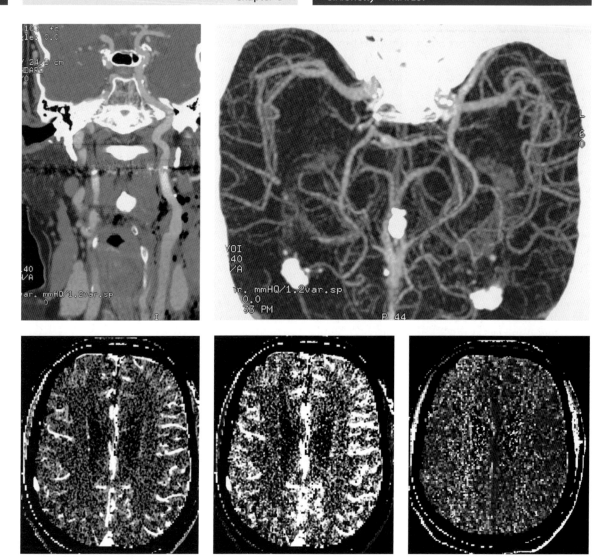

Figure 5.10

CTP was performed 3 h following left carotid endarterectomy (*CEA*) showing reperfusion hyperemia. *Top row*: CTA shows preserved flow in the left carotid artery at the site of CEA. *Bottom row*: CBV/CBF/MTT shows increased CBF and shortened MTT on the *left*, consistent with reperfusion hyperemia

5.10 Imaging Predictors of Clinical Outcome

Predicting outcome is perilous. The penumbra is dynamic, and several factors influence its fate, including time post-ictus, residual and collateral blood flow, admission glucose, temperature, hematocrit, systolic blood pressure, and treatment, including hyperoxia [129]. As already mentioned, CTA/CTP has the potential to serve as a surrogate marker of stroke severity, likely exceeding the NIHSS score or ASPECTS as a predictor of outcome [26, 50–57].

Infarct Core and Clinical Outcome. As noted earlier, measuring the penumbra is technically challenging. Flow thresholds for various states of tissue perfusion vary considerably among studies and techniques applied [130]. Despite this, a number of consistent messages emerge from a review of the literature regarding imaging outcome prediction in acute ischemic stroke. The most important of these messages is that "core" is crucial. Multiple studies, examining heterogeneous cohorts of patients receiving varied treatments, consistently find that ultimate clinical outcome is strongly correlated with admission "core" lesion volume – be it measured by DWI, CT-CBV, subthreshold xenon CT-CBF, or unenhanced CT [131–135]. One of these studies is especially noteworthy, because results were stratified by degree of recanalization at 24 h. This study revealed "that 2 factors mainly influenced clinical outcome: (1) recanalization ($P=0.0001$) and (2) day-0 DWI lesion volume ($P=0.03$)" [136]. In a study of CTP in patients with MCA stem occlusions, patients with admission whole-brain CT perfusion lesions volumes >100 ml (equal to approximately one-third the volume of the MCA territory) had poor clinical outcomes, regardless of recanalization status. Moreover, in those patients from the same cohort who had early complete MCA recanalization, final infarct volume was closely approximated by the size of the initial whole-brain CT perfusion lesion [36].

Risk of Hemorrhage. The degree of early CBF reduction in acute stroke may also help predict hemorrhagic risk. Preliminary results from our group suggest that severe hypoattenuation, relative to normal tissue, on whole-brain CTP images, may also identify ischemic regions more likely to bleed following i.a. thrombolysis [45]. In a SPECT study of 30 patients who had complete recanalization within 12 h of stoke onset, those with less than 35% of normal cerebellar flow at infarct core were at a significantly higher risk for hemorrhage [125]. Indeed, multiple studies have suggested that severely ischemic regions with early reperfusion are at the highest risk for hemorrhagic transformation [133, 137]. Of note, there is a suggestion that the presence of punctate microhemorrhage is correlated with the risk of hemorrhagic transformation; these small foci of hemorrhage are seen on gradient echo (susceptibility-weighted) MR sequences and are not visible on unenhanced CT [138]. It remains to be seen, however, whether these microbleeds will serve as a contraindication to thrombolytic therapy.

5.11 Experimental Applications of CTP in Stroke

The additional information about capillary-level hemodynamics afforded by CTP could be particularly important in future clinical trials of acute stroke therapy, in which CTP could refine the selection of subjects to include only those patients most likely to benefit from treatment; this imaging-guided patient selection may help to demonstrate beneficial effects that would be obscured if patients without salvageable tissue were included. CTA combined with CTP could be used to identify patients with proximal large vessel occlusive thrombus, who are the most appropriate candidates for i.a. treatment [14, 29, 139]. The ability of perfusion imaging to quantitatively determine ischemic brain regions that are viable but at risk for infarction if blood flow is not quickly restored – so called ischemic penumbra – might provide a more rational basis for establishing the maximum safe time window for administering thrombolytic agents than the current, arbitrary cutoffs of 3 h post-ictus for i.v. and 6 h post-ictus for i.a. thrombolysis [50, 140] (Table 5.6). MRP has already been used to support extending the therapeutic time window in a subset of patients with a DWI–MR-PWI mismatch: the DIAS trial of patients with an NIHSS of 4–20 and an MR diffusion–perfusion mismatch (where the perfusion abnormality was defined using MTT) showed significantly improved rates of reperfusion and clinical outcome when i.v. desmoteplase was administered between 3 and 9 h of ictus onset in an escalating dose range of 62–125 µg/kg [101]. CTP could serve a similar role in rationally extending the therapeutic time window for stroke intervention.

Despite a multitude of animal studies that have demonstrated a benefit from neuroprotective agents, the only therapy proven in humans to improve outcome has been thrombolysis (both i.v. and i.a.) [2, 3, 140]. There is growing literature positing that ischemic, potentially salvageable "penumbral" tissue is an ideal target for neuroprotective agents [55, 111, 141], suggesting that CTP or other perfusion techniques may be suited to selection of patients in trials of these agents. Kidwell and Warach [142] argue that enrollment in clinical trials should require a definitive diagnosis of stroke, confirmed by imaging and lab studies.

5.12 Conclusion

As new treatments are developed for stroke, the potential clinical applications of CTP imaging in the diagnosis, triage, and therapeutic monitoring of these diseases are certain to increase.

Technical advances in scanner hardware and software will no doubt continue to increase the speed, coverage, and resolution of CTP imaging. CTP offers the promise of efficient utilization of imaging resources, and, potentially, of decreased morbidity. Most importantly, current CT technology already permits the incorporation of CTP as part of an all-in-one acute stroke examination to quickly and accurately answer the four fundamental questions of stroke triage, further increasing the contribution of imaging to the diagnosis and treatment of acute stroke.

References

1. American Heart Association (2003) Heart disease and stroke statistics – 2004 update. American Heart Association, Dallas, Tex.
2. Furlan A, Higashida R, Wechsler L et al (1999) Intra-arterial Prourokinase for Acute Ischemic Stroke: The PROACT II Study: A Randomized Controlled Trial. J Am Med Assoc 282:2003–2011
3. Furlan A, Higashida R, Wechsler L et al (1999) Intra-arterial prourokinase for acute ischemic stroke. J Am Med Assoc 282:2003–2011
4. Marler JR, Tilley BC, Lu M et al (2000) Early stroke treatment associated with better outcome: the NINDS rt-PA stroke study. Neurology 55:1649–1655
5. Del Zoppo GJ, Poeck K, Pessin MS et al (1992) Recombinant tissue plasminogen activator in acute thrombotic and embolic stroke. Ann Neurol 32:78–86
6. Hacke W, Kaste M, Fieschi C et al (1995) Intravenous thrombolysis with recombinant tissue plasminogen activator for acute hemispheric stroke. The European Cooperative Acute Stroke Study (ECASS). J Am Med Assoc 274:1017–1025
7. Madden KP, Karanjia PN, Adams HP Jr., Clarke WR (1995) Accuracy of initial stroke subtype diagnosis in the TOAST study. Trial of ORG 10172 in Acute Stroke Treatment. Neurology 45:1975–1979
8. Ezzeddine MA, Lev MH, McDonald CT et al (2202) CT angiography with whole brain perfused blood volume imaging: added clinical value in the assessment of acute stroke. Stroke 33:959–966
9. Dubey N, Bakshi R, Wasay M, Dmochowski J (2001) Early computed tomography hypodensity predicts hemorrhage after intravenous tissue plasminogen activator in acute ischemic stroke. J Neuroimaging 11:184–188
10. Lev MH, Nichols SJ (2000) Computed tomographic angiography and computed tomographic perfusion imaging of hyperacute stroke. Top Magn Reson Imaging 11:273–287
11. Wardlaw J, Dorman P, Lewis S, Sandercock P (1999) Can stroke physicians and neuroradiologists identify signs of early cerebral infarction on CT? J Neurol Neursosurg Psychiatry 67:651–653
12. Schaefer PW, Romero JM, Grant PE et al (2002) Diffusion magnetic resonance imaging of acute ischemic stroke. Semin Roentgenol 37:219–229
13. Schaefer PW, Grant PE, Gonzalez G (2000) Diffusion-weighted MR imaging of the Brain. Radiology 217:331–345
14. Lev MH, Farkas J, Rodriguez VR et al (2001) CT angiography in the rapid triage of patients with hyperacute stroke to intraarterial thrombolysis: accuracy in the detection of large vessel thrombus. J Comput Assist Tomogr 25:520–528
15. Lev MH, Gonzalez RG (2002) CT angiography and CT perfusion imaging. In: Toga AW, Mazziotta JC (eds) Brain mapping: the methods, 2nd edn. Academic Press, San Diego, Calif., pp 427–484

16. Wildermuth S, Knauth M, Brandt T, Winter R, Sartor K, Hacke W (1998) Role of CT angiography in patient selection for thrombolytic therapy in acute hemispheric stroke. Stroke 29:935–938

17. Knauth M, von Kummer R, Jansen O, Hahnel S, Dorfler A, Sartor K (1997) Potential of CT angiography in acute ischemic stroke. Am J Neuroradiol 18:1001–1010

18. Schellinger PD, Fiebach JB, Hacke W (2003) Imaging-based decision making in thrombolytic therapy for ischemic stroke: present status. Stroke 34:575–583

19. Warach S (2001) Tissue viability thresholds in acute stroke: the 4-factor model. Stroke 32:2460–2461

20. Roberts HC, Roberts TP, Dillon WP (2001) CT perfusion flow assessment: "up and coming" or "off and running"? Am J Neuroradiol 22:1018–1019

21. Hamberg LM, Hunter GJ, Halpern EF, Hoop B, Gazelle GS, Wolf GL (1996) Quantitative high resolution measurement of cerebrovascular physiology with slip-ring CT. Am J Neuroradiol 17:639–650

22. Hamberg LM, Hunter GJ, Kierstead D, Lo EH, Gilberto Gonzalez R, Wolf GL (1996) Measurement of cerebral blood volume with subtraction three-dimensional functional CT. Am J Neuroradiol 17:1861–1869

23. Fox SH, Tanenbaum LN, Ackelsberg S, He HD, Hsieh J, Hu H (1998) Future directions in CT technology. Neuroimaging Clin North Am 8:497–513

24. Smith WS, Roberts HC, Chuang NA et al (2003) Safety and feasibility of a CT protocol for acute stroke: combined CT, CT angiography, and CT perfusion imaging in 53 consecutive patients. Am J Neuroradiol 24:688–690

25. Gleason S, Furie KL, Lev MH et al (2001) Potential influence of acute CT on inpatient costs in patients with ischemic stroke. Acad Radiol 8:955–964

26. Berzin T, Lev M, Goodman D et al (2001) CT perfusion imaging versus MR diffusion weighted imaging: prediction of final infarct size in hyperacute stroke (abstract). Stroke 32:317

27. Bove P, Lev M, Chaves T et al (2001) CT perfusion imaging improves infarct conspicuity in hyperacute stroke. Stroke 32:325b

28. Cenic A, Nabavi DG, Craen RA, Gelb AW, Lee TY (1999) Dynamic CT measurement of cerebral blood flow: a validation study. Am J Neuroradiol 20:63–73

29. Hunter GJ, Hamberg LM, Ponzo JA et al (1998) Assessment of cerebral perfusion and arterial anatomy in hyperacute stroke with three-dimensional functional CT: early clinical results. Am J Neuroradiol 19:29–37

30. Klotz E, Konig M (1999) Perfusion measurements of the brain: using the dynamic CT for the quantitative assessment of cerebral ischemia in acute stroke. Eur J Radiol 30:170–184

31. Koenig M, Klotz E, Luka B, Venderink DJ, Spittler JF, Heuser L (1998) Perfusion CT of the brain: diagnostic approach for early detection of ischemic stroke. Radiology 209:85–93

32. Koroshetz WJ, Gonzales RG (1999) Imaging stroke in progress: magnetic resonance advances but computed tomography is poised for counterattack. Ann Neurol 46:556–558

33. Koroshetz WJ, Lev MH (2002) Contrast computed tomography scan in acute stroke: "You can't always get what you want but you get what you need". Ann Neurol 51:415–416

34. Lee KH, Lee SJ, Cho SJ et al (2000) Usefulness of triphasic perfusion computed tomography for intravenous thrombolysis with tissue-type plasminogen activator in acute ischemic stroke. Arch Neurol 57:1000–1008

35. Lee KH, Cho SJ, Byun HS et al (2000) Triphasic perfusion computed tomography in acute middle cerebral artery stroke: a correlation with angiographic findings. Arch Neurol 57:990–999

36. Lev MH, Segal AZ, Farkas J et al (2001) Utility of perfusion-weighted CT imaging in acute middle cerebral artery stroke treated with intra-arterial thrombolysis: prediction of final infarct volume and clinical outcome. Stroke 32:2021–2028

37. Nabavi DG, Cenic A, Dool J et al (1999) Quantitative assessment of cerebral hemodynamics using CT: stability, accuracy, and precision studies in dogs. J Comput Assist Tomogr 23:506–515

38. Nabavi DG, Cenic A, Craen RA et al (1999) CT assessment of cerebral perfusion: experimental validation and initial clinical experience. Radiology 213:141–149

39. Nabavi DG, Cenic A, Henderson S, Gelb AW, Lee TY (2001) Perfusion mapping using computed tomography allows accurate prediction of cerebral infarction in experimental brain ischemia. Stroke 32:175–183

40. Ponzo J, Hunter G, Hamburg L et al (1998) Evaluation of collateral circulation in acute stroke patients using CT angiography (abstract). Stroke, Orlando, Fla.

41. Roberts HC, Dillon WP, Smith WS (2000) Dynamic CT perfusion to assess the effect of carotid revascularization in chronic cerebral ischemia. Am J Neuroradiol 21:421–425

42. Roberts HC, Roberts TP, Smith WS, Lee TJ, Fischbein NJ, Dillon WP (2001) Multisection dynamic CT perfusion for acute cerebral ischemia: the "toggling-table" technique. Am J Neuroradiol 22:1077–1080

43. Rother J, Jonetz-Mentzel L, Fiala A et al (2000) Hemodynamic assessment of acute stroke using dynamic single-slice computed tomographic perfusion imaging. Arch Neurol 57:1161–1166

44. Shrier D, Tanaka H, Numaguchi Y, Konno S, Patel U, Shibata D (1997) CT angiography in the evaluation of acute stroke. Am J Neuroradiol 18:1011–1020

45. Swap C, Lev M, McDonald C et al (2002) Degree of oligemia by perfusion-weighted CT and risk of hemorrhage after IA thrombolysis. Stroke – Proceedings of the 27th International Conference on Stroke and Cerebral Circulation. San Antonio, Tex.

46. Wintermark M, Maeder P, Verdun FR et al (2000) Using 80 kVp versus 120 kVp in perfusion CT measurement of regional cerebral blood flow. Am J Neuroradiol 21:1881–1884

47. Wintermark M, Thiran JP, Maeder P, Schnyder P, Meuli R (2001) Simultaneous measurement of regional cerebral blood flow by perfusion CT and stable xenon CT: a validation study. Am J Neuroradiol 22:905–914

48. Wintermark M, Reichhart M, Thiran JP et al (2002) Prognostic accuracy of cerebral blood flow measurement by perfusion computed tomography, at the time of emergency room admission, in acute stroke patients. Ann Neurol 51:417–432

49. Eastwood JD, Lev MH, Azhari T et al (2002) CT perfusion scanning with deconvolution analysis: pilot study in patients with acute middle cerebral artery stroke. Radiology 222:227–236

50. Albers GW (1999) Expanding the window for thrombolytic therapy in acute stroke. The potential role of acute MRI for patient selection. Stroke 30:2230–2237

51. Barber PA, Demchuk AM, Zhang J, Buchan AM (2000) Validity and reliability of a quantitative computed tomography score in predicting outcome of hyperacute stroke before thrombolytic therapy. ASPECTS Study Group. Alberta Stroke Programme Early CT Score. Lancet 355:1670–1674

52. Broderick JP, Lu M, Kothari R et al (2000) Finding the most powerful measures of the effectiveness of tissue plasminogen activator in the NINDS tPA stroke trial. Stroke 31:2335–2341

53. Schellinger PD, Jansen O, Fiebach JB et al (2000) Monitoring intravenous recombinant tissue plasminogen activator thrombolysis for acute ischemic stroke with diffusion and perfusion MRI. Stroke 31:1318–1328

54. Tong D, Yenari M, Albers G, O'Brien M, Marks M, Moseley M (1998) Correlation of perfusion- and diffusion weighted MRI with NIHSS Score in acute (<6.5 hour) ischemic stroke. Stroke 29:2673

55. Warach S (2001) New imaging strategies for patient selection for thrombolytic and neuroprotective therapies. Neurology 57:S48–S52

56. Von Kummer R, Holle R, Grzyska U, Hofmann E et al (1996) Interobserver agreement in assessing early CT signs of middle cerebral artery infarction. Am J Neuroradiol 17:1743–1748

57. Grotta JC, Chiu D, Lu M et al (1999) Agreement and variability in the interpretation of early CT changes in stroke patients qualifying for intravenous rtPA therapy (see comments). Stroke 30:1528–1533

58. Lev MH (2003) CT versus MR for acute stroke imaging: is the "obvious" choice necessarily the correct one? Am J Neuroradiol 24:1930–1931

59. Lev MH, Koroshetz WJ, Schwamm LH, Gonzalez RG (2002) CT or MRI for imaging patients with acute stroke: visualization of "tissue at risk"? Stroke 33:2736–2737

60. Von Kummer R, Allen KL, Holle R et al (1997) Acute stroke: usefulness of early CT findings before thrombolytic therapy. Radiology 205:327–333

61. Von Kummer R (2003) Early major ischemic changes on computed tomography should preclude use of tissue plasminogen activator. Stroke 34:820–821

62. Fiorelli M, von Kummer R (2002) Early ischemic changes on computed tomography in patients with acute stroke. J Am Med Assoc 287:2361–2362 [author reply 2362]

63. Mullins ME, Lev MH, Schellingerhout D, Koroshetz WJ, Gonzalez RG (2002) Influence of availability of clinical history on detection of early stroke using unenhanced CT and diffusion-weighted MR imaging. Am J Roentgenol 179:223–228

64. Lev M, Farkas J, Gemmete J et al (1999) Acute stroke: improved nonenhanced CT detection – benefits of soft-copy interpretation by using variable window width and center level settings. Radiology 213:150–155

65. Fiorelli M, Toni D, Bastianello S et al (2000) Computed tomography findings in the first few hours of ischemic stroke: implications for the clinician. J Neurol Sci 173:10–17

66. Axel L (1980) Cerebral blood flow determination by rapid-sequence computed tomography. Radiology 137:679–686

67. Bae KT, Tran HQ, Heiken JP (2000) Multiphasic injection method for uniform prolonged vascular enhancement at CT angiography: pharmacokinetic analysis and experimental porcine model. Radiology 216:872–880

68. Fleischmann D, Rubin GD, Bankier AA, Hittmair K (2000) Improved uniformity of aortic enhancement with customized contrast medium injection protocols at CT angiography. Radiology 214:363–371

69. Bae KT, Tran HQ, Heiken JP (2004) Uniform vascular contrast enhancement and reduced contrast medium volume achieved by using exponentially decelerated contrast material injection method. Radiology 231:732–736

70. Fleischmann D, Hittmair K (1999) Mathematical analysis of arterial enhancement and optimization of bolus geometry for CT angiography using the discrete fourier transform. J Comput Assist Tomogr 23:474–484

71. Aksoy FG, Lev MH (2000) Dynamic contrast-enhanced brain perfusion imaging: technique and clinical applications. Semin Ultrasound CT MR 21:462–477

72. Eastwood JD, Lev MH, Provenzale JM (2003) Perfusion CT with iodinated contrast material. Am J Roentgenol 180:3–12

73. Wintermark M, Maeder P, Thiran JP, Schnyder P, Meuli R (2001) Quantitative assessment of regional cerebral blood flows by perfusion CT studies at low injection rates: a critical review of the underlying theoretical models. Eur Radiol 11:1220–1230

74. Lev MH, Kulke SF, Weisskoff RM et al (1997) Dose dependence of signal to noise ratio in functional MRI of cerebral blood volume mapping with sprodiamide. J MRI 7:523–527

75. Coutts SB, Simon JE, Tomanek AI et al (2003) Reliability of assessing percentage of diffusion-perfusion mismatch. Stroke 34:1681–1683

76. Roccatagliata L, Lev MH, Mehta N, Koroshetz WJ, Gonzalez RG, Schaefer PW (2003) Estimating the size of ischemic regions on CT perfusion maps in acute stroke: is freehand visual segmentation sufficient? Proceedings of the 89th Scientific Assembly and Annual Meeting of the Radiological Society of North America. Chicago, Ill., p 1292

77. Mullins ME, Lev MH, Bove P et al (2004) Comparison of image quality between conventional and low-dose nonenhanced head CT. Am J Neuroradiol 25:533–538

78. Kendell B, Pullicono P (1980) Intravascular contrast injection in ischemic lesions, II. Effect on prognosis. Neuroradiology 19:241–243

79. Doerfler A, Engelhorn T, von Kommer R, Weber J et al (1998) Are iodinated contrast agents detrimental in acute cerebral ischemia? An experimental study in rats. Radiology 206:211–217

80. Palomaki H, Muuronen A, Raininko R, Piilonen A, Kaste M (2003) Administration of nonionic iodinated contrast medium does not influence the outcome of patients with ischemic brain infarction. Cerebrovasc Dis 15:45–50

81. Aspelin P, Aubry P, Fransson SG, Strasser R, Willenbrock R, Berg KJ (2003) Nephrotoxic effects in high-risk patients undergoing angiography. N Engl J Med 348:491–499

82. Fiorella D, Heiserman J, Prenger E, Partovi S (2004) Assessment of the reproducibility of postprocessing dynamic CT perfusion data. Am J Neuroradiol 25:97–107

83. Kealey SM, Loving VA, Delong DM, Eastwood JD (2004) User-defined vascular input function curves: influence on mean perfusion parameter values and signal-to-noise ratio. Radiology 231:587–593

84. Sanelli PC, Lev MH, Eastwood JD et al (2004) The effect of varying user-selected input parameters on quantitative values in CT perfusion maps. Acad Radiol 11:1085–1092

85. Villringer A, Rosen BR, Belliveau JW et al (1988) Dynamic imaging with lanthanide chelates in normal brain: contrast due to magnetic susceptibility effects. Magn Reson Med 6:164–174

86. Zilkha E, Ladurner G, Iliff LD, Du Boulay GH, Marshall J (1976) Computer subtraction in regional cerebral blood-volume measurements using the EMI-Scanner. Br J Radiol 49:330–334

87. Shih TT, Huang KM (1988) Acute stroke: detection of changes in cerebral perfusion with dynamic CT scanning. Radiology 169:469–474

88. Meier P, Zieler K (1954) On the theory of the indicator-dilution method for measurement of blood flow and volume. J Appl Physiol 6:731–744

89. Roberts G, Larson K (1973) The interpretation of mean transit time measurements for multi-phase tissue systems. J Theor Biol 39:447–475

90. Wirestam R, Andersson L, Ostergaard L et al (2000) Assessment of regional cerebral blood flow by dynamic susceptibility contrast MRI using different deconvolution techniques. Magn Reson Med 43:691–700

91. Cenic A, Nabavi DG, Craen RA, Gelb AW, Lee TY (2000) A CT method to measure hemodynamics in brain tumors: validation and application of cerebral blood flow maps. Am J Neuroradiol 21:462–470

92. Ostergaard L et al (1996) High resolution of cerebral blood flow using intravascular tracer bolus passages, part I: mathematical approach ad statistical analysis. Magn Reson Imaging Med 36(5):715–725

93. Ostergaard L, Chesler DA, Weisskoff RM, Sorensen AG, Rosen BR (1999) Modeling cerebral blood flow and flow heterogeneity from magnetic resonance residue data. J Cereb Blood Flow Metab 19:690–699

94. Furukawa M, Kashiwagi S, Matsunaga N, Suzuki M, Kishimoto K, Shirao S (2002) Evaluation of cerebral perfusion parameters measured by perfusion CT in chronic cerebral ischemia: comparison with xenon CT. J Comput Assist Tomogr 26:272–278

95. Gillard JH, Antoun NM, Burnet NG, Pickard JD (2001) Reproducibility of quantitative CT perfusion imaging. Br J Radiol 74:552–555

96. Eastwood JD, Lev MH, Wintermark M et al (2003) Correlation of early dynamic CT perfusion imaging with whole-brain MR diffusion and perfusion imaging in acute hemispheric stroke. Am J Neuroradiol 24:1869–1875

97. Wintermark M, Reichhart M, Cuisenaire O et al (2002) Comparison of admission perfusion computed tomography and qualitative diffusion- and perfusion-weighted magnetic resonance imaging in acute stroke patients. Stroke 33:2025–2031

98. Schramm P, Schellinger PD, Klotz E et al (2004) Comparison of perfusion computed tomography and computed tomography angiography source images with perfusion-weighted imaging and diffusion-weighted imaging in patients with acute stroke of less than 6 hours' duration. Stroke 35(7):1652–1658

99. Rose SE, Janke AL, Griffin M, Strudwick MW, Finnigan S, Semple J, Chalk JB (2004) Improving the prediction of final infarct size in acute stroke with bolus delay-corrected perfusion MRI measures. J Magn Reson Imaging 20(6):941–947

100. Serena J, Davalos A, Segura T, Mostacero E, Castillo J (2003) Stroke on awakening: looking for a more rational management. Cerebrovasc Dis 16:128–133

101. Hacke W, Albers G, Al-Rawi Y et al (2005) The Desmoteplase in Acute Stroke Trial (DIAS): A Phase II MRI-Based 9-hour Window Acute Stroke Thrombolysis Trial with Intravenous Desmoteplase. Stroke 36:66–73

102. Rother J (2003) Imaging-guided extension of the time window: ready for application in experienced stroke centers? Stroke 34:575–583

103. Rother J, Schellinger PD, Gass A et al (2002) Effect of intravenous thrombolysis on MRI parameters and functional outcome in acute stroke <6 hours. Stroke 33: 2438–2445

104. Parsons MW, Barber PA, Chalk J et al (2002) Diffusion- and perfusion-weighted MRI response to thrombolysis in stroke. Ann Neurol 51:28–37

105. Schramm P, Schellinger PD, Fiebach JB et al (2002) Comparison of CT and CT angiography source images with diffusion-weighted imaging in patients with acute stroke within 6 hours after onset. Stroke 33:2426–2432

106. Alpert NM, Berdichevsky D, Levin Z, Thangaraj V, Gonzalez G, Lev MH (2001) Performance evaluation of an automated system for registration and postprocessing of CT scans. J Comput Assist Tomogr 25:747–752

107. Schellingerhout D, Lev MH, Bagga RJ et al (2003) Coregistration of head CT comparison studies: assessment of clinical utility. Acad Radiol 10:242–248

108. Kidwell CS, Saver JL, Mattiello J et al (2000) Thrombolytic reversal of acute human cerebral ischemic injury shown by diffusion/perfusion magnetic resonance imaging. Ann Neurol 47:462–469

109. Kidwell CS, Saver JL, Starkman S et al (2002) Late secondary ischemic injury in patients receiving intraarterial thrombolysis. Ann Neurol 52:698–703

110. Hunter GJ, Silvennoinen HM, Hamberg LM et al (2003) Whole-brain CT perfusion measurement of perfused cerebral blood volume in acute ischemic stroke: probability curve for regional infarction. Radiology 227:725–730

111. Warach S (2003) Measurement of the ischemic penumbra with MRI: it's about time. Stroke 34:2533–2534

112. Wu O, Koroshetz WJ, Ostergaard L et al (2001) Predicting tissue outcome in acute human cerebral ischemia using combined diffusion- and perfusion-weighted MR imaging. Stroke 32:933–942

113. Barber PA, Darby DG, Desmond PM et al (1998) Prediction of stroke outcome with echoplanar perfusion- and diffusion-weighted MRI. Neurology 51:418–426

114. Astrup J, Siesjo BK, Symon L (1981) Thresholds in cerebral ischemia – the ischemic penumbra. Stroke 12:723–725

115. Sorensen AG, Buonanno FS, Gonzalez RG et al (1996) Hyperacute stroke: evaluation with combined multisection diffusion-weighted and hemodynamically weighted echo-planar MR imaging. Radiology 199:391–401

116. Sunshine JL, Tarr RW, Lanzieri CF, Landis DMD, Selman WR, Lewin JS (1999) Hyperacute stroke: ultrafast MR imaging to triage patients prior to therapy. Radiology 212:325–332

117. Schlaug G, Benfield A, Baird AE et al (1999) The ischemic penumbra: operationally defined by diffusion and perfusion MRI. Neurology 53:1528–1537

118. Mehta N, Lev MH, Mullins ME et al (2003) Prediction of final infarct size in acute stroke using cerebral blood flow/cerebral blood volume mismatch: added value of quantitative first pass CT perfusion imaging in successfully treated versus unsuccessfully treated/untreated patients. Proceedings of the 41st Annual Meeting of the American Society of Neuroradiology, Washington DC

119. Aksoy FG, Lev MH, Eskey CJ, Eastwood JD, Koroshetz WJ, Gonzalez RG (2000) CT perfusion imaging of acute stroke: how well do CBV, CBF, and MTT maps predict final infarct size? Proceedings of the 86th Scientific Assembly and Annual Meeting of the Radiological Society of North America, Chicago, Ill.

120. Rohl L, Ostergaard L, Simonsen CZ et al (2001) Viability thresholds of ischemic penumbra of hyperacute stroke defined by perfusion-weighted MRI and apparent diffusion coefficient. Stroke 32:1140–1146

121. Grandin CB, Duprez TP, Smith AM et al (2001) Usefulness of magnetic resonance-derived quantitative measurements of cerebral blood flow and volume in prediction of infarct growth in hyperacute stroke. Stroke 32:1147–1153

122. Schaefer PW, Ozsunar Y, He J et al (2003) Assessing tissue viability with MR diffusion and perfusion imaging. Am J Neuroradiol 24:436–443

123. Lev MH, Hunter GJ, Hamberg LM et al (2002) CT versus MR imaging in acute stroke: comparison of perfusion abnormalities at the infarct core. Proceedings of the 40th Annual Meeting of the American Society of Neuroradiology. Vancouver, Canada

124. Sasaki O, Takeuchi S, Koizumi T, Koike T, Tanaka R (1996) Complete recanalization via fibrinolytic therapy can reduce the number of ischemic territories that progress to infarction. Am J Neuroradiol 17:1661–1668

125. Ueda T, Sakaki S, Yuh W, Nochide I, Ohta S (1999) Outcome in acute stroke with successful intra-arterial thrombolysis procedure and predictive value of initial single-photon emission-computed tomography. J Cereb Blood Flow Metab 19:99–108

126. Liu Y, Karonen JO, Vanninen RL et al (2000) Cerebral hemodynamics in human acute ischemic stroke: a study with diffusion- and perfusion-weighted magnetic resonance imaging and SPECT. J Cereb Blood Flow Metab 20:910–920

127. Hatazawa J, Shimosegawa E, Toyoshima H et al (1999) Cerebral blood volume in acute brain infarction: a combined study with dynamic susceptibility contrast MRI and 99mTc-HMPAO-SPECT. Stroke 30:800–806

128. Shimosegawa E, Hatazawa J, Inugami A et al (1994) Cerebral infarction within six hours of onset: prediction of completed infarction with technetium-99m-HMPAO SPECT. J Nucl Med 35:1097–1103

129. Koennecke HC (2003) Editorial comment – challenging the concept of a dynamic penumbra in acute ischemic stroke. Stroke 34:2434–2435

130. Heiss WD (2000) Ischemic penumbra: evidence from functional imaging in man. J Cereb Blood Flow Metab 20:1276–1293

131. Jovin TG, Yonas H, Gebel JM et al (2003) The cortical ischemic core and not the consistently present penumbra is a determinant of clinical outcome in acute middle cerebral artery occlusion. Stroke 34:2426–2433

132. Lev MH, Roccatagliata L, Murphy EK et al (2004) A CTA based, multivariable, "benefit of recanalization" model for acute stroke triage: core infarct size on CTA source images independently predicts outcome. Proceedings of the 42nd Annual Meeting of the American Society of Neuroradiology, Seattle, Washington

133. Suarez J, Sunshine J, Tarr R et al (1999) Predictors of clinical improvement, angiographic recanalization, and intracranial hemorrhage after intra-arterial thromblysis for acute ischemic stroke. Stroke 30:2094–2100

134. Molina CA, Alexandrov AV, Demchuk AM, Saqqur M, Uchino K, Alvarez-Sabin J (2004) Improving the predictive accuracy of recanalization on stroke outcome in patients treated with tissue plasminogen activator. Stroke 35:151–156

135. Baird AE, Dambrosia J, Janket S et al (2001) A three-item scale for the early prediction of stroke recovery. Lancet 357:2095–2099

136. Nighoghossian N, Hermier M, Adeleine P et al (2003) Baseline magnetic resonance imaging parameters and stroke outcome in patients treated by intravenous tissue plasminogen activator. Stroke 34:458–463

137. Ogasawara K, Ogawa A, Ezura M, Konno H, Suzuki M, Yoshimoto T (2001) Brain single-photon emission CT studies using 99mTc-HMPAO and 99mTc-ECD early after recanalization by local intraarterial thrombolysis in patients with acute embolic middle cerebral artery occlusion. Am J Neuroradiol 22:48–53

138. Kidwell CS, Chalela JA, Saver JL et al (2003) Hemorrhage Early MRI Evaluation (HEME Study): Preliminary Results of a Multicenter Trial of Neuroimaging in Patients with Acute Stroke Symptoms Within 6 Hours of Onset (abstract). Stroke 34:239

139. Del Zoppo G (1995) Acute stroke- on the threshold of a therapy. N Engl J Med 333:1632–1633

140. Muir KW, Grosset DG (1999) Neuroprotection for acute stroke: making clinical trials work. Stroke 30:180–182

141. Grotta J (2002) Neuroprotection is unlikely to be effective in humans using current trial designs. Stroke 33:306–307

142. Kidwell CS, Warach S (2003) Acute ischemic cerebrovascular syndrome: diagnostic criteria. Stroke 34:2995–2998

143. Calamante F, Gadian DG, Connelly A (2000) Delay and dispersion effects in dynamic susceptibility contrast MRI: simulations using singular value decomposition. Magn Reson Med 44(3):466–473

Conventional MRI and MR Angiography of Stroke

David Vu, R. Gilberto González,
Pamela W. Schaefer

Contents

Stroke can be evaluated with both conventional MRI and MR angiography (MRA) sequences. The first section of this chapter discusses the appearance of stroke on conventional MR sequences (i.e., not diffusion or perfusion), while the second section discusses MRA and its role in evaluating stroke etiologies.

6.1 Conventional MRI and Stroke

Strokes have a characteristic appearance on conventional MRI that varies with infarct age. Temporal evolution of strokes is typically categorized into hyperacute (0–6 h), acute (6–24 h), subacute (24 h to approximately 2 weeks), and chronic stroke (>2 weeks old).

6.1.1 Hyperacute Infarct

In the hyperacute stage of infarct, there is occlusion or slow flow in the vessels supplying the area of infarcted tissue. Within minutes of the infarct, the signal flow void on T2-weighted images is lost (Fig. 6.1). FLAIR (fluid attenuated inversion recovery), an inversion recovery sequence that suppresses the CSF signal, can show high intravascular signal against the surrounding low-signal subarachnoid space [1] (Fig. 6.2). In one study, 65% of infarcts <6 h old showed a FLAIR high signal within vessels, and, in some cases, the finding of a FLAIR high signal in vessels preceded changes in the diffusion-weighted images [2].

Gradient recalled echo (GRE) T2*-weighted images can detect an intraluminal thrombus (deoxyhemoglobin) in hyperacute infarcts as a linear low signal region of magnetic susceptibility (Fig. 6.2). In one

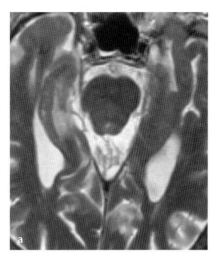

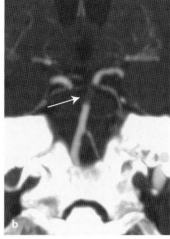

Fig. 6.1 a, b

Basilar occlusion. **a** The T2-weighted image shows loss of the signal flow void in the basilar artery in this patient with basilar occlusion and hyperacute pontine infarct. No parenchymal abnormality is noted at this early time point. **b** Coronal maximal intensity projection (*MIP*) image from the CT angiogram demonstrates the occlusion as a filling defect (*arrow*)

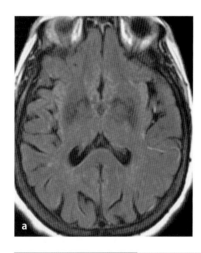

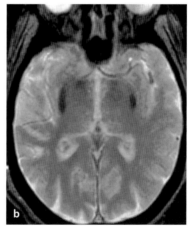

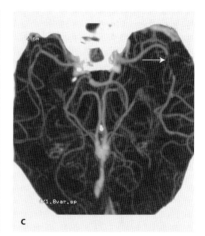

Fig. 6.2 a–c

Left middle cerebral artery (*MCA*) thrombus. The left MCA shows high signal from an intraluminal clot on FLAIR-weighted images (**a**) but low signal on gradient recalled echo (*GRE*) T2*-weighted images (**b**). This corresponds to a filling defect (*arrow*) on CT angiogram (**c**). A subtle FLAIR high signal is present at the left insula

study of 30 patients with MCA thrombus, gradient echo had 83% sensitivity in detecting the thrombus, compared with 52% sensitivity for noncontrast CT in detecting a dense MCA sign [3].

Contrast-enhanced T1-weighted images show arterial enhancement in 50% of hyperacute strokes [1] (Fig. 6.3). This arterial enhancement is thought to be secondary to slow flow, collateral flow or hyperperfu-sion following early recanalization. It may be detected as early as 2 h after stroke onset and can persist for up to 7 days. During this period, there is usually no parenchymal enhancement because inadequate collateral circulation prevents contrast from reaching the infarcted tissue. Rarely, early parenchymal enhancement may occur when there is early reperfusion or good collateralization.

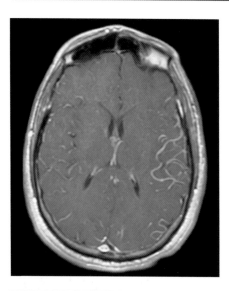

Figure 6.3

Arterial enhancement from infarct. T1-weighted post-contrast image shows increased enhancement of the left middle cerebral artery (*MCA*) vessels in this hyperacute infarct

In the hyperacute period (first 6 h), there is shift of water from the extracellular to the intracellular space but there may be little increase in overall tissue water. Therefore, while the development of altered signal intensity on FLAIR- or T2-weighted images may occur as early as 2–3 h after stroke onset, conventional MRI is not sensitive enough for evaluation of infarcts in the hyperacute stage; one study found an 18% sensitivity of T2-weighted images in detecting infarct in the first 6 h and a false-negative rate of 30–50% [4]. FLAIR-weighted sequences are slightly more sensitive than T2-weighted images in the detection of parenchymal changes in acute infarcts but have an estimated sensitivity of only 29% in the first 6 h [5].

6.1.2 Acute Infarct

By 24 h, as the overall tissue water content increases due to vasogenic edema following blood–brain barrier disruption, conventional MRI becomes more sensitive for the detection of parenchymal infarcts. Signal changes during the first 24 h are best appreciated

in the cortical and deep gray matter. Infarcts in the acute stage usually demonstrate focal or confluent areas of T2 and FLAIR hyperintensity with sulcal effacement. During this time, the white matter may be hyperintense, but also may show no abnormality or demonstrate hypointensity. Proposed etiologies for the subcortical white matter hypointensity are free radicals, sludging of deoxygenated red blood cells, and iron deposition [6]. Because cerebrospinal fluid (CSF) is hypointense, FLAIR has improved detection of small infarctions in brain parenchyma, such as cortex and periventricular white matter, adjacent to CSF. By 24 h, T2-weighted and FLAIR-weighted images detect 90% of infarcts [1]. An increase in tissue water also leads to hypointensity on T1-weighted images. However, in the acute period, T1-weighted images are relatively insensitive at detecting parenchymal changes compared with T2-weighted images. At 24 h, sensitivity is still only approximately 50%.

6.1.3 Subacute Infarct

In the subacute phase of infarct (1 day to 2 weeks), the increase in vasogenic edema results in increased T2 and FLAIR hyperintensity, increased T1 hypointensity, and better definition of the infarction and swelling (Fig. 6.4). The brain swelling is manifest as gyral thickening, effacement of sulci and cisterns, effacement of adjacent ventricles, midline shift, and brain herniation. The swelling reaches a maximum at about 3 days and resolves by 7–10 days [7]. There is increased T2 and FLAIR signal within the first week that usually persists but there may be "MR fogging" [8]. MR fogging occurs when the infarcted tissue becomes difficult to see because it has developed a signal intensity similar to that of normal tissue. This is thought to result from infiltration of the infarcted tissue by inflammatory cells. One study of 7- to 10-day-old strokes identified 88% of subacute strokes on T2-weighted images, and another determined that T2- and FLAIR-weighted images were equally sensitive at detecting 10-day-old infarcts [7].

In the subacute phase, arterial enhancement peaks at 1–3 days. Large infarcts will also demonstrate meningeal enhancement that may represent reactive

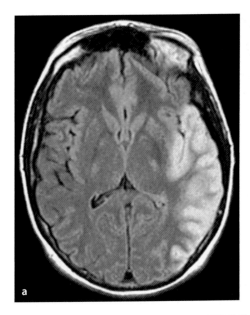
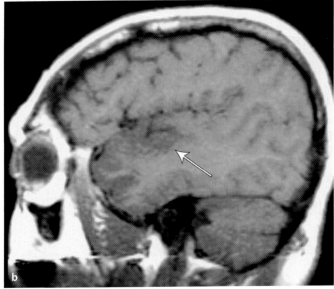

Fig. 6.4 a, b

Cortical edema in a subacute infarct. a The axial FLAIR-weighted image shows high signal, gyral swelling, and sulcal effacement. b There is subtle low signal and gyral swelling (*arrow*) seen on the T1-weighted sagittal image

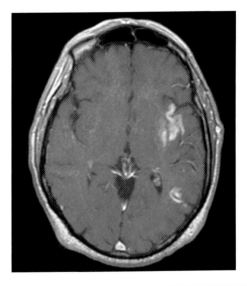

Figure 6.5

Enhancing infarcts. Postcontrast T1-weighted image shows gyriform enhancement at the left insula and posterior parietal lobe from a subacute left MCA infarct

hyperemia, which peaks at 2–6 days. Arterial and meningeal enhancement both typically resolve by 1 week [9]. In addition, parenchymal enhancement occurs during this phase. Gray matter enhancement can appear band-like or gyriform (Fig. 6.5). This is secondary to disruption of the blood–brain barrier and restored tissue perfusion from a recanalized occlusion or collateral flow. This parenchymal enhancement may be visible at 2–3 days but is consistently present at 6 days and persists for 6–8 weeks [9]. Some infarcts, such as watershed and noncortical infarcts, may enhance earlier.

6.1.4 Chronic Infarcts

After 2 weeks, the mass effect and edema within infarcts decrease and the parenchyma develops tissue loss and gliosis. During this time, parenchymal enhancement peaks at 1–4 weeks and then gradually fades [9]. The chronic stage of infarction is well es-

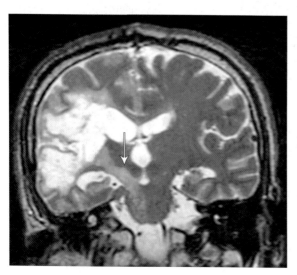

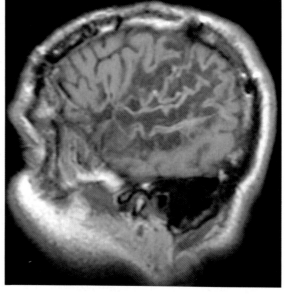

Figure 6.6

Wallerian degeneration. Coronal T2-weighted image shows encephalomalacia of the right frontal and temporal lobes and T2 high signal extending into the right cerebral peduncle (*arrow*) from Wallerian degeneration

Figure 6.7

Laminar necrosis. This sagittal noncontrast T1-weighted image shows gyriform T1 high signal in a chronic left MCA infarct. Mild enlargement of the sulci is consistent with encephalomalacia

tablished by 6 weeks. At this point, necrotic tissue and edema are resorbed, the gliotic reaction is complete, the blood–brain barrier is intact, and reperfusion is established [9]. There is no longer parenchymal, meningeal or vascular enhancement, and the vessels are no longer hyperintense on FLAIR images. There is tissue loss with ventricular, sulcal, and cisternal enlargement. There is increased T2 hyperintensity and T1 hypointensity due to increased water content associated with cystic cavitation. With large middle cerebral artery (MCA) territory infarctions, there is Wallerian degeneration, characterized by T2 hyperintensity and tissue loss, of the ipsilateral cortical spinal tract [10] (Fig. 6.6).

Chronic infarcts can demonstrate peripheral gyriform T1 high signal from petechial hemorrhage or from laminar necrosis [11] (Fig. 6.7).

6.1.5 Hemorrhagic Transformation

Hemorrhagic transformation (HT) of brain infarction represents secondary bleeding into ischemic tissue, varying from small petechiae to parenchymal hematoma. It has a natural incidence of 15% to 26% during the first 2 weeks and up to 43% over the first month after cerebral infarction [12, 13]. Predisposing factors include stroke etiology (HT is more frequent with embolic strokes), reperfusion, good collateral circulation, hypertension, anticoagulant therapy, and thrombolytic therapy. In patients treated with intra-arterial (i.a.) thrombolytic therapy, a higher National Institutes of Health Stroke Scale (NIHSS) score, longer time to recanalization, lower platelet count and a higher glucose level are associated with HT [14].

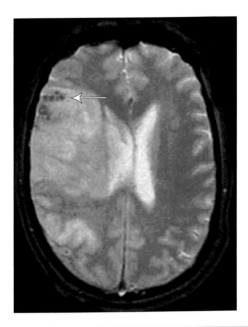

Figure 6.8

Petechial hemorrhage. Gyriform low signal in the right frontal lobe (*arrow*) on this GRE T2* image corresponds to susceptibility from petechial hemorrhage in an acute infarct

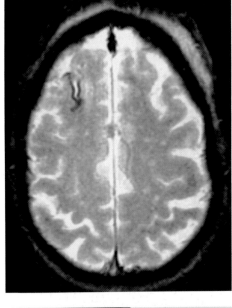

Figure 6.9

Hemosiderin in chronic infarct. The low signal from the gyriform on this GRE T2*-weighted image at the right frontal lobe is from hemosiderin in an old petechial bleed

Because T1-, T2-, and FLAIR-weighted images are insensitive at detecting acute blood products (deoxyhemoglobin), GRE T2* sequences should be used to detect hemorrhage in the acute stroke setting (Fig. 6.8). GRE T2* sequences have increased sensitivity to blood breakdown products due to their paramagnetic properties. One study demonstrated GRE images to be as sensitive as CT at detecting parenchymal hemorrhage in acute strokes [15]. Another study observed that in detecting acute blood products, GRE T2*-weighted images were more sensitive than T2-, FLAIR-, or echo planar T2-weighted images [16]. Some data suggest that microbleeds detected by susceptibility predict symptomatic hemorrhage following tissue plasminogen activator (t-PA) treatment [17].

As blood products evolve into methemoglobin, T1-weighted sequences become more sensitive at detecting blood products [18]. Chronic hemorrhages are best detected on GRE T2* images as areas of susceptibility (Fig. 6.9).

6.1.6 Conclusion

Conventional MRI can diagnose infarcts at all stages of temporal evolution but are most sensitive after the hyperacute stage (see Table 6.1). During the hyperacute stage, the predominant findings are loss of flow voids on T2-weighted images, FLAIR hyperintensity in affected vessels, and vascular enhancement. In the acute to chronic stage, FLAIR and T2 parenchymal abnormalities are evident and Wallerian degeneration develops. The subacute stage is also marked by parenchymal swelling followed by parenchymal enhancement. The detection of acute hemorrhagic infarct requires the use of a T2* GRE susceptibility sequence since other conventional MRI sequences are not sensitive enough for acute bleeds.

Table 6.1. The appearance of arterial infarcts on conventional MRI

Stage	Conventional MR appearance	Evolution
Hyperacute (0–6 h)	T2 shows loss of signal flow void	Occurs within minutes of the infarct
	FLAIR shows vessel high signal	Occurs within minutes of the infarct
	GRE T2* shows blooming susceptibility	Occurs within minutes of the infarct
	T1 post-contrast shows arterial enhancement	Occurs at 2 hours and can last 7 days
	There are no reliable parenchymal findings for infarct at this stage	
Acute (6–24 hours)	Vascular abnormalities from the hyperacute stage persist	
	T2 and FLAIR show gyriform high signal and sulcal effacement	Appears by 24 h (90% sensitivity)
	T2 can show subcortical low signal	
	GRE T2* show gyriform susceptibility from petechial bleed	Can occur at any time in the acute to subacute stage
	No parenchymal enhancement is present	
Subacute (1 day to 2 weeks)	T2 and FLAIR show gyriform high signal and sulcal effacement from mass effect	Reaches a maximum at 3–5 days and decreases by 1 week. Rarely, "MR fogging" appears at 2 weeks
	T1 can show gyriform high signal from petechial bleed	Appears once methemoglobin develops
	T1 post-contrast shows arterial enhancement	Peaks at 1–3 days and resolves by 1 week
	T1 post-contrast shows meningeal enhancement	Peaks at 2–6 days and resolves by 1 week
	T1 post-contrast show parenchymal enhancement as vessels recanalize	Can be seen at 2–3 days, consistently seen at 6 days and persists for 6–8 weeks
Chronic	T2 shows high signal from gliosis and Wallerian degeneration	Persists indefinitely
	Volume loss is present	Persists indefinitely
	T1 shows low signal from cavitation	Persists indefinitely
	GRE T2* shows low signal hemosiderin from petechial bleeds	Persists indefinitely

6.2 MR Angiogram and Stroke

Magnetic resonance angiography (MRA) is a set of vascular imaging techniques capable of depicting the extracranial and intracranial circulation. In the setting of acute stroke, these techniques are useful for determining stroke etiology and assessing vascular flow dynamics. Specifically, they are used to evaluate the severity of stenosis or occlusion as well as collateral flow. A typical stroke protocol includes two-dimensional (2D) and/or three-dimensional (3D) time-of-flight (TOF) and contrast-enhanced MRA images through the neck and 3D TOF MRA images through the Circle of Willis. For dissection, a fat saturated pregadolinium axial T1 sequence through the neck is added. This section discusses the major MRA techniques, including the advantages and disadvantages of each, as well as how MRA is used to evaluate the specific disease processes that lead to stroke.

6.2.1 Noncontrast MRA

MRA is broadly divided into noncontrast and contrast-enhanced techniques. Noncontrast MRA can be acquired with phase contrast (PC) or TOF techniques, and both can be acquired as 2D slabs or 3D volumes.

6.2.1.1 TOF MRA

TOF MRA is a gradient echo sequence that depicts vascular flow by repeatedly applying a radio frequency (RF) pulse to a volume of tissue, followed by dephasing and rephasing gradients. Stationary tissues in this volume become saturated by the repeated RF pulses and have relatively low signal. By contrast, flowing blood in vessels has relatively increased signal because it continuously carries unsaturated spins into the imaging volume. The vessel contrast or flow-related enhancement is proportional to the velocity. Signal from venous blood is minimized by placing a saturation band above the imaging volume [19].

Two-dimensional TOF MRA is typically performed in the neck region with a relatively large flip angle (60°). Multiple sequential, 1-mm-thick axial slices are obtained. Blood flowing perpendicular to the multiple thin slices is well imaged because it is not exposed to enough RF pulses to become saturated. However, blood flowing in the imaging plane (in-plane flow) is exposed to more RF pulses and may become saturated and lose signal; this artifact can often be seen at the horizontal turns of the vertebral arteries as well as the petrous segments of the internal carotid arteries (Fig. 6.10) [19].

Three-dimensional TOF MRA is typically performed in the head region with a smaller flip angle (20°). A volume of tissue covering the skull base to the Circle of Willis is obtained and then divided into 1-mm-thick slices using an additional phase encoding step [20]. While the smaller flip angle reduces saturation artifacts, any flowing blood that remains

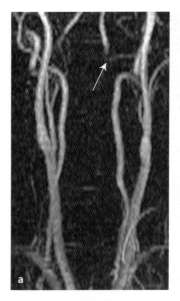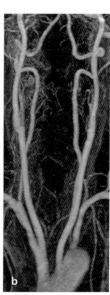

Fig. 6.10 a, b

Normal neck MRA. a MIP image of 2D TOF of the neck shows artifactual signal loss at the horizontal turn of the left vertebral artery (*arrow*). b This area has normal flow on MIP images from the contrast-enhanced MRA. The contrast-enhanced MRA gives excellent depiction of the origins of the neck vessels

in the imaging volume for long enough is exposed to multiple RF pulses and can artifactually lose signal. This signal loss is usually seen in the distal Circle of Willis vessels (Fig. 6.11). The smaller flip angle also decreases the background saturation. Typically, a ramped flip angle is used to minimize vascular saturation effects while maximizing the suppression of the background signal. Magnetization transfer is additionally applied in 3D TOF MRA to further decrease the background signal.

Compared with 2D TOF, the 3D TOF technique has better spatial resolution, a better signal-to-noise ratio and less intravoxel dephasing, but it is more limited by the vascular saturation artifact and therefore can cover only a small volume. A hybrid technique between 2D and 3D TOF known as MOTSA (multiple overlapping thin slab acquisition) acquires partially overlapping thin 3D volumes. The ends of the 3D volume have saturation artifact and are discarded while

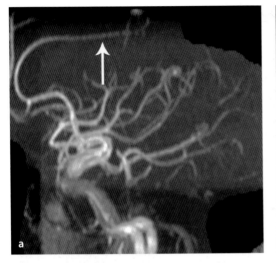
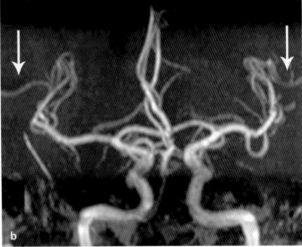

Fig. 6.11 a,b

Normal 3D TOF MRA of the head. Segmented MIP images from a frontal (a) and lateral (b) projection show normal vessels with decreased flow-related enhancement in the distal anterior cerebral artery (*ACA*) (*arrow* in **a**) and distal MCA vessels (*arrows* in **b**)

Fig. 6.12 a–c

Internal carotid artery (*ICA*) stenosis. **a** Time-of-flight (*TOF*) MRA shows a segment of signal loss at the proximal ICA. **b** The length of this focal signal loss is overestimated when compared with contrast-enhanced MRA. **c** This could represent stenosis or occlusion, but was shown to be a high-grade stenosis on CT angiogram

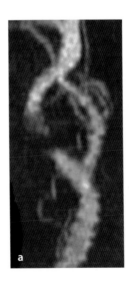
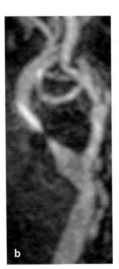
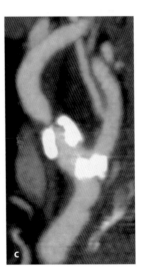

central portions are assembled into a single MRA. MOTSA has higher spatial resolution than 2D TOF while covering a larger area than 3D TOF MRA, because it is less susceptible to saturation artifact.

TOF MRA, especially 2D TOF, is also vulnerable to artifactual signal loss from flow turbulence. This causes phase dispersion so that the rephasing gradient is unable to generate a strong echo. This artifact can be seen at vessel bifurcation points or distal to stenoses and can result in overestimates of the degree or length of vascular stenoses (Fig. 6.12).

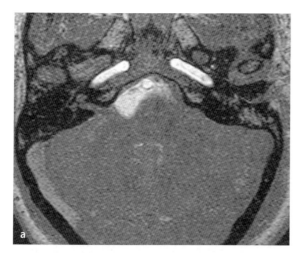

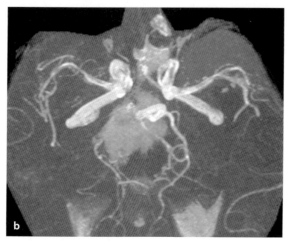

Fig. 6.13 a, b

TOF MRA artifact. **a** Blood (methemoglobin) in the pre-pontine cistern has high signal on the TOF MRA because the signal from substances with a short T1 is not adequately suppressed. **b** On the MIP images, this high signal obscures portions of the basilar artery and left posterior cerebral artery

TOF MRA can have artifact from poor background suppression. Signal from stationary tissues are in theory suppressed with repeated RF pulses, but substances with a short T1, such as fat or methemoglobin in hematomas, are not usually fully saturated. Consequently, these substances demonstrate high signal on TOF MRA and can mimic areas of flow or obscure

vessels (Fig. 6.13). This artifact can sometimes be overcome by segmenting out areas of high signal, and high fat signal can be reduced by setting the echo time (TE) to 2.3 or 6.9 ms, to place fat and water out of phase.

6.2.1.2 Phase-Contrast MRA

Phase-contrast MRA (PC MRA) is a gradient echo sequence that depicts blood flow by quantifying differences in the transverse magnetization between stationary and moving tissue [19]. Following a RF pulse, pairs of symmetric but opposed phase encoding gradients are applied in one direction within the imaging volume; the first gradient dephases and the second rephases the transverse magnetization. Stationary tissues have no net change in phase because they experience equal but opposite magnetic field environments during the dephasing and then the rephasing gradients. Moving blood, however, experiences different magnetic field environments as each gradient is applied. The spins in moving blood acquire a phase shift during the dephasing pulse, which is not completely reversed during the rephasing pulse. The net phase shift, either positive or negative, determines direction of flow, and the amount of phase shift (in degrees) is proportional to the velocity or magnitude of blood flow.

PC MRA is acquired in three orthogonal directions, and the direction of flow is depicted as a relatively high or low signal against a gray background (Fig. 6.14). Orthogonal maps can also be combined to form an overall flow-related enhancement map without directionality. Like TOF MRA, PC MRA can be obtained with 2D or 3D techniques. Clinically, PC MRA is used to evaluate intracranial collateral flow distal to a stenosis.

An artifact unique to PC MRA is that phase shifts exceeding 180° are interpreted as slow flow in the opposite direction. This aliasing artifact leads to incorrect determination of flow direction. In order to avoid this, a velocity encoding parameter (VENC) is selected which represents the maximum expected flow velocity in the imaging volume. This value adjusts the strength of the bipolar gradients to prevent phase shifts from exceeding 180°.

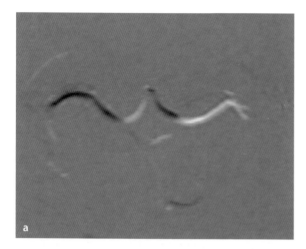

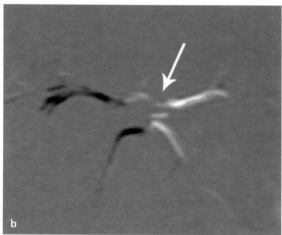

Normal and abnormal phase-contrast MRA (*PC MRA*) of the circle of Willis. **a** Normal 2D PC MRA with direction encoding in the right/left direction (vessel is bright if flowing right to left and dark if flowing left to right). Normally the signal in the A1 branch is opposite that in the M1 branches. **b** Two-dimensional PC MRA from a 4-year-old with severe stenosis in the left internal carotid artery (*ICA*) shows retrograde flow in the left A1 (*arrow*) via the anterior communicating artery (*ACoA*). The left A1 and M1 therefore have the same high signal

PC MRA has several advantages over TOF MRA. As mentioned above, PC MRA can demonstrate flow direction. Also, since PC MRA shows only moving tissues, stationary tissues with short T1 such as fat or methemoglobin do not demonstrate high signal. Another advantage is that PC MRA can image very slowly moving blood since it does not suffer the saturation effects of TOF imaging. Finally, PC MRA can be obtained after i.v. gadolinium administration without image degradation because PC MRA does not rely on T1 values to generate the MRA image. Following contrast, TOF MRA is usually limited because gadolinium shortens the T1 and veins become hyperintense.

The major disadvantage of PC MRA is that it uses a longer TE than TOF MRA. This results in increased intravoxel dephasing and signal loss around stenoses and areas of turbulence. Also, 3D PC MRA has similar spatial resolution but is a longer sequence compared to 3D TOF MRA and is therefore more susceptible to motion artifacts. Consequently, 3D TOF MRA is usually employed to image the head. However, if there is concern that a subacute clot may mimic flow-related enhancement, 3D PC MRA should be performed. Also, because 3D TOF MRA cannot determine flow direction, 2D PC MRA (a much shorter sequence compared to 3D PC MRA) is frequently used to assess collateral retrograde flow in the anterior or posterior communicating arteries in association with severe internal carotid artery (ICA) stenosis or to assess retrograde flow in the basilar artery due to severe stenosis.

In the neck, TOF techniques are preferred over PC techniques due to the latter's longer scan times, which are needed to provide the same coverage and spatial resolution. Two-dimensional TOF MRA provides superior flow-related enhancement and allows coverage of the entire neck. Compared to 2D TOF MRA, 3D TOF MRA provides superior spatial resolution and is less susceptible to phase dispersion artifacts, but it is more susceptible to saturation effects and cannot cover a large area. Three-dimensional TOF techniques are therefore used to delineate the bifurcation only. Two-dimensional PC techniques are used to evaluate flow direction in the vertebral arteries when subclavian steal is suspected. Also, since compared to TOF, 2D PC techniques are more sensitive to the detection of very slow flow, they can be used to differentiate high-grade stenosis with a string sign from occlusion.

6.2.2 Contrast-Enhanced MRA

Contrast-enhanced MRA (CE MRA) is performed with a rapid, short repetition time (TR, 10 ms) gradient echo sequence following an i.v. bolus of gadolinium. The gadolinium shortens the T1 to less than 10 ms so that opacified vessels are hyperintense. Background tissues, including normally T1-hyperintense structures such as fat and methemoglobin in hematomas, have low signal because they have intrinsic T1 relaxation times of much greater than 10 ms [19].

CE MRA is usually obtained from the arch to the skull base in the coronal plane and is often obtained with a first-pass technique (Fig. 6.10). This requires obtaining the MRA during peak arterial enhancement to avoid venous enhancement. The timing of this arterial phase can be determined by a test bolus or by automatic bolus detection. k-space is filled during peak arterial enhancement in order to maximize image contrast. Another technique known as time-resolved CE MRA acquires the MRA and fills k-space before, during, and after the arterial bolus. This does not require synchronization of the MRA with the injection. In theory, this technique can depict flow dynamics but is limited by the trade-off between temporal and spatial resolution [19].

CE MRA is a reliable modality to image neck vessels but can have poor signal-to-noise ratio at the edge of the imaging volume or have respiratory motion artifact. Respiratory motion artifact limits adequate visualization of the major vessel origins off the arch as well as the origins of the right common, right subclavian, and bilateral vertebral arteries.

CE MRA has several advantages over noncontrast MRA (i.e., PC and TOF MRA): CE MRA can cover a much larger area of anatomy (from the arch to the skull base) in a much shorter acquisition time and is less susceptible to patient motion. CE MRA also has a greater signal-to-noise ratio and less dephasing from turbulence and does not suffer signal loss from satu-

ration effects. CE MRA images the contrast within a vessel lumen and is therefore a more anatomic evaluation, while noncontrast MRA depicts physiology, and anatomy must be inferred from blood flow. This can be misleading when a vessel is not seen on TOF techniques due to reversal of flow or very slow flow (Fig. 6.15).

The disadvantages of CE MRA compared to noncontrast MRA is that the CE MRA data must be obtained during the narrow time window of arterial enhancement and cannot be repeated until the intravascular gadolinium agent is cleared. Thus improper timing (scanning too early or late) results in poor arterial enhancement and an inadequate study that cannot immediately be repeated. Also, the spatial resolution of CE techniques is inferior to that of TOF techniques, and contrast MRA is also minimally invasive as it typically requires a 20-ml power injection of gadolinium contrast at 2 ml/s.

In clinical practice, CE MRA is routinely used to image the great vessel origins and the neck. In general, it does not overestimate carotid bifurcation and other stenoses as much as TOF techniques because it is less susceptible to dephasing from turbulence and does not suffer signal loss from saturation effects. However, many institutions continue to image the neck with both CE and TOF techniques. Due to poorer spatial resolution, CE MRA may underestimate carotid stenosis. TOF techniques are also useful when the arterial bolus is timed incorrectly and when there is unsuspected reversal of flow. For example, in Fig. 6.15, the left vertebral artery appears normal on the CE image and one would assume antegrade flow. However, the vessel is not seen on the 2D TOF flight images, suggesting retrograde flow with saturation of spins due to a superior saturation pulse.

A comparison of the MRA techniques and their typical clinical applications is presented in Table 6.2.

6.2.3 Image Processing

Noncontrast and contrast MRA can be postprocessed as a maximum intensity projection (MIP) image. This technique first creates a 3D model of the vessels from the MRA raw data. A set of parallel rays is then drawn from the model and the highest inten-

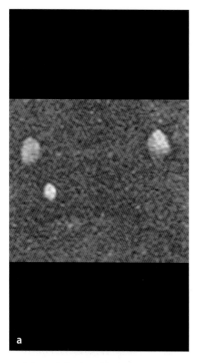
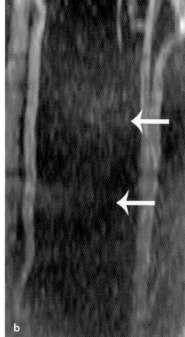
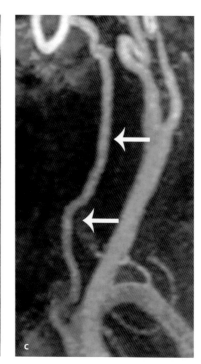

Fig. 6.15 a–c

Slow flow or subclavian steal syndrome. Two-dimensional TOF MRA source image (a) and MIP image of the TOF MRA (b) show absent flow and possible occlusion of the left vertebral artery (*arrows* in b). CE MRA (c), however, shows flow in this vessel (*arrows*). This discrepancy can occur from slow flow leading to signal saturation on 2D TOF or from reversed flow in subclavian steal syndrome

sity along each ray is projected to form a 2D MIP image. Multiple projections of the model are created from different vantage points so that viewing sequential MIP images gives the illusion of observing a rotating 3D MRA model.

6.2.4 Extracranial Atherosclerosis and Occlusions

MRA of neck vessels is important in stroke management because extracranial atherosclerosis causes an estimated 20–30% of strokes. The North American Symptomatic Carotid Endarterectomy Trial (NASCET) trial demonstrated that carotid endarterectomy improves survival in symptomatic patients with carotid stenosis of 70–99% [21]. The Asymptomatic Carotid

Atherosclerosis Study also suggested that asymptomatic patients with a stenosis of 60% could benefit from endarterectomy [22]. Since then, multiple studies have evaluated the ability of CE and noncontrast MRA to distinguish between nonsurgical (<70%) and surgical (70–99%) stenoses.

CE MRA is generally accurate in evaluation of stenoses. A 2003 study comparing CE MRA and digital subtraction angiography (DSA) showed a sensitivity of 97% and specificity of 95% for stratifying nonsurgical from surgical stenoses [23]. However, a 2004 prospective study also comparing DSA and CE MRA showed a sensitivity of 93% and specificity of 81% for detecting severe stenosis [24]. This poorer performance of CE MRA was attributed to interobserver variability, and this study noted that using CE

Table 6.2. MRA techniques and applications. (*CE MRA* Contrast-enhanced MRA, *PC* phase contrast, *TOF* time of flight)

	Advantages	Disadvantages	Clinical applications
2D TOF	Is noninvasive	Typically overestimates vessel stenosis	Is used routinely as the "back up" MRA of the neck in case the CE MRA is suboptimal
	Can image slow flow	Has in-plane artifactual signal loss	is used routinely in MR venography
	Can image a large volume of tissue	Is susceptible to signal loss from flow turbulence	can sometimes suggest subclavian steal if combined with CE MRA
	Can be repeated if suboptimal	Has low spatial resolution	
	Can be obtained after contrast administration but is slightly degraded by venous signal	Has misregistration artifact on MIP reconstructions	
3D TOF	Is noninvasive	Can image only a small volume due to saturation artifact	Is used routinely to evaluate the circle of Willis to detect intracranial stenoses and occlusions
	Has high spatial resolution	Has poor background suppression; fat or blood may appear bright on the MRA	Can estimate carotid bifurcation stenoses
	Shows complex vascular flow	Cannot image slow flow because of saturation effects	
	Is less susceptible to intravoxel dephasing	Is time consuming and susceptible to patient motion	
	Can be repeated if suboptimal		
	Can be obtained after contrast administration but is slightly degraded by venous signal		
2D PC MRA	Is able to show the direction and magnitude of flow	Has low spatial resolution	Is used occasionally to determine collateral flow around the circle of Willis
	Does not show high signal artifact from fat or blood	Is more susceptible to turbulent dephasing than TOF MRA	Is used occasionally to determines subclavian steal and abnormal flow direction in the neck
	Can show very slow moving blood and helps differentiate occlusion from near occlusion	Can have aliasing artifact if an incorrect VENC is used	Can detect slow flow if near-occlusion is suspected
	Can be obtained after gadolinium administration	2D PC of the neck takes longer than 2D TOF of the neck with similar coverage	Is used occasionally in MR venography
	Can be repeated if suboptimal		
	2D PC of the circle of Willis is faster than 3D TOF or PC MRA		

Table 6.2. (continued)

	Advantages	Disadvantages	Clinical applications
3D PC MRA	Has high spatial resolution	Is time consuming; 3D TOF MRA is faster with similar spatial resolution	Is rarely used
	Does not show high signal artifact from fat or blood		Used if intravascular clot will confuse 3D TOF MRA interpretation
CE MRA	Is fast, thus minimizing patient motion artifact	Has lower spatial resolution than 3D TOF MRA	Is used routinely to evaluate stenoses and occlusions of the neck vessels and neck vessel origins at the aortic arch
	Is less susceptible to signal loss from flow turbulence	Occasionally underestimates stenosis	
	Has no saturation artifact	Must be obtained in arterial phase	
	Has good signal-to-noise ratio	Cannot be repeated until i.v. contrast has cleared	
	Images a large volume of tissue	Is minimally invasive, requiring rapid power injection of contrast	
	Does not show high signal artifact from fat or blood		
	Accurate in estimating stenoses		
	Helps differentiate occlusion from near-occlusion		

MRA alone would have misclassified 15% of cases and would have altered clinical decision-making in 6.0% of cases [24]. The authors concluded that this was a sufficiently low error rate to support use of CE MRA, but noted that catheter angiography was still the gold standard.

A 2003 study observed that stenoses measured by CE MRA and DSA are tightly correlated by a linear regression analysis ($r=0.967$ with a 95% confidence interval of 2.8%) [25]. While this was true for the study overall, the study warned that stenosis measurements by a single CE MRA exam for an individual patient have a larger confidence interval and may not reliably discriminate between small increments of stenosis (e.g., between a 69% and 71% stenosis). Nevertheless, in most patients, CE MRA is accurate for stratifying stenoses into the broad categories of surgical versus nonsurgical lesions.

Some reports suggest that noncontrast MRA of the neck is less accurate than CE MRA in discriminating surgical from nonsurgical stenoses. One 2002 study comparing 2D and 3D TOF MRA to DSA reported that 23% of their patients would have received unindicated endarterectomies while another 33% would have been improperly denied endarterectomies had noncontrast MRA results been used alone [26]. Several studies from 1992 to 1994 also reported that 2D TOF MRA overestimated up to 48% of moderate stenoses, erroneously categorizing them as surgical lesions [27] and one study demonstrated that 2D TOF MRA has a sensitivity of 84% and specificity of 75% in differentiating surgical from nonsurgical stenoses [28]. However, a number of studies suggest that 3D TOF MRA has a sensitivity and specificity of grading carotid artery stenosis similar to those of CE MRA. One study demonstrated a sensitivity of 94%

and specificity of 85% for 3D TOF MRA in distinguishing surgical from nonsurgical stenoses [28]. Another study demonstrated Pearson correlation coefficients of 0.94 for CE MRA versus DSA, 0.95 for 3D TOF MRA versus DSA and 0.94 for CE MRA versus 3D TOF MRA [29]. Also, a 2003 meta-analysis combining 4 contrast and 17 noncontrast MRA studies published from 1994 to 2001 reported a pooled sensitivity of 95% and pooled specificity of 90% for MRA's ability to discriminate between stenoses greater than or equal to 70% [30].

In general, both noncontrast and CE MRA overestimate stenoses when compared with DSA, and this leads to a decrease in specificity. For noncontrast MRA, this is primarily related to signal loss from dephasing and saturation artifacts. Pixel exclusion on MIP images and motion degradation can also artifactually exaggerate the degree of stenosis on both noncontrast and CE MRA [24]. Nearly all studies evaluating MRA rely on DSA as a gold standard since this was used in the NASCET and ACAS trials. Some papers, however, question the accuracy of DSA in grading stenoses, pointing to underestimation of stenosis by DSA compared with 3D rotational catheter angiography [31, 32]. Some have suggested that the specificity measured on MRA studies may be falsely low from using a suboptimal gold standard [31].

Discriminating near occlusion from total occlusion is critical, as the former can indicate urgent surgery while the latter contraindicates surgical treatment. Several studies show that MRA has high sensitivity and specificity for making this differentiation [30, 33, 34]. El-Saden et al. [33], in a retrospective study using noncontrast and CE MRA together, reported a 92% sensitivity for detecting 37 total occlusions and a 100% sensitivity for detecting 21 near-occlusions [33]. A meta-analysis of both CE MRA and noncontrast MRA studies reported a pooled sensitivity of 98% and pooled specificity of 100% in differentiating high-grade stenosis from occlusion [30]. Other studies, however, do not report such high accuracies [35] and many practices still rely on DSA to differentiate definitively occlusion from near-occlusion.

6.2.5 Intracranial Atherosclerosis and Occlusions

In the setting of acute stroke, intracranial MRA can detect areas of stenosis and occlusion as well as determine collateral flow (Fig. 6.16). Defining the location of intracranial vessel pathology is clinically important since an estimated 38% of patients with acute strokes have arterial occlusion seen on DSA [36] (and distal clots are more likely than proximal clots to recanalize following tissue plasminogen activator (t-PA) [37]. As a result, proximal clots are treated more aggressively, sometimes using intra-arterial techniques. In the acute setting, localizing intracranial occlusions is often performed by CT angiogram, but MRA can also depict these findings (Fig. 6.17).

Several studies report that intracranial MRA has a variable reliability of detecting occlusion and stenoses in the acute stroke setting. A 1994 study of TOF MRA compared to DSA in stroke reported 100% sensitivity and 95% specificity for detecting intracranial occlusion [38], and another demonstrated 88% sensitivity and 97% specificity for detecting MCA lesions compared with DSA [39]. A 2002 study, however, showed that, with the addition of contrast to TOF MRA, 21% of vessels initially thought to be occluded on noncontrast TOF MRA were actually patent on CE TOF MRA [40]. Few studies have determined the clinical significance of these MRA findings in stroke, but a recent 2004 study using phase-contrast MRA in acute stroke showed that absent flow in the M1 segment can help predict infarct growth [41].

The degree of collateral flow seen on DSA is an independent radiologic predictor of favorable outcome following thrombolytic treatment [42]. TOF MRA, however, is limited in evaluation of collateral flow. One study found a negative predictive value as low as 53% for TOF MRA's ability to detect collateral flow when compared with transcranial Doppler [43]. A 2004 study showed that, on TOF MRA, prominence of distal PCA vessels ipsilateral to an M1 occlusion represents collateral blood flow via leptomeningeal vessels [44]. The significance of this finding remains uncertain.

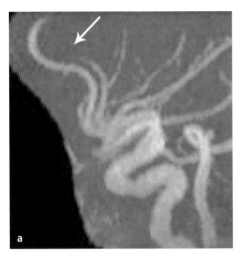
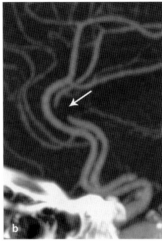
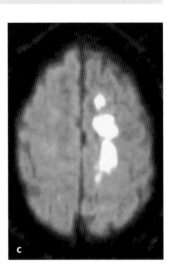

Fig. 6.16 a–c

Anterior cerebral artery occlusion and infarct. a MIP of 3D TOF MRA shows absent flow-related enhancement of the distal A2 segment of the left anterior cerebral artery (*ACA, arrow*). b This corresponds to a focal filling defect on CT angiography (*CTA, arrow*). Note that MRA cannot image the slow collateral flow in the distal left ACA. c Diffusion-weighted image (*DWI*) shows the left ACA territory infarct

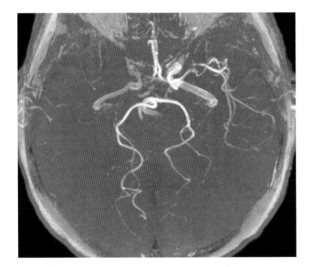

Figure 6.17

Right MCA occlusion. Three-dimensional TOF MRA MIP image shows absent flow-related enhancement in the right MCA from embolic occlusion. Note the decreased signal in the right petrous ICA from a saturation effect secondary to slow flow. There is also severe stenosis of the distal left MCA

6.2.6 Dissection

Vascular dissection is an important etiology of acute infarction, causing up to 20% of infarcts in young patients and an estimated 2.5% of infarcts in the overall population [45]. Dissection occurs when blood extends into the wall of a vessel through an intimal tear. This may occur in the extracranial or intracranial vessels, the carotid or vertebral arteries, and may be spontaneous or post-traumatic in etiology [46, 47]. Dissection most frequently occurs in the carotid artery as it enters the skull base and in the vertebral artery segment from C2 to the foramen magnum. Dissections cause stroke primarily through embolization rather than through flow limitation [48].

Acute dissections show luminal narrowing on MRA and a flap can occasionally appear as a linear low signal defect on MRA. The signal of the intramural blood follows that of parenchymal hematomas, but hemosiderin deposition is not typically seen. Once methemoglobin develops, the wall of the vessel appears hyperintense on fat-saturated T1-weighted images [49] (Fig. 6.18). Chronically, the vessel can occlude, recanalize, show pseudoaneurysms, or become dilated [50].

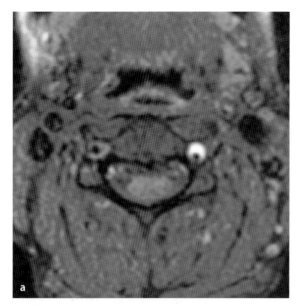

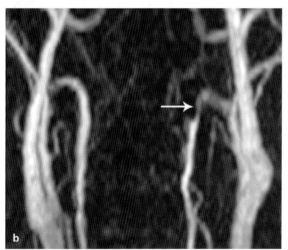

Fig. 6.18 a, b

Left vertebral artery dissection. **a** Axial T1 fat-saturated image of the neck shows a crescent of high signal at the left vertebral artery from intramural hemoglobin. **b** Contrast-enhanced MRA shows a narrowed left vertebral artery (*arrow*)

In a study of 19 internal carotid and five vertebral artery dissections, the MR appearance alone had an estimated 84% sensitivity and 99% specificity for diagnosing carotid dissections and a 60% sensitivity and 98% specificity for diagnosing vertebral artery dissection [51]. Noncontrast MRA (TOF) has low sensitivity (20%) for detecting vertebral artery dissection, but preliminary data suggest that CE MRA may improve the evaluation of vertebral artery dissection [52]. Recently, case reports of false-negatives have been reported for CE MRA in diagnosing dissection [53].

6.2.7 Other Infarct Etiologies

MRA can help determine other etiologies of arterial infarct, including moya moya disease, vasculitis, and fibromuscular dysplasia.

6.2.7.1 Moya Moya

The term moya moya refers to primary moya moya disease and moya moya pattern, associated with an underlying disease such as atherosclerosis or radiation therapy. There is an increased incidence of primary moya moya disease in Asians and in patients with neurofibromatosis or sickle cell disease. Pathologically, there is a progressive occlusive vasculopathy of the supraclinoid internal carotid artery with extension into the proximal anterior and middle cerebral arteries associated with characteristic dilated prominent collateral vessels. Pediatric patients with moya moya disease tend to develop symptoms from acute infarction while adults with moya moya disease more frequently present with symptoms from intracranial hemorrhage into the deep gray nuclei. MRA can depict stenoses and occlusion of the internal carotid, middle cerebral, and anterior cerebral arteries (Fig. 6.19) [54, 55], and the estimated sensitivity and specificity of MRA in diagnosing moya moya disease in one study of 26 patients were 73% and 100% respectively [56]. Furthermore, one recent study reported that MRA depiction of moya moya collaterals in patients with sickle cell anemia was correlated with future cerebrovascular events [57]. MRA is also frequently used in planning vascular by-pass surgery and following response to treatment.

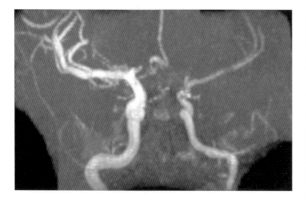

Figure 6.19

Moya moya disease. Three-dimensional TOF MRA shows decreased flow-related enhancement in the left ICA at the skull base. There is high-grade stenosis or occlusion at the left supraclinoid ICA in this patient with sickle cell anemia

6.2.7.2 Vasculitis

Vasculitis affecting the central nervous system (CNS) represents a heterogeneous group of inflammatory diseases that may be idiopathic or associated with autoimmune diseases, infections, drug exposure, radiation or cancer. Vessel walls are infiltrated by inflammatory cells, and there is increased vasomotor reactivity related to the release of neuropeptides. These properties lead to vessel narrowing. There is also loss of normal endothelial anticoagulant properties and vessels have increased susceptibility to thrombosis. Consequently, patients with vasculitis develop ischemic and thrombotic infarctions. There is also altered wall competence, which can result in dissection or vessel wall disruption with intracranial hemorrhage. MRA is clinically used to screen for vasculitis, but is less sensitive than DSA (Fig. 6.20). One study of 14 patients with suspected vasculitis reported that MRA could detect distal stenoses in vasculitis with a sensitivity of 62–79% and a specificity of 83–87% when compared with a DSA gold standard [58].

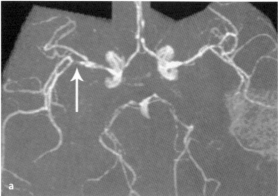

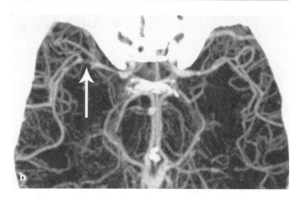

Fig. 6.20 a, b

Vasculitis. **a** MIP of 3D TOF MRA shows scattered areas of narrowing in the right MCA (*arrow*), bilateral posterior cerebral artery (*PCA*), and anterior cerebral artery (*ACA*) in this patient with primary CNS vasculitis. **b** MIP from CT angiogram also shows scattered vessel narrowing, especially at the right MCA (*arrow*)

6.2.7.3 Fibromuscular Dysplasia

Fibromuscular dysplasia (FMD) is an uncommon idiopathic vasculopathy causing stenoses most often in the renal and internal carotid arteries, and patients with FMD of the neck vessels can present with infarcts or transient ischemic attacks. MRA in FMD can show alternating areas of stenosis (Fig. 6.21) but one study noted that 2D TOF MRA is limited in evaluation of FMD, as slice misregistration artifacts can mimic alternating stenoses [59]. In practice, MRA is useful is distinguishing FMD from vessel dissection or hypoplasia [60].

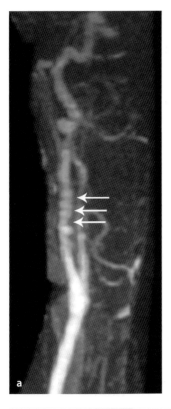
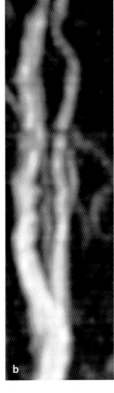

Fig. 6.21 a, b

Fibromuscular dysplasia. **a** CE MRA of the left internal carotid artery shows alternating stenoses (*arrows*) in this patient with fibromuscular dysplasia. **b** 2D TOF MIP image also demonstrates the stenoses but these can be confused with slice misregistration artifacts

6.2.8 Venous Infarct

Venous occlusion can lead to infarct through a reduction in cerebral blood flow. Venous infarcts are under-recognized and tend to develop into a hemorrhage [61]. Parenchymal findings on MR include imaging cerebral swelling, venous infarctions, and in-

tracranial hemorrhage. The MR appearance of intravascular clot is variable depending on the age of thrombus and the degree of residual flow. In general, methemoglobin demonstrates hyperintensity on T1-weighted images and there is usually the absence of a flow void on T2-weighted images.

MR venography greatly aids in diagnosing cerebral venous thrombosis and in determining the extent of thrombosis. Typically, a 2D TOF sequence is obtained in the coronal plane [62]. If flow-related enhancement is not seen within a sinus, there should be a high suspicion of sinus thrombosis (Fig. 6.22). However, MRV must be interpreted alongside standard MR sequences because the absence of flow-related enhancement can also be seen in atretic sinuses, in regions of complex flow due to complex geometry or where there is in-plane flow [63]. In addition, T1 hyperintense clot can be confused with flow-related enhancement on TOF techniques but the flow-related enhancement usually has higher signal intensity. Preliminary data also support the use of first-pass contrast-enhanced venography [64].

6.2.9 Conclusion

In the setting of acute stroke, MRA is useful for determining the severity of stenosis, vascular occlusion, and collateral flow. CE MRA and 3D TOF techniques have relatively high sensitivity and specificity in differentiating surgical from nonsurgical carotid stenoses. Three-dimensional TOF MRA is quite sensitive and specific for the evaluation of intracranial proximal stenoses and occlusions. Two-dimensional PC MRA is useful for determining collateral flow patterns in the circle of Willis. MRA is also useful in the determination of stroke etiologies such as dissection, fibromuscular dysplasia, vasculitis, and moya moya. Currently, MRA is relatively insensitive to the detection of stenoses in distal intracranial vessels but this detection will improve with new MR hardware and software.

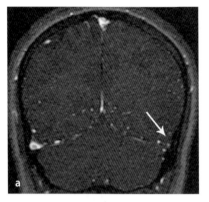
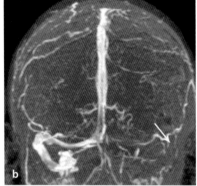
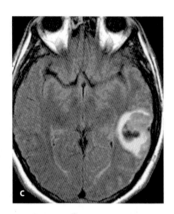

Fig. 6.22 a–c

Venous thrombus and venous infarct. 2D TOF MRV (a) and MIP image of the MR venogram (b) show absent flow in the left transverse sinus corresponding to thrombus (*arrow*). c FLAIR image shows high and low signal at the posterior left temporal lobe corresponding to hemorrhagic infarct

References

1. Yuh WT et al (1991) MR imaging of cerebral ischemia: findings in the first 24 hours. Am J Neuroradiol 12(4):621–629
2. Maeda M et al (2001) Time course of arterial hyperintensity with fast fluid-attenuated inversion-recovery imaging in acute and subacute middle cerebral arterial infarction. J Magn Reson Imaging 13(6):987–990
3. Flacke S et al (2000) Middle cerebral artery (MCA) susceptibility sign at susceptibility-based perfusion MR imaging: clinical importance and comparison with hyperdense MCA sign at CT. Radiology 215(2):476–482
4. Shimosegawa E et al (1993) Embolic cerebral infarction: MR findings in the first 3 hours after onset. Am J Roentgenol 160(5):1077–1082
5. Perkins CJ et al (2001) Fluid-attenuated inversion recovery and diffusion- and perfusion-weighted MRI abnormalities in 117 consecutive patients with stroke symptoms. Stroke 32(12):2774–2781
6. Ida M et al (1994) Subcortical low intensity in early cortical ischemia. Am J Neuroradiol 15(7):1387–1393
7. Ricci PE et al (1999) A comparison of fast spin-echo, fluid-attenuated inversion-recovery, and diffusion-weighted MR imaging in the first 10 days after cerebral infarction. Am J Neuroradiol 20(8):1535–1542
8. Asato R, Okumura R., Konishi J (1991) "Fogging effect" in MR of cerebral infarct. J Comput Assist Tomogr 15(1):160–162
9. Crain MR et al (1991) Cerebral ischemia: evaluation with contrast-enhanced MR imaging. Am J Neuroradiol 12(4):631–639
10. Kuhn MJ, Mikulis DJ, Ayoub DM, Kosofsky BE, Davis KR, Taveras JM (1989) Wallerian degeneration after cerebral infarction: evaluation with sequential MR imaging. Radiology 172(1):179–182
11. Boyko OB et al (1992) Non-heme mechanisms for T1 shortening: pathologic, CT, and MR elucidation. Am J Neuroradiol 13(5):1439–1445
12. Hornig CR, Dorndorf W, Agnoli AL (1986) Hemorrhagic cerebral infarction – a prospective study. Stroke 17(2):179–185
13. Hakim AM, Ryder-Cooke A, Melanson D (1983) Sequential computerized tomographic appearance of strokes. Stroke 14(6):893–897
14. Kidwell CS et al (2002) Predictors of hemorrhagic transformation in patients receiving intra-arterial thrombolysis. Stroke 33(3):717–724
15. Hermier M et al (2001) MRI of acute post-ischemic cerebral hemorrhage in stroke patients: diagnosis with T2*-weighted gradient-echo sequences. Neuroradiology 43(10):809–815
16. Lin DD et al (2001) Detection of intracranial hemorrhage: comparison between gradient-echo images and b(0) images obtained from diffusion-weighted echo-planar sequences. Am J Neuroradiol 22(7):1275–1281
17. Hermier M, Nighoghossian N. Contribution of susceptibility-weighted imaging to acute stroke assessment. Stroke 35(8):1989–1994
18. Bradley WG Jr (1993) MR appearance of hemorrhage in the brain. Radiology 189(1):15–26
19. Jewells V, Castillo M (2003) MR angiography of the extracranial circulation. Magn Reson Imaging Clin North Am 11(4):585–597, vi

20. Sohn CH, Sevick RJ, Frayne R (2003) Contrast-enhanced MR angiography of the intracranial circulation. Magn Reson Imaging Clin North Am 11(4):599–614

21. Barnett HJ et al (1998) Benefit of carotid endarterectomy in patients with symptomatic moderate or severe stenosis. North American Symptomatic Carotid Endarterectomy Trial Collaborators. N Engl J Med 339(20):1415–1425

22. Executive Committee for the Asymptomatic Carotid Atherosclerosis Study (1995) Endarterectomy for asymptomatic carotid artery stenosis. J Am Med Assoc 273(18):1421–1428

23. Alvarez-Linera J et al (2003) Prospective evaluation of carotid artery stenosis: elliptic centric contrast-enhanced MR angiography and spiral CT angiography compared with digital subtraction angiography. Am J Neuroradiol 24(5):1012–1019

24. U-King-Im JM, Trivedi RA, Graves MJ et al (2004) Contrast-enhanced MR angiography for carotid disease: diagnostic and potential clinical impact. Neurology 62(8):1282–1290

25. Hathout GM, Duh MJ, El-Saden SM (2003) Accuracy of contrast-enhanced MR angiography in predicting angiographic stenosis of the internal carotid artery: linear regression analysis. Am J Neuroradiol 24(9):1747–1756

26. Wardlaw JM et al (2002) Interobserver variability of magnetic resonance angiography in the diagnosis of carotid stenosis – effect of observer experience. Neuroradiology 44(2):126–132

27. Stark DWB (1999) Magnetic resonance imaging. Elsevier, New York

28. Patel MR et al (1995) Preoperative assessment of the carotid bifurcation. Can magnetic resonance angiography and duplex ultrasonography replace contrast arteriography? Stroke 26(10):1753–1758

29. Nederkoorn PJ et al (2003) Carotid artery stenosis: accuracy of contrast-enhanced MR angiography for diagnosis. Radiology 228(3):677–682

30. Nederkoorn PJ, van der Graaf Y, Hunink MG (2003) Duplex ultrasound and magnetic resonance angiography compared with digital subtraction angiography in carotid artery stenosis: a systematic review. Stroke 34(5):1324–1332

31. Elgersma OE et al (2000) Multidirectional depiction of internal carotid arterial stenosis: three-dimensional time-of-flight MR angiography versus rotational and conventional digital subtraction angiography. Radiology 216(2):511–516

32. Elgersma OE et al (1999) Maximum internal carotid arterial stenosis: assessment with rotational angiography versus conventional intraarterial digital subtraction angiography. Radiology 213(3):777–783

33. El-Saden SM et al (2001) Imaging of the internal carotid artery: the dilemma of total versus near total occlusion. Radiology 221(2):301–308

34. Heiserman JE et al (1992) Carotid artery stenosis: clinical efficacy of two-dimensional time-of-flight MR angiography. Radiology 182(3):761–768

35. Modaresi KB et al (1999) Comparison of intra-arterial digital subtraction angiography, magnetic resonance angiography and duplex ultrasonography for measuring carotid artery stenosis. Br J Surg 86(11):1422–1426

36. Furlan A et al (1999) Intra-arterial prourokinase for acute ischemic stroke. The PROACT II study: a randomized controlled trial. Prolyse in acute cerebral thromboembolism. J Am Med Assoc 282(21):2003–2011

37. Del Zoppo GJ et al (1992) Recombinant tissue plasminogen activator in acute thrombotic and embolic stroke. Ann Neurol 32(1):78–86

38. Stock KW et al (1995) Intracranial arteries: prospective blinded comparative study of MR angiography and DSA in 50 patients. Radiology 195(2):451–456

39. Korogi Y et al (1994) Intracranial vascular stenosis and occlusion: diagnostic accuracy of three-dimensional, Fourier transform, time-of-flight MR angiography. Radiology 193(1):187–193

40. Yang JJ et al (2002) Comparison of pre- and postcontrast 3D time-of-flight MR angiography for the evaluation of distal intracranial branch occlusions in acute ischemic stroke. Am J Neuroradiol 23(4):557–567

41. Liu Y et al (2004) Acute ischemic stroke: predictive value of 2D phase-contrast MR angiography–serial study with combined diffusion and perfusion MR imaging. Radiology 231(2):517–527

42. Kucinski T et al (2003) Collateral circulation is an independent radiological predictor of outcome after thrombolysis in acute ischaemic stroke. Neuroradiology 45(1):11–18

43. Hoksbergen AW et al (2003) Assessment of the collateral function of the circle of Willis: three-dimensional time-of-flight MR angiography compared with transcranial color-coded duplex sonography. Am J Neuroradiol 24(3):456–462

44. Uemura A et al (2004) Prominent laterality of the posterior cerebral artery at three-dimensional time-of-flight MR angiography in M1-segment middle cerebral artery occlusion. Am J Neuroradiol 25(1):88–91

45. Provenzale JM (1995) Dissection of the internal carotid and vertebral arteries: imaging features. Am J Roentgenol 165(5):1099–1104

46. Shin JH et al (2000) Vertebral artery dissection: spectrum of imaging findings with emphasis on angiography and correlation with clinical presentation. Radiographics 20(6):1687–1696

47. Fisher CM, Ojemann RG, Roberson GH (1978) Spontaneous dissection of cervico-cerebral arteries. Can J Neurol Sci 5(1):9–19

48. Benninger DH et al (2004) Mechanism of ischemic infarct in spontaneous carotid dissection. Stroke 35(2):482–485

49. Ozdoba C, Sturzenegger M, Schroth G (1996) Internal carotid artery dissection: MR imaging features and clinical-radiologic correlation. Radiology 199(1):191–198

50. Mokri B et al (1986) Spontaneous dissection of the cervical internal carotid artery. Ann Neurol 19(2):126–138

51. Levy C et al (1994) Carotid and vertebral artery dissections: three-dimensional time-of-flight MR angiography and MR imaging versus conventional angiography. Radiology 190(1):97–103

52. Leclerc X et al (1999) Preliminary experience using contrast-enhanced MR angiography to assess vertebral artery structure for the follow-up of suspected dissection. Am J Neuroradiol 20(8):1482–1490

53. Khan R, Smith JK, Castillo M (2002) False-negative contrast MRA in the setting of carotid artery dissection. Emerg Radiol 9(6):320–322

54. Yamada I, Matsushima Y, Suzuki S (1992) Moyamoya disease: diagnosis with three-dimensional time-of-flight MR angiography. Radiology 184(3):773–778

55. Yamada I et al (2001) High-resolution turbo magnetic resonance angiography for diagnosis of Moyamoya disease. Stroke 32(8):1825–1831

56. Yamada I, Suzuki S, Matsushima Y (1995) Moyamoya disease: comparison of assessment with MR angiography and MR imaging versus conventional angiography. Radiology 196(1):211–2128

57. Steen RG et al (2003) Brain imaging findings in pediatric patients with sickle cell disease. Radiology 228(1):216–225

58. Demaerel P et al (2004) Magnetic resonance angiography in suspected cerebral vasculitis. Eur Radiol 14(6):1005–1012

59. Heiserman JE et al (1992) MR angiography of cervical fibromuscular dysplasia. Am J Neuroradiol 13(5):1454–1457

60. Furie DM, Tien RD (1994) Fibromuscular dysplasia of arteries of the head and neck: imaging findings. Am J Roentgenol 162(5):1205–1209

61. Tsai FY et al (1995) MR staging of acute dural sinus thrombosis: correlation with venous pressure measurements and implications for treatment and prognosis. Am J Neuroradiol 16(5):1021–1029

62. Liauw L et al (2000) MR angiography of the intracranial venous system. Radiology 214(3):678–682

63. Ayanzen RH et al (2000) Cerebral MR venography: normal anatomy and potential diagnostic pitfalls. Am J Neuroradiol 21(1):74–78

64. Farb RI et al (2003) Intracranial venous system: gadolinium-enhanced three-dimensional MR venography with auto-triggered elliptic centric-ordered sequence–initial experience. Radiology 226(1):203–209

Diffusion MR of Acute Stroke

Pamela W. Schaefer, A. Kiruluta,
R. Gilberto González

Contents

7.1 Introduction

Diffusion magnetic resonance imaging provides unique information on the state of living tissue because it gives image contrast that is dependent on the molecular motion of water. The method was introduced into clinical practice in the mid 1990s, but because of its demanding MR engineering requirements, primarily high-performance magnetic field gradients, it has only recently undergone widespread dissemination. Because it employs ultrafast, echo planar MRI scanning, it is highly resistant to patient motion, and imaging times range from a few seconds to 2 minutes. Diffusion MRI is the most reliable method for detecting acute ischemia and has assumed an essential role in the detection of acute ischemic brain infarction and in differentiating acute infarction from other disease processes.

7.2 Basic Concepts/Physics of Diffusion MRI

The term diffusion refers to the general transport of matter whereby molecules or ions mix through normal agitation in a random way. Even though diffusion is a random process, there is an underlying driving mechanism. When describing the mixing of different liquids or gases, diffusion is described in terms of a concentration gradient of the diffusing substance: from areas of high concentration to areas of low concentration. In biological tissues, however, concentration is not the driving force, and instead the process of interest is the motion of water within water driven by thermal agitation, commonly referred to as Brownian motion or self-diffusion. For example, the

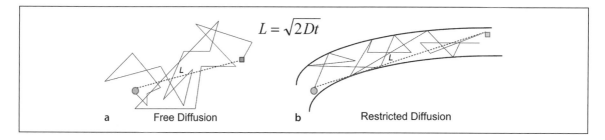

$$L = \sqrt{2Dt}$$

a   Free Diffusion   b   Restricted Diffusion

Figure 7.1 a, b

Comparison of unrestricted or free diffusion (**a**) of a particle with restricted diffusion (**b**). Biological structures have barriers such as cell membranes, which restrict diffusion to a specific bounded path. In the latter case, directional structures such as axons have free diffusion along their principle axes and restricted diffusion perpendicular to that axis. This directional dependency is called anisotropy

path of a pollen grain suspended in water provides good visualization of Brownian motion of all liquid water molecules whether in pure water, a porous medium or biological tissue. After each displacement, there is a collision and then a new random orientation for the next displacement. Hence, the particles take a random walk consisting of a succession of n random displacements. In the case of unrestricted diffusion, the particle wanders freely in all directions throughout the medium as shown in Fig. 7.1a. The distance traversed by the particle in time t, referred to as the mean free path L, is the direct line connecting its initial to its final position and it is proportional to the square root of the diffusion constant D (Fig. 7.1). Since there is no directional (spatial) variation in the free diffusion rate D, the diffusion is called isotropic. For water at 37 °C, the diffusion constant D is approximately 3.2×10^{-3} mm$^2 \cdot$ s^{-1}.

In biological tissues, water molecules encounter a number of complex semi-permeable structures in the intracellular, extracellular, and vascular compartments. As a result, water diffusion through such structures exhibits directionality in the orientation of preferred motion. The measured diffusion is thus greater parallel to the barriers (Fig. 7.1b) than perpendicular to them. This directional dependence is known as anisotropy [1].

In vivo measurement of water diffusion using MRI exploits the fact that spins moving through a magnetic field gradient acquire phase at a rate depending on both the gradient strength and the velocity of the spins. The basic sequence for measuring diffusion is a spin echo pulse sequence shown in Fig. 7.2. The method utilizes a pair of equal but opposite strong gradient pulses placed symmetrically around the 180° refocusing pulse. The effect of the spin echo is to reverse this dephasing (loss of signal due to a fanning out of the spin vectors which do not add coherently) in the interval TE/2 (where TE is echo time) so that an echo, a coherent sum of all spin vectors into a single vector, is formed at a time TE/2 after the application of the 180° pulse. The effect on the spin system of the first gradient lobe before the 180° pulse is to increase the rate at which the various spin vectors fan out, resulting in faster signal decay. The gradient lobe after the 180° pulse is in effect polarity reversed relative to the first lobe so that the total gradient dephasing is zero. Thus, the first gradient lobe increases the fanning out of the various spin vectors while the second lobe fans them back inwards to create the echo.

However, this is only true for static tissues which see both these gradients in their entirety so that the two phase shifts are identical in magnitude and cancel each other out. If the spins are moving, such as spins in flowing blood, then the amount of signal dephasing will be both spatial and time-dependent. During the second gradient pulse, this phase is unwound at the same rate as it was wound by the first gradient pulse but, since the spins are moving, they undergo a different overall phase change as they are

Figure 7.2

Stejskal–Tanner diffusion spin echo sequence [138]. Spins accumulate phase shift during the first gradient pulse. The 180° pulse inverts the phase of all spins. The second gradient lobe induces another phase shift that is effectively opposite to the first gradient pulse due to the effect of the spin echo. The phase shifts are identical in magnitude and cancel each other out. For moving or diffusing spins, the translation of the spins to different locations in time t results in an incomplete refocusing and hence the attenuation of the resulting echo. $b=\gamma^2G^2\delta^2(\Delta-\delta/3)$, and D is the diffusion coefficient. γ is the gyromagnetic ratio. G is the magnitude of, δ the width of, and Δ the time between, the two balanced diffusion gradient pulses

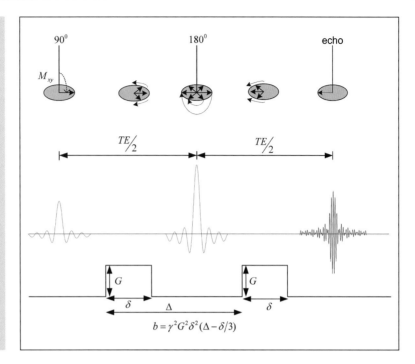

now in a different magnetic field from where they were during the first pulse. The result is a weaker echo compared to stationary tissue since the rephasing of the MR signal is incomplete.

Spins undergoing diffusion also dephase, but because their motion is random, each spin within a voxel ends up with a different amount of phase at the end of the second gradient lobe. Since the magnetization vectors of all spins in the voxel are added to form the acquired echo, the spread in spin vectors due to the random motion results in an overall reduction of the echo signal. The exponential loss in signal in the diffusion case is significantly higher than in a simple flow case due to the inherent randomness. The measured MR signal loss due to diffusion is given by:

$$S = S_0 e^{-bD} \tag{7.1}$$

where S is the diffusion-weighted (DW) signal intensity, S_0 is the signal with no diffusion gradients applied, b characterizes the diffusion-sensitizing gradi-

ent pulses (timing, amplitude, shape, and spacing – see Fig. 7.2) and D is the diffusion constant. The apparent diffusion coefficient (ADC) for a given direction is calculated on a pixel-by-pixel basis by fitting signal intensities to Eq. 7.1 so that:

$$D = b \cdot \ln\frac{S_0}{S} \tag{7.2}$$

where ln is the natural logarithm function. The reference to an ADC is because the actual diffusion coefficient is complicated by other factors such as variations in anisotropy in tissue, choice of parameters in the b value, and some confounding factors due to inherent perfusion and motion, which result in an estimate rather than the actual value. The effects due to motion are mitigated by using single-shot echo planar (EPI) acquisition to minimize the imaging time.

Acquiring multiple DW images for a series of b values allows the determination of the apparent diffusion coefficient ($D \approx$ ADC) by a pixel-by-pixel least-squares fit of Eq. 7.2 as shown in Fig. 7.3 for a specific gradient direction. In the simplest case, two images

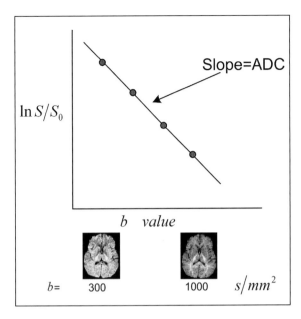

Figure 7.3

The ADC for a given gradient direction is calculated on a pixel-by-pixel basis by fitting signal intensities to the diffusion equation for at least two diffusion-weighted images corresponding to two separate *b* values. The slope of the fit corresponds to the ADC value for that particular gradient direction

are obtained: one averaged diffusion-weighted image for a specific *b* value (for example, diffusion gradients applied along the *x*-axis) followed by a reference T2 image (*b*=0) so that ADC_{xx} is obtained from the fit as shown in Fig. 7.3. The process is repeated to obtain ADC_{yy} and ADC_{zz}.

The diffusion-weighted image (DWI), also known as the isotropic image, is calculated as the geometrical mean of the three diffusion-weighted T2 images derived from the three orthogonal gradient directions (*x*, *y*, *z*) and it is given by:

$$DWI_{\text{avg}} = \left(DWI_x \cdot DWI_y \cdot DWI_z \right)^{1/3} \tag{7.3}$$

The resulting DWI image has not only diffusion contrast but also T2 contrast (also known as "T2 shine through"). In order to remove the T2 weighting, the

DWI *S* is divided by the T2 image S_0 (*b*=0). The exponential image is easily thus derived from Eq. 7.1 as:

$$EXP = \frac{S}{S_0} = e^{-b \cdot ADC} \tag{7.4}$$

7.2.1 Diffusion Tensor Imaging (DTI)

The preceding discussion of DWI assumed that diffusion could be represented as a single quantity. However, in the presence of highly oriented biological structures, such as white matter, this is not the case. Diffusion tensor imaging (DTI) is the term used to describe the extension of DWI to the three spatial directions by applying the sensitizing gradients in all three directions (*x*, *y*, and *z*). The measured diffusion properties of anisotropic tissues will differ when the diffusion gradients are applied along different directions. The complete characterization of the diffusion properties of an anisotropic structure requires that the full effective diffusion tensor be measured. The diffusion coefficient thus becomes:

$$D = \begin{bmatrix} D_{xx} & D_{xy} & D_{xz} \\ D_{yx} & D_{yy} & D_{yz} \\ D_{zx} & D_{zy} & D_{zz} \end{bmatrix} \tag{7.5}$$

For example to obtain D_{xy}, both the *x* and *y* gradients must be applied simultaneously. DWI only gives information concerning three orthogonal diffusion directions, and its full matrix is thus given as:

$$D = \begin{bmatrix} D_{xx} & 0 & 0 \\ 0 & D_{yy} & 0 \\ 0 & 0 & D_{zz} \end{bmatrix} \tag{7.6}$$

where the off-diagonal elements are zero and hence the method is biased towards a particular orientation. In an anisotropic environment, an ellipsoid is elongated as shown in Fig. 7.4b, c, preferentially in one direction. The longest, middle, and shortest of the ellipsoid principal axes are denoted by λ_1, λ_2, and λ_3 and are referred to as eigenvalues. Each has a corresponding eigenvector representing its respective diffusion direction. When these principal axes are aligned with the physical measurement coordinate

Figure 7.4 a–c

Relationship between anisotropic diffusion, diffusion ellipsoids, and diffusion tensor. a In an isotropic environment, diffusion is equal in all directions and can be characterized by diagonal elements (D_{xx}, D_{yy}, and D_{zz}), all of which have the same value D. b, c In anisotropic diffusion, the diffusion tensor is geometrically equivalent to an ellipsoid, with the three eigenvectors of the tensor matrix set as the minor and major axis of the ellipsoid

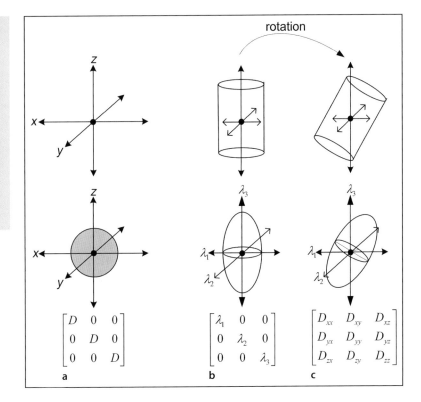

system (x, y, z), as in the isotropic case in Fig. 7.4a, λ_1, λ_2, and λ_3 can be directly measured since they lie on this frame of reference. However, for the anisotropic case, they are never aligned and the diffusion tensor matrix in Eq. 7.4 has nine nonzero values that need to be determined to fully characterized the full 3D diffusion tensor.

The appropriate gradient amplitude and direction are applied to obtain the desired diffusion orientation for the necessary tensor matrix value. For example, to obtain D_{xx}, only G_x is employed. Similarly, for D_{xy}, both $0.707G_x$ and $0.707G_y$ are employed and a DWI image is obtained (Fig. 7.5). With increasing number of diffusion encoding gradient directions, data sampling becomes more uniform and less biased to any particular direction. High angular resolution DTI schemes are typically generated uniformly on a spherical surface divided by the diffusion encoding gradients.

To visualize the tensor, it iss important that the scalar metrics are rotationally invariant, which means that they do not depend on the coordinate system in which the tensor was measured. A rotationally invariant measure of isotropic diffusion is the mean of the principal diffusivity (D) and is given by:

$$ADC = \frac{Trace(D)}{3} = \frac{D_{xx} + D_{yy} + D_{zz}}{3} \tag{7.7}$$

Imaging time can be reduced by measuring the diagonal elements of the diffusion tensor that will provide a rotationally invariant measure of isotropic diffusion as is the case for a simple diffusion weighted image (DWI) .

For a scalar measurement of the amount of anisotropy in tissue, rotationally invariant metrics from the diffusion tensor have been proposed by Basser et al. [2]. The fractional anisotropy (FA) map is defined as the proportion of the diffusion tensor D that can be assigned to anisotropic diffusion. It is given by:

$$FA = \sqrt{\frac{3}{2}} \frac{\sqrt{\left(\lambda_1 - \langle\lambda\rangle\right)^2 + \left(\lambda_2 - \langle\lambda\rangle\right)^2 + \left(\lambda_3 - \langle\lambda\rangle\right)^2}}{\sqrt{\lambda_1^2 + \lambda_2^2 + \lambda_3^2}} \tag{7.8}$$

$$\begin{bmatrix} DD_{xx} & DD_{xy} & DD_{xz} \\ DD_{yx} & DD_{yy} & DD_{yz} \\ DD_{zx} & DD_{zy} & DD_{zz} \end{bmatrix} \longrightarrow$$

notice symmetry along diagonal

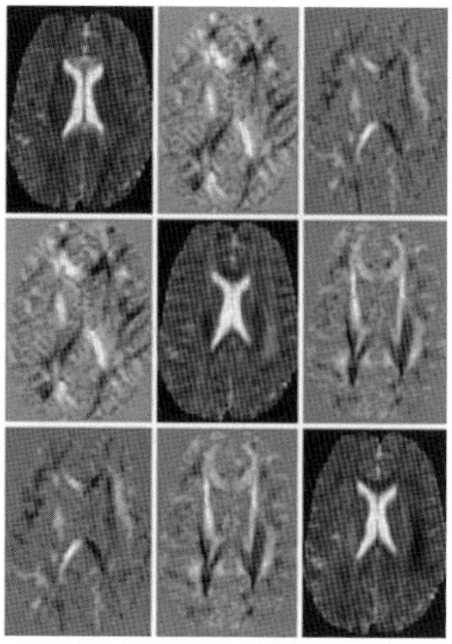

Figure 7.5

Sample display of axial brain images with the different gradient sensitization of the tensor matrix. The off-diagonal elements provide information about the interactions between the x, y, and z directions. For example, ADC_{yx} gives information about the correlation between displacements in the x and y directions. A geometric pixel-by-pixel mean (Eq. 7.3) of the images in the main diagonal is the DWI image as in the isotropic diffusion case

where the $\langle \lambda \rangle = \dfrac{Trace(D)}{3}$ is the mean diffusivity. FA is very easy to interpret, having a great visual impact as white matter is white, while grey matter is grey. FA is equal to zero for perfectly isotropic diffusion and 1 for the hypothetical case of an infinite cylinder.

7.3 Diffusion MR Images for Acute Stroke

For acute stroke studies, DWI images, exponential images, ADC maps and T2-weighted images should be reviewed (Fig. 7.6). In lesions such as acute ischemic strokes, the T2 and diffusion effects both cause increased signal on the DWI and we identify regions of decreased diffusion best on DWI. The exponential image and ADC maps are used to exclude "T2 shine through" as the cause of the increased signal on DWI. Truly decreased diffusion will be hypointense on ADC and hyperintense on exponential images. The exponential image and ADC map are also useful for detecting areas of increased diffusion that may be masked by T2 effects on the DWI. On DWI, regions with elevated diffusion may be slightly hypointense, isointense, or slightly hyperintense, depending on the strength of the diffusion and T2 components. Regions with elevated diffusion are hyperintense on ADC maps and hypointense on exponential images.

7.4 Theory for Decreased Diffusion in Acute Stroke

The biophysical basis for the rapid decrease in ADC values of acutely ischemic brain tissue is complex (Table 7.1). Cytotoxic edema induced by acute hyponatremic encephalopathy is associated with decreased diffusion [3], and is therefore thought to contribute to the decreased diffusion associated with acute stroke. Furthermore, there is decreased $Na^+/K^+ATPase$ activity without a significant increase in brain water [4] when decreased diffusion is present in acutely ischemic rat brain tissue. Ouabain, a $Na^+/K^+ATPase$ inhibitor, is associated with ADC reduction in rat cortex [5]. These findings suggest that ischemia leads to energy metabolism disruption with failure of the $Na^+/K^+ATPase$ and other ionic pumps. This leads to loss of ionic gradients and a net transfer of water from the extracellular to the intracellular compartment where water mobility is relatively decreased.

Furthermore, changes in the extracellular space may contribute to decreased diffusion associated with acute stroke. With cellular swelling, there is reduced extracellular space volume and a decrease in the diffusion of low molecular weight tracer molecules in animal models [6, 7], suggesting increased tortuosity of extracellular space pathways. In addition, intracellular metabolite ADCs are significantly

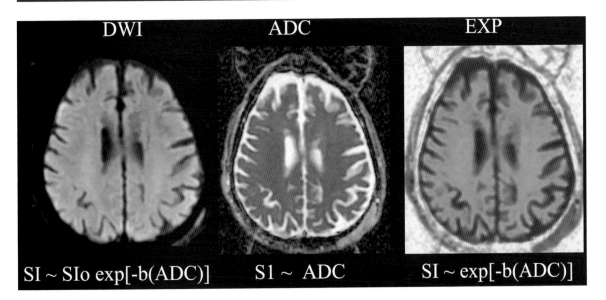

DWI
ADC
EXP

$SI \sim SIo \, exp[-b(ADC)]$ $S1 \sim ADC$ $SI \sim exp[-b(ADC)]$

Figure 7.6

Typical diffusion MR maps. The appearances on the DWI, exponential (*EXP*) image, and ADC map, as well as the corresponding mathematic expressions for their signal intensities, are shown. Image parameters are $b=1000$ s/mm^2; effective gradient, 25 mT/m; repetition time, 7500 ms; minimum echo time; matrix, 128×128; field of view, 200×200 mm; section thickness, 5 mm with 1 mm gap. (*SI* Signal intensity, *SIo* signal intensity on T2-weighted image)

Table 7.1. Theories for decreased diffusion in acute stroke

Number	Theory
1	Failure of Na$^+$/K$^+$ATPase and other ionic pumps with loss of ionic gradients and net transfer of water from the extracellular to the intracellular compartment
2	Reduced extracellular space volume and increased tortuosity of extracellular space pathways due to cell swelling
3	Increased intracellular viscosity from microtubule dissociation and fragmentation of other cellular components
4	Increased intracellular space tortuosity
5	Decreased cytoplasmic mobility.
6	Temperature decrease
7	Increased cell membrane permeability

reduced in ischemic rat brain [8–10]. Proposed explanations are increased intracellular viscosity due to microtubule dissociation, and fragmentation of other cellular components due to collapse of the energy-dependent cytoskeleton, increased tortuosity of the intracellular space, and decreased cytoplasmic mobility. It is noteworthy that the normal steady-state function of these structures requires ATP. Other factors, such as temperature decrease [11, 12] and cell membrane permeability [13, 14], play a minor role in explaining ADC decreases in ischemic brain tissue.

7.5 Time Course of Diffusion Lesion Evolution in Acute Stroke

In animals following middle cerebral artery occlusion, ischemic tissue ADCs decrease to 16–68% below those of normal tissue at 10 min to 2 h [15–21]. In animals, diffusion coefficients pseudonormalize (the ADCs are similar to those of normal brain tissue but

Table 7.2. Diffusion MRI findings in stroke. (*ADC* Apparent diffusion coefficient, *DWI* diffusion-weighted image, *EXP* exponential image, *FA* fractional anisotropy)

Pulse sequence	Hyperacute (0–6 h)	Acute (6–24 h)	Early subacute (1–7 days)	Late subacute	Chronic
Reason for ADC changes	Cytotoxic edema	Cytotoxic edema	Cytotoxic edema with small amount of vasogenic edema	Cytotoxic and vasogenic edema	Vasogenic edema, then gliosis and neuronal loss
DWI	Hyperintense	Hyperintense	Hyperintense, gyral hypointensity from petechial hemorrhage	Hyperintense (due to T2 component)	Isointense to hypointense
ADC	Hypointense	Hypointense	Hypointense	Isointense	Hyperintense
EXP	Hyperintense	Hyperintense	Hyperintense	Isointense	Hypointense
Low B T2	Isointense	Hyperintense	Hyperintense, gyral hypointensity from petechial hemorrhage	Hyperintense	Hyperintense
FA	Hyperintense	Hyperintense to hypointense	Hypointense	Hypointense	Hypointense

the tissue is not viable) at approximately 48 hours and are elevated thereafter. In humans, the time course is longer (Table 7.2; Fig. 7.7). Decreased diffusion in ischemic brain tissue is observed as early as 30 min after vascular occlusion [22–25]. The ADC continues to decrease with peak signal reduction at 1–4 days. This decreased diffusion is markedly hyperintense on DWI (a combination of T2 and diffusion weighting), less hyperintense on exponential images, and hypointense on ADC images. The ADC returns to baseline at 1–2 weeks. This is consistent with the persistence of cytotoxic edema (associated with decreased diffusion) as well as cell membrane disruption, and the development of vasogenic edema (associated with increased diffusion). At this point, a stroke is usually mildly hyperintense on the DWI images due to the T2 component and isointense on the ADC and exponential images. Thereafter, the ADC is elevated secondary to increased extracellular water, tissue cavitation, and gliosis. There is slight hypointensity, isointensity or hyperintensity on the DWI images (depending on the strength of the T2 and diffusion components), in-

creased signal intensity on ADC maps, and decreased signal on exponential images.

The time course is influenced by a number of factors including infarct type and patient age [26]. Minimum ADC is reached more slowly and transition from decreasing to increasing ADC is later in lacunes versus other stroke types (nonlacunes) [27]. In nonlacunes, the subsequent rate of ADC increase is more rapid in younger versus older patients. Early reperfusion may also alter the time course. Early reperfusion causes pseudonormalization as early as 1–2 days in humans who receive intravenous recombinant tissue plasminogen activator (rtPA) within 3 hours after stroke onset [28]. Furthermore, there are different temporal rates of tissue evolution toward infarction within a single ischemic lesion. Nagesh et al. [29] demonstrated that, while the average ADC of an ischemic lesion is depressed within 10 hours, different zones within an ischemic lesion may demonstrate low, pseudonormal or elevated ADCs. In the absence of thrombolysis, in spite of these variations, tissue with reduced ADC nearly always progresses to infarction.

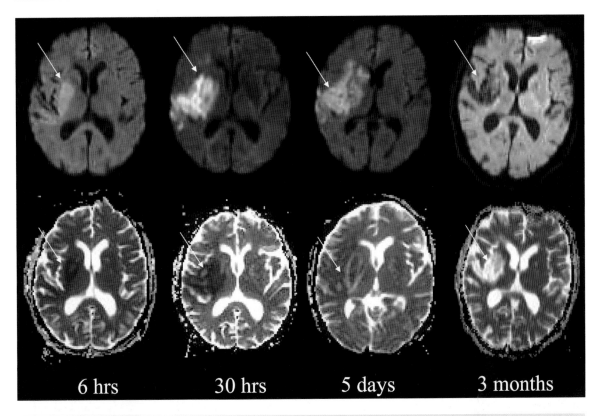

6 hrs   30 hrs   5 days   3 months

Figure 7.7

DWI and ADC time course of stroke evolution. Patient is a 72-year-old female with a history of atrial fibrillation with acute left hemiparesis. At 6 h, the right middle cerebral artery (*MCA*) infarction is mildly hyperintense on DWI and mildly hypointense on ADC images secondary to early cytotoxic edema. At 30 h, the DWI hyperintensity and ADC hypointensity are pronounced secondary to increased cytotoxic edema. This is the ADC nadir. At 5 days, the ADC hypointensity is mild, indicating that the ADC has nearly pseudonormalized. This is secondary to cell lysis and the development of vasogenic edema. The lesion remains markedly hyperintense on the DWI images because the T2 and diffusion components are combined. At 3 months, the infarction is DWI hypointense and ADC hyperintense, secondary to the development of gliosis and tissue cavitation

7.6 Reliability

Conventional CT and MR imaging cannot reliably detect infarction at early time points (less than 6 h) because detection of hypoattenuation on CT and hyperintensity on T2-weighted and fluid attenuated inversion recovery (FLAIR) MR images requires substantial increases in tissue water. For infarctions imaged within 6 h after stroke onset, reported sensitivities are 38–45% for CT and 18–46% for MRI [30, 31]. For infarctions imaged within 24 h, one study reported a sensitivity of 58% for CT and 82% for MRI [32].

Unlike conventional images, diffusion-weighted images are highly sensitive and specific in the detection of hyperacute and acute infarctions [30, 33–35] (Table 7.3). They are very sensitive to the decreased diffusion of water that occurs early in ischemia, and they have a much higher contrast-to-noise ratio compared with CT and conventional MRI. Reported sen-

Table 7.3. Reliability of DWI for the detection of acute ischemic infarction in hyperacute stroke

Pulse sequence	Sensitivity	Specificity
CT	38–45%	82–96%
Conventional MR	18–46%	70–94%
DWI	88–100%	88–100%
DWI – false-negative lesions	1. Brainstem or deep gray nuclei lacunes 2. DWI-negative, perfusion-positive lesions that eventually infarct	
DWI – false-positive lesions	1. T2 shine through 2. Other entities with decreased diffusion – usually demyelinative lesion or nonenhancing tumor	

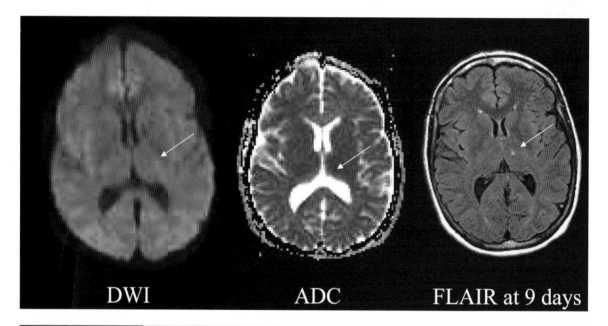

DWI   ADC   FLAIR at 9 days

Figure 7.8

Thalamic lacune without an acute DWI abnormality. Patient is a 45-year-old female with patent foramen ovale. Initial DWI and ADC images demonstrate no definite acute infarction. Follow-up FLAIR image demonstrates a punctate hyperintense left thalamic lacunar infarction (*white arrow*)

sitivities range from 88% to 100% and reported specificities range from 86% to 100%. A lesion with decreased diffusion correlates highly with infarction.

Most false-negative DWI images occur with punctate lacunar brainstem or deep gray nuclei infarctions [30, 33, 34, 36] (Fig. 7.8). Some lesions were presumed on the basis of an abnormal neurologic exam while others were are seen on follow-up DWI. False-negative DWI images also occur in patients with regions of decreased perfusion (increased mean transit time and decreased relative cerebral blood flow) that are hyperintense on follow-up DWI; that is, they

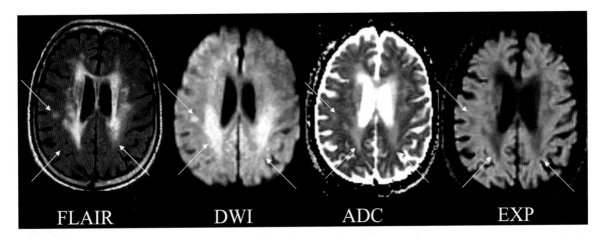

FLAIR   DWI   ADC   EXP

Figure 7.9

T2 "shine through". Patient is a 78-year-old male with dizziness. DWI hyperintense lesions in the right posterior frontal subcortical white matter and bilateral posterior corona radiata are hyperintense on FLAIR images and ADC maps, and hypointense on exponential images. These findings are consistent with elevated diffusion secondary to microangiopathic change rather than acute infarction suggested by the DWI images alone

initially had brain regions with ischemic but viable tissue that eventually infarcted. These findings stress the importance of obtaining early follow-up imaging in patients with normal DWI images and persistent stroke-like deficits so that appropriate treatment is initiated as early as possible.

False-positive DWI images occur in patients with a subacute or chronic infarction with "T2 shine through" (Fig. 7.9). In other words, a lesion appears hyperintense on the DWI images due to an increase in the T2 signal rather than a decrease in diffusion. If the DW images are interpreted in combination with ADC maps or exponential images, this pitfall can be avoided. All acute lesions should demonstrate hypointense signal on ADC maps and increased signal on exponential images, while subacute to chronic lesions should demonstrate increased signal on ADC maps and decreased signal on exponential images. False-positive DWI images have also been reported with cerebral abscess (restricted diffusion due to increased viscosity), and tumor (restricted diffusion due to dense cell packing) [33]. Other entities with decreased diffusion that may be confused with acute infarction are venous infarctions, demyelinative le-

sions (decreased diffusion due to myelin vacuolization), hemorrhage, herpes encephalitis (decreased diffusion due to cell necrosis), and diffuse axonal injury (decreased diffusion due to cytotoxic edema or axotomy with retraction ball formation) [37]. When these lesions are reviewed in combination with routine T1, FLAIR, T2, and gadolinium-enhanced T1-weighted images, they are usually readily differentiated from acute infarctions.

Although after 24 h, CT, FLAIR and T2-weighted images are reliable at detecting acute infarctions, diffusion imaging continues to improve stroke diagnosis in the subacute setting. Older patients commonly have FLAIR and T2 hyperintense white matter abnormalities that are indistinguishable from acute infarctions. However, the acute infarctions are hyperintense on DWI and hypointense on ADC maps while the chronic foci are usually isointense on DWI and hyperintense on ADC maps due to elevated diffusion (Fig. 7.10). In one study of indistinguishable acute and chronic white matter lesions on T2-weighted images in 69% of patients, the sensitivity and specificity of DWI for detecting the acute subcortical infarction were 94.9% and 94.1%, respectively [38].

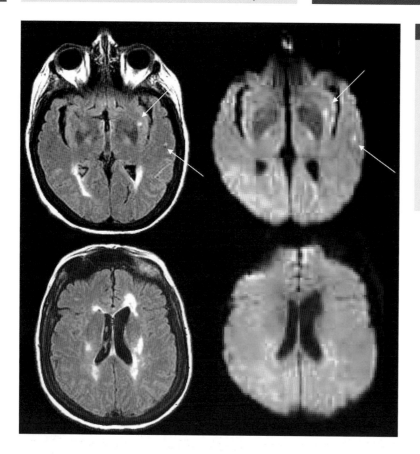

Figure 7.10

Periventricular nonspecific white matter changes versus acute infarction. Patient is a 61-year-old female with hypertension. FLAIR-weighted images demonstrate multiple hyperintense white matter foci of unclear chronicity. Diffusion-weighted images demonstrate that lesions in the left external capsule and left temporal subcortical white matter (*white arrows*) are acute

7.7 Reversibility of DWI Stroke Lesions

In the absence of thrombolysis, reversibility (abnormal on initial DWI but normal on follow-up images) of DWI hyperintense lesions is very rare (Table 7.4). Grant et al. [39] could identify only 21 out of thousands of DWI hyperintense lesions that demonstrated reversibility and most etiologies were not ischemic. The etiologies were acute stroke or transient ischemic attack (TIA) (3 patients), transient global amnesia (7 patients), status epilepticus (4 patients), hemiplegic migraine (3 patients), and venous sinus thrombosis (4 patients) (Fig. 7.11). ADC ratios (ipsilateral abnormal over contralateral normal-appearing brain) were similar to those in patients with acute stroke. Gray matter ADC ratios were 0.64–0.79; white matter ADC ratios were 0.20–0.87 [39].

In the setting of intravenous and/or intra-arterial thrombolysis, DWI reversibility is more common and was seen in 33% of initially DWI-abnormal tissue in one study [40] (Fig. 7.12). However, determining whether tissue with an initial diffusion abnormality is normal at follow-up is complicated. A normal appearance on follow-up DWI, ADC or T2-weighted images may not reflect complete tissue recovery. Kidwell et al. [40], in the same study, reported a decrease in size from the initial DWI abnormality to the follow-up DWI abnormality immediately after intra-arterial thrombolysis in 8/18 patients, but a subsequent increase in DWI lesion volume was observed in 5 patients. A number of studies have demonstrated that ADCs are significantly higher in DWI-reversible tissue compared with DWI-abnormal tissue that infarcts. Mean ADCs range from 663×10^{-6} mm$^2 \cdot$ s^{-1} to 732×10^{-6} mm$^2 \cdot$ s^{-1} in DWI-reversible regions com-

Table 7.4. Reversibility of DWI stroke lesions

Definition	DWI abnormal tissue that appears normal at follow-up imaging
Entities associated with DWI reversibility	Acute stroke – usually following thrombolysis
	Venous infarction
	Hemiplegic migraine
	Transient global amnesia
	Status epilepticus
Lesion location	White matter more often than gray matter
Amount of DWI reversible tissue in arterial strokes following tPA	12–33%
ADC values	Higher in DWI-reversible versus DWI-nonreversible tissue
	$(663–732) \times 10^{-6}$ mm^2/s in DWI-reversible regions
	$(608–650) \times 10^{-6}$ mm^2/s in DWI-abnormal regions that infarct

pared with 608×10^{-6} mm$^2 \cdot$ s^{-1} to 650×10^{-6} mm$^2 \cdot$ s^{-1} in DWI-abnormal regions that infarct [40, 41]. Animal models have also shown high correlation between threshold ADCs of 550×10^{-6} mm$^2 \cdot$ s^{-1} and tissue volume with histologic infarction.

Other studies question the existence of an ADC threshold. In one study, the final T2 lesion volume on day 7 was less than half the tissue volume with an initial ADC of less than 60% of normal in two patients with early reperfusion [42]. This is well below the threshold ADCs of approximately 80% of normal tissue, discussed above. It is likely that the duration and severity of ischemia rather than the absolute ADC value determine ADC normalization and tissue recovery. For example, the degree of ADC decrease correlates strongly with the severity of perfusion deficits, and the cerebral blood flow (CBF) threshold for tissue infarction increases with increasing occlusion time [43]. Jones et al. [44] demonstrated that the CBF threshold for tissue infarction was 10–12 ml 100 g^{-1} min^{-1} for 2–3 h of occlusion but 17–18 ml 100 g^{-1} min^{-1} for permanent occlusion of the MCA in monkeys [44].

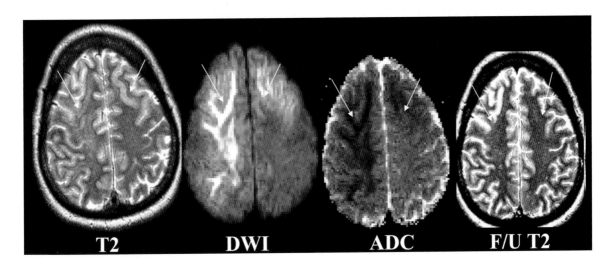

T2   **DWI**   **ADC**   **F/U T2**

Figure 7.11

A 31-year-old female with seizures and superior sagittal sinus thrombosis and reversible DWI abnormalities. In the bilateral frontal and right parietal lobes, there is T2 and DWI hyperintensity and ADC hypointensity (*arrows*). These findings are consistent with cytotoxic edema. On follow-up T2-weighted images (*F/U T2*), following thrombolysis, the lesions have nearly completely resolved

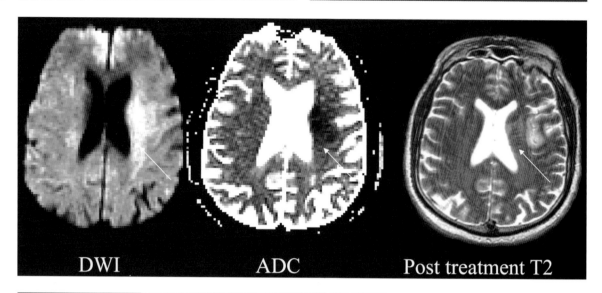

DWI   ADC   Post treatment T2

Figure 7.12

Acute ischemic stroke with DWI reversibility. Patient is a 69-year-old male with sudden onset of speech difficulties and right-sided weakness. MRA demonstrated MCA occlusion. He was treated with intra-arterial (*i.a.*) rtPA with complete recanalization. DWI images and ADC maps demonstrate acute ischemia involving the left caudate body, corona radiata, and frontal subcortical white matter. Follow-up T2-weighted images demonstrate hyperintensity, consistent with infarction in the frontal subcortical white matter and part of the caudate body and corona radiata. However, part of the corona radiata (*white arrow*) and caudate body appear normal on the follow-up T2-weighted images

7.8 Prediction of Hemorrhagic Transformation

Hemorrhagic transformation (HT) of brain infarction represents secondary bleeding into ischemic tissue with a natural incidence of 15% to 26% during the first 2 weeks and up to 43% over the first month after cerebral infarction [45–48] (Table 7.5). Predisposing factors include stroke etiology (HT is more frequent with embolic strokes), reperfusion, good collateral circulation, hypertension, anticoagulant therapy, and thrombolytic therapy. In patients treated with intra-arterial (i.a.) thrombolytic therapy, a higher National Institutes of Health Stroke Scale (NIHSS) score, a longer time to recanalization, a lower platelet count, and a higher glucose level are associated with HT [49].

The most commonly proposed pathophysiological mechanism for HT is that severe ischemia leads to greater disruption of the cerebral microvasculature and greater degradation of the blood–brain barrier. Reperfusion into the damaged capillaries following clot lysis leads to blood extravasation with the development of petechial hemorrhage or hematoma. However, multiple studies describe HT in spite of persistent arterial occlusion [45, 50]. HT in this setting may result from preservation of collateral flow. rtPA thrombolytic therapy may aggravate ischemia-induced microvascular damage by activation of the plasminogen-plasmin system with release and activation of metalloproteinases [51–53] that are thought to cause degradation of the basal lamina during an ischemic insult.

Table 7.5. Factors associated with hemorrhagic transformation. (*CBF* Cerebral blood flow, *MCA* middle cerebral artery, *NIHSS* National Institutes of Health Stroke Scale)

Clinical	High NIHSS
	Low platelets
	High glucose
	Hypertension
Vascular	Good collateral vessels
	Early reperfusion
	Embolic stroke
Therapy	Anticoagulation
	Thrombolytic therapy
Imaging parameters	Larger volume of the initial DWI abnormality
	Higher percentage of pixels with ADC <550×10^{-6} mm^2/s
	Hypodensity in greater than one-third of the MCA territory on CT
	Early parenchymal enhancement
	Prior microbleeds detected on T2* gradient echo images
	Very low CBF on SPECT and MR perfusion imaging

Since ADC values can mark the severity and extent of ischemia, a number of investigators have assessed the value of the ADC in predicting HT (Fig. 7.13). Selim et al. [54] demonstrated that the volume of the initial DWI lesion and the absolute number of voxels with ADC value ≤550 × 10^{-6} mm^{2}s correlated with HT of infarctions treated with intravenous t-PA [54]. Tong et al. [55] demonstrated that the mean ADC of ischemic regions that experienced HT was significantly lower than the overall mean ADC of all ischemic areas analyzed [(510±140)×10^{-6} mm^2 · s^{-1} versus (623±113)×10^{-6} mm^2 · s^{-1}]. There was also a significant difference when comparing the HT-destined ischemic areas with non-HT-destined areas within the same ischemic lesion (P=0.02). Oppenheim et al. [56] demonstrated 100% sensitivity and 71% specificity for predicting hemorrhagic transfor-

mation when they divided infarcts into those with a mean ADC core of less than 300×10^{-6} mm^2 · s^{-1} versus those with a mean ADC core of greater than 300×10^{-6} mm^2 · s^{-1}) [56]. Other imaging parameters predictive of HT include

1. Hypodensity in greater than one-third of the MCA territory on CT [57].
2. Early parenchymal enhancement on gadolinium-enhanced T1-weighted images [58].
3. Ischemic brain tissue with a CBF less than 35% of the normal cerebellar blood flow on SPECT imaging [59].
4. CBF ratio of less than 0.18 on MR perfusion imaging [60].
5. Prior microbleeds detected on T2* gradient echo [61].

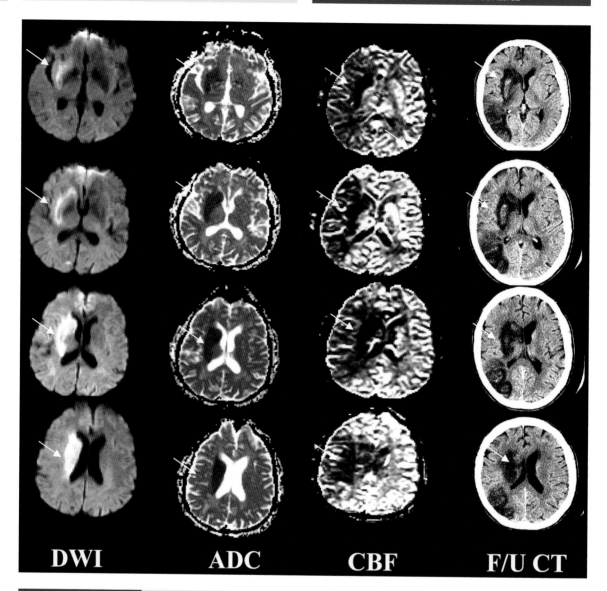

DWI ADC CBF F/U CT

Figure 7.13

Acute ischemic stroke with hemorrhagic transformation. Patient is 76-year-old male with left-sided hemiplegia, treated with i.a. rtPA. There is an acute stroke (DWI hyperintense, ADC hypointense) involving the right insula, subinsular region, basal ganglia, and deep white matter. Note the profound reduction in ADC and cerebral blood flow (*CBF*) in the basal ganglia and deep white matter (*white arrows*) where there is hemorrhagic transformation on follow-up CT (*F/U CT*). Follow-up CT also demonstrates extension of the infarction into the right parietal but not into the right frontal portion of the ischemic penumbra

Table 7.6. Diffusion tensor imaging

Parameters measured	1. Trace of the diffusion tensor [Tr(ADC)] or the average diffusivity calculates overall diffusion in a tissue region, independent of direction
	2. Indices of diffusion anisotropy – fractional anisotropy (*FA*) and lattice index (*LI*), calculate the degree of differences in diffusion in different directions
	3. Fiber orientation mapping provides information on white matter tract structure, integrity and connectivity
Tr(ADC)	Discriminates differences in gray versus white matter diffusion
	<D> decreases greater in WM versus GM in acute and subacute periods
	<D> increases much more in white matter than in gray matter in the chronic period
FA	Correlates with stroke onset time
	Elevated for up to 12 hours and then decreases over time
	Correlates inversely with T2 change
	Three temporal stages in stroke evolution: Increased FA and reduced ADC Decreased FA and decreased ADC Decreased FA and elevated ADC
Fiber orientation mapping	Can detect Wallerian degeneration prior to conventional images
	May be useful in predicting motor function at outcome

7.9 Diffusion Tensor Imaging

The physical principles of diffusion tensor imaging (DTI) are discussed in the Section 7.2.1 above. DTI allows the calculation of three parameters that all may be useful in the evaluation of acute ischemic stroke (Table 7.6).

1. The trace of the diffusion tensor [Tr(ADC)] or the average diffusivity, <D> ($<D> = (\lambda_1 + \lambda_2 + \lambda_3)/3$ where λ_1, λ_2, and λ_3 are the eigenvalues of the diffusion tensor] that calculates the overall diffusion in a tissue region, independent of direction [62].
2. Indices of diffusion anisotropy, such as fractional anisotropy (FA) or the lattice index (LI), that calculate of the degree of differences in diffusion in different directions [2, 63].
3. Fiber orientation mapping that provides information on white matter tract structure, integrity, and connectivity [64–66].

Because DTI has a relatively high signal-to-noise ratio, measurement of average diffusivity, <D>, has provided new information on differences between gray and white matter diffusion that were not appreciable with the measurement of diffusion along three orthogonal directions [67, 68]. A number of studies have demonstrated that <D> decreases are greater in white matter versus gray matter in the acute and subacute periods and that <D> increases are much higher in white matter versus gray matter in the chronic period. Furthermore, <D> images may detect regions of reduced white matter diffusion that appeared normal on diffusion-weighted images. While gray matter is typically considered to be more vulnerable to ischemia than white matter, recent animal experiments have demonstrated that severe histopathologic changes can occur in white matter as early as 30 min after acute stroke onset. Also, reduced bulk water motion from cytoskeletal collapse and disruption of fast axonal transport, which do not exist in gray matter, may occur in white matter.

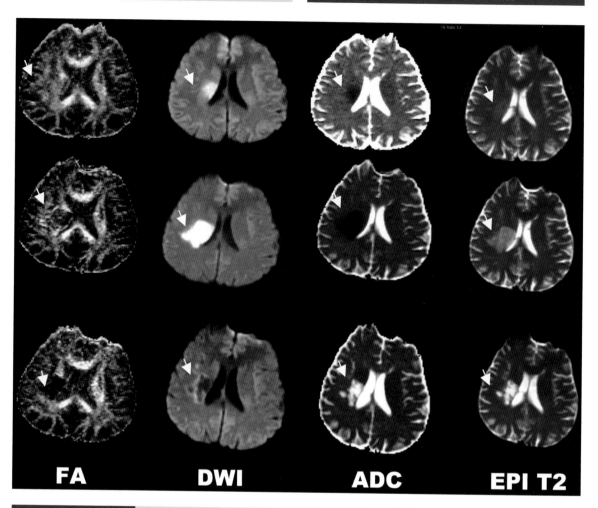

Figure 7.14

Temporal evolution of fractional anisotropy (*FA*) changes in acute ischemic stroke. A 50-year-old male with left hemiparesis was examined at 5 h, 3 days, and 3 months after onset. At 5 h (*row 1*), the right putamen stroke (*arrow*) is hyperintense on FA images, hyperintense on DWI images, hypointense on ADC images and is not seen on echo planar T2-weighted images (*EPI T2*). These findings are consistent with the first stage of FA changes in stroke described by Yang et al. [76]. After 3 days (*row 2*), the lesion is hypointense on FA images, hyperintense on DWI images, hypointense on ADC images, and hyperintense on T2-weighted images. These findings are consistent with the second stage of FA changes in stroke described by Yang et al. [76]. At 3 months (*row 3*), the lesion is hypointense on FA images, hypointense on DWI images, hyperintense on ADC images, and hyperintense on T2-weighted images. These findings are consistent with third stage of FA changes in stroke described by Yang et al. [76]

Diffusion anisotropy refers to the principle that water diffusion is different in different directions due to tissue structure [69, 70]. Gray matter has relatively low diffusion anisotropy. In white matter, diffusion is much greater parallel than perpendicular to white matter tracts, in part because white matter has highly organized tract bundles [62, 69, 71, 72]. Oligodendrocyte concentration and fast axonal transport may

Figure 7.15

Wallerian degeneration in the right corticospinal tract 3 months after an infarction in the right MCA territory. Fractional anisotropy (*FA*) images demonstrate hypointensity secondary to reduced FA in the right corticospinal tract (*arrow*)

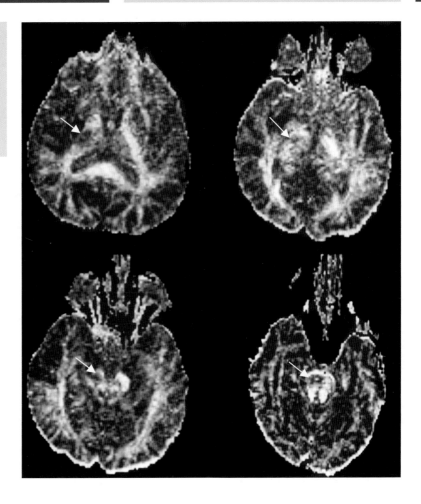

also contribute to diffusion anisotropy. In addition, it is thought that the intracellular compartment is more anisotropic while the extracellular compartment is less anisotropic [73]. Sources of anisotropy in the intracellular compartment could be the presence of microtubules, organelles, and intact membranes [74].

In the acute stroke setting, FA correlates with time of stroke onset [75, 76]. In general, FA is elevated in the hyperacute and early acute periods, becomes reduced at 12–24 h and progressively decreases over time. However, there are different temporal rates of stroke progression and a number of investigators have demonstrated that there is heterogeneity between lesions and within lesions of FA evolution [75, 76]. Yang et al. [76] described three temporally relat-

ed different phases in the relationship between FA and ADC (Fig. 7.14). Increased FA and reduced ADC characterize the initial phase, reduced FA and reduced ADC characterize the second phase, and reduced FA with elevated ADC characterize the more chronic third phase [76]. Furthermore, FA inversely correlates with T2 signal change [77].

These changes can be explained as follows. As cytotoxic edema develops, there is shift of water from the extracellular to the intracellular space, but cell membranes remain intact and there is yet to be an overall increase in tissue water. This would explain elevated FA, reduced ADC, and normal T2. As the ischemic insult progresses, cells lyse, the glial reaction occurs and there is degradation of the blood–brain

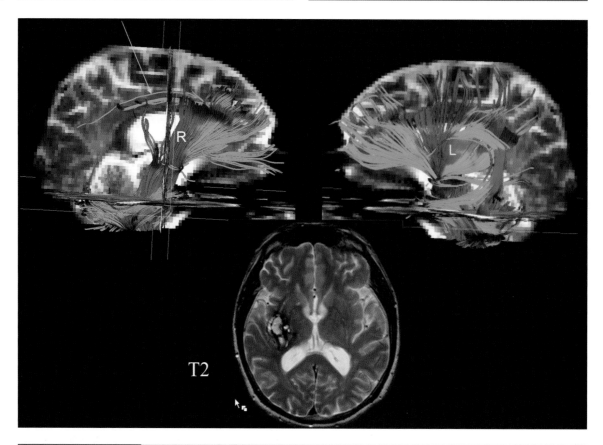

Figure 7.16

A 70-year-old male with acute left hemiparesis secondary to hypertensive hemorrhage. Diffusion tensor tractography images demonstrate disruption of the right corticospinal tract

barrier, and an overall increase in tissue water, predominantly in the extracellular space. This would explain reduced FA, elevated ADC, and elevated T2. Reduced FA, reduced ADC, and elevated T2 may occur when there is an overall increase in tissue water but the intracellular fraction is still high enough to cause reduced ADCs and the extracellular portion is high enough to cause reduced FAs. Other factors, such as loss of axonal transport, loss of cellular integrity, and decreases in interstitial fluid flow, may contribute to decreases in FA over time.

A number of studies have demonstrated that the decreases in FA associated with ischemia are significantly greater in white matter compared with gray matter [68, 76]. The reason for these differences likely relates to the structural differences between gray and white matter. In the white matter extracellular space, there are dense arrays of parallel white matter tracts. With acute ischemia, the diffusion decrease is much greater in λ_1, the eigenvalue that coincides with the long axis of white matter fiber tracts, compared with the other eigenvalues. In the gray matter extracellular space there is a meshwork. With acute ischemia, the diffusion decrease is similar between eigenvalues.

Investigators are beginning to evaluate how strokes affect adjacent white matter tracts. Fiber orientation mapping can detect Wallerian degeneration prior to conventional images and may be useful in predicting motor function at outcome (Figs. 7.15, 7.16). One study demonstrated that FA is significantly decreased in the internal capsules and corona radiata in acute stroke patients with moderate to severe hemiparesis versus patients with no or mild hemiparesis [78]. Another study of subacute stroke patients demonstrated a significant reduction in the eigenvalues perpendicular to the axial imaging plane at 2–3 weeks in eight patients with poor recovery following acute stroke, but not in eight patients with good recovery [79]. In the chronic period, DTI can distinguish between a primary stroke and a region of Wallerian degeneration. A primary chronic stroke has reduced FA and elevated mean diffusivity, while the corticospinal tract has reduced FA but preserved or only slightly elevated mean diffusivity [80].

7.10 Correlation with Clinical Outcome

A number of studies have shown how DWI can be used to predict clinical outcome. Some studies have demonstrated statistically significant correlations between the acute anterior circulation DWI and ADC lesion volume and both acute and chronic neurological assessment tests including the NIHSS, the Canadian Neurological Scale, the Glasgow Outcome Score, the Barthel Index, and the Modified Rankin Scale [25, 81–87]. Correlations between DWI and ADC volume and clinical outcome range from $r=0.65$ to 0.78. In general, correlations are stronger for cortical strokes than for penetrator artery strokes [25, 83]. Lesion location may explain this difference. For example, a small ischemic lesion in the brainstem could produce a worse neurologic deficit than a cortical lesion of the same size. In fact, one study of posterior circulation strokes showed no correlation between initial DWI lesion volume and NIHSS [88]. A significant correlation has also been reported between the acute ADC ratio (ADC of lesion/ADC of normal contralateral brain) and chronic neurologic assessment scales [25, 81]. Furthermore, one study demonstrated that patients with a mismatch between the initial NIHSS score (>8) and the initial DWI lesion volume (<25 ml) had a higher probability of infarct growth

and early neurologic deterioration [89]. Another demonstrated that, for ICA and MCA strokes, a DWI volume greater than $89\,cm^3$ was highly predictive [receiver operating characteristic (ROC) curve with 85.7% sensitivity and 95.7% specificity] of early neurologic deterioration [90].

7.11 Stroke Mimics

These syndromes generally fall into four categories: (1) nonischemic lesions with no acute abnormality on routine or diffusion-weighted images; (2) ischemic lesions with reversible clinical deficits which may have imaging abnormalities; (3) vasogenic edema syndromes which may mimic acute infarction clinically and on conventional imaging; (4) other entities with decreased diffusion.

7.12 Nonischemic Lesions with No Acute Abnormality on Routine or Diffusion-Weighted Images

Nonischemic syndromes that present with signs and symptoms of acute stroke but have no acute abnormality identified on DWI or routine MR images include peripheral vertigo, migraines, seizures, dementia, functional disorders, and metabolic disorders. The clinical deficits associated with these syndromes are usually reversible. If initial imaging is normal and a clinical deficit persists, repeat DWI should be obtained [36]. False-negative DWI and perfusion-weighted images (PWI) occur in patients with small brainstem or deep gray nuclei lacunar infarctions.

7.13 Syndromes with Reversible Clinical Deficits that may have Decreased Diffusion

7.13.1 Transient Ischemic Attack

An acute neurologic deficit of presumed vascular etiology that resolves within 24 h is defined as a transient ischemic attack (TIA). Of patients with TIAs, 21–48% have DWI hyperintense lesions, consistent with small infarctions [91–94] (Fig. 7.17). These le-

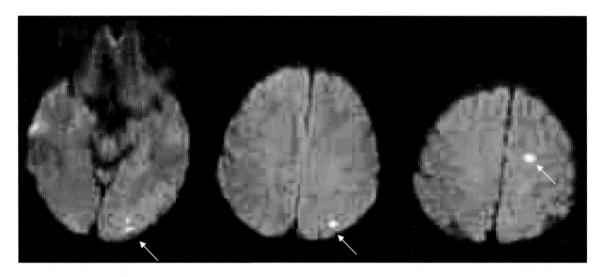

Figure 7.17

Transient ishcemic attack. Patient is 57-year-old male with transient right hand, arm and leg weakness and numbness. DWI images demonstrate punctate hyperintense lesions, consistent with acute infarctions, in the left occipital, parietal and frontal lobes (*white arrows*)

sions are usually less than 15 mm in size and are in the clinically appropriate vascular territory. In one study, 20% of the lesions were not seen at follow-up; the lesions could have been too small to see on follow-up conventional MRI due to atrophy or they could have been reversible [92]. The small DWI lesions are most likely not the cause of the patient's symptoms, but may represent markers of a more widespread reversible ischemia. Reported statistically significant independent predictors of lesions with decreased diffusion on DWI are previous nonstereotypic TIA, cortical syndrome, an identified stroke mechanism, TIA duration greater than 30 min, aphasia, motor deficits, and disturbance of higher brain function [91, 92, 94, 95]. One study demonstrated an increased stroke risk in patients with TIAs and abnormalities on DWI [93]. In another study, the information obtained from DWI changed the suspected localization of the ischemic lesion as well as the suspected etiologic mechanism in over one-third of patients [92].

7.13.2 Transient Global Amnesia

Transient global amnesia (TGA) is a clinical syndrome characterized by sudden onset of profound memory impairment resulting in both retrograde and anterograde amnesia without other neurological deficits. The symptoms typically resolve in 3–4 h. Many patients with TGA have no acute abnormality on conventional or diffusion-weighted images [96]. A number of studies, however, have reported punctate lesions with decreased diffusion in the medial hippocampus, the parahippocampal gyrus, and the splenium of the corpus callosum [97–100] (Fig. 7.18). Follow-up T2-weighted sequences in some patients have shown persistence of these lesions that the authors concluded were small infarctions. One study, however, reported more diffuse and subtle DWI hyperintense lesions in the hippocampus that resolved on follow-up imaging [101]. The authors concluded that this phenomenon might be secondary to spreading depression rather than reversible ischemia. One more recent study demonstrated that the detection of DWI changes in TGA is delayed [102]; the authors ob-

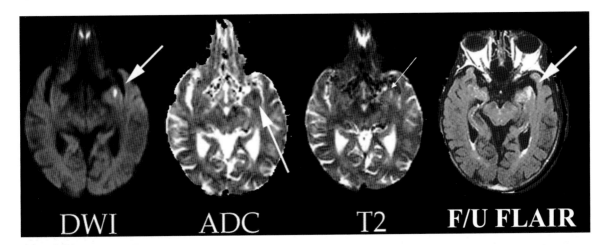

Figure 7.18

Transient global amnesia. Patient is 77-year-old female with acute global amnesia that resolved within 24 h. There is a punctate DWI and T2 hyperintense and ADC hypointense lesion in the left medial temporal lobe (*arrows*). The lesion persists on follow-up FLAIR images

served DWI abnormalities in only 2/31 patients with TGA in the hyperacute phase, but at 48 hours, 26/31 patients had DWI abnormalities in the hippocampus. It is currently unclear whether the TGA patients with DWI abnormalities have a different prognosis, or different etiologic mechanism or whether they should be managed differently compared to TGA patients without DWI abnormalities.

7.14 Vasogenic Edema Syndromes

Patients with these syndromes frequently present with acute neurologic deficits, which raise the question of acute ischemic stroke (Table 7.7). Furthermore, conventional imaging cannot reliably differentiate cytotoxic from vasogenic edema because both types of edema produce T2 hyperintensity in gray and/or white matter. Diffusion MR imaging has become essential in differentiating these syndromes from acute stroke because it can reliably distinguish vasogenic from cytotoxic edema. While cytotoxic edema is characterized by decreased diffusion, vaso-

genic edema is characterized by elevated diffusion due to a relative increase in water in the extracellular compartment [103–105]. Vasogenic edema is characteristically hypointense to slightly hyperintense on DWI images because these images have both T2 and diffusion contributions. Vasogenic edema is hyperintense on ADC maps and hypointense on exponential images while cytotoxic edema is hypointense in ADC maps and hyperintense on exponential images.

7.14.1 Posterior Reversible Encephalopathy Syndrome (PRES)

PRES is a syndrome that occurs secondary to loss of cerebral autoregulation and capillary leakage in association with a variety of clinical entities [106]. These include acute hypertension; treatment with immunosuppressive agents such as cyclosporin and tacrolimus; treatment with chemotherapeutic agents such as intrathecal methotrexate, cisplatin and interferon alpha interferon; and hematologic disorders such as hemolytic uremic syndrome, thrombotic thrombocytopenia purpura, acute intermittent por-

Table 7.7. Stroke mimics

Nonischemic syndromes that present with signs and symptoms of acute stroke but have no acute abnormality identified on DWI or routine MR images

Peripheral vertigo
Migraines
Seizures
Dementia
Functional disorders
Amyloid angiopathy
Metabolic disorders

Syndromes with reversible clinical deficits that may have decreased diffusion

Transient ischemic attacks
  – 21–48% with DWI-hyperintense lesions
  – DWI-hyperintense lesions associated with increased stroke risk
  – DWI-hyperintense lesions change the suspected localization of the ischemic lesion as well as the suspected etiologic mechanism in over one-third of patients
Transient global amnesia
  – Punctate lesions with decreased diffusion in the hippocampus, the parahippocampal gyrus, and the splenium of the corpus callosum
  – Some lesions appear at later time points
  – Some lesions resolve
  – Question of ischemic versus spreading depression mechanism

Vasogenic edema/capillary leak syndromes

Syndromes
  – Posterior reversible encephalopathy syndrome
  – Hyperperfusion syndrome post carotid endarterectomy
Conventional MR imaging findings
  – T2 hyperintensity in gray and/or white matter that may mimic acute stroke
DWI findings
  – Elevated diffusion secondary to vasogenic edema
  – May have peripheral cytotoxic edema due to mass effect and capillary compression
  – Occasionally have vasogenic edema followed by cytotoxic edema in the whole lesion

phyria and cryoglobulinemia [107–118]. Typical presenting features are headaches, decreased alertness, altered mental status, seizures, and visual loss including cortical blindness.

The pathophysiology is not entirely clear [105, 119]. The predominant hypothesis is that markedly increased pressure and/or toxins damage endothelial tight junctions. This leads to extravasation of fluid and the development of vasogenic edema. Another less likely possibility, based on angiographic findings of narrowings in medium- and large-sized vessels, is that vasospasm is the major pathophysiologic mechanism.

T2- and FLAIR-weighted sequences typically demonstrate bilateral symmetric hyperintensity and swelling in subcortical white matter and overlying cortex in the occipital, parietal, and posterior temporal lobes as well as the posterior fossa. The posterior circulation predominance is thought to result from the fact that there is less sympathetic innervation (which supplies vasoconstrictive protection to the brain in the setting of acute hypertension) in the posterior compared with the anterior circulation. However, anterior circulation lesions are not uncommon, and are frequently in a borderzone distribution.

Acutely, DWI usually show elevated and less frequently normal diffusion (Fig. 7.19). Rarely, there are small foci of decreased diffusion. This is helpful since posterior distribution lesions can mimic basilar tip occlusion with arterial infarctions, and borderzone anterior circulation lesions can mimic watershed infarctions both clinically and on T2-weighted sequences. Arterial and watershed infarctions are characterized by decreased diffusion. The clinical deficits and MR abnormalities are typically reversible. However, rare small areas of decreased diffusion that progress to infarction have been observed and, in some cases, tissue initially characterized by elevated or normal diffusion progresses to infarction [120].

7.14.2 Hyperperfusion Syndrome Following Carotid Endarterectomy

In rare cases following carotid endarterectomy, patients may develop a hyperperfusion syndrome [121]. Patients typically present with seizures, but may have focal neurologic deficits. T2-weighted images demonstrate hyperintensity in frontal and parietal cortex and subcortical white matter that may mimic arterial infarction. However, unlike

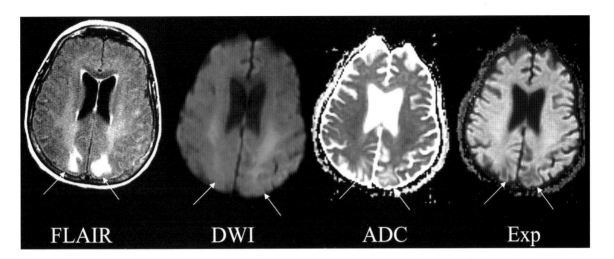

FLAIR   DWI   ADC   Exp

Figure 7.19

Posterior reversible encephalopathy syndrome. Patient is 64-year-old female with mental status changes. FLAIR images demonstrate hyperintense lesions in the bilateral parietal occipital regions that suggest acute infarctions (*arrows*). The lesions are isointense on DWI images, hyperintense on ADC images, and hypointense on exponential images. These diffusion MR characteristics are consistent with vasogenic edema

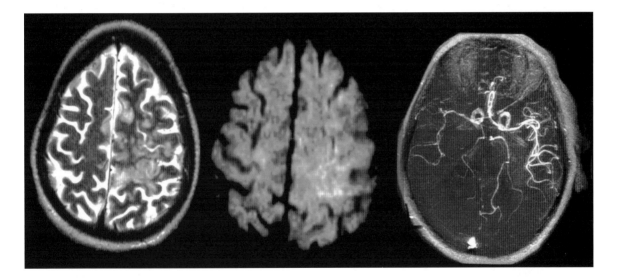

Figure 7.20

Hyperperfusion syndrome following carotid endarterectomy (CEA). Patient is 79-year-old female 1 week after CEA, with status epilepticus. T2-weighted image demonstrates gray and white matter hyperintensity in the left frontal lobe, suggestive of acute infarction. There is no decreased diffusion on the DWI images. ADC maps (not shown) demonstrated elevated diffusion, consistent with vasogenic edema. 3D time-of-flight MRA demonstrates increased flow-related enhancement in the left middle cerebral artery territory

Table 7.8. Other entities that may show restricted diffusion

Disease	Possible pathophysiologic basis for decreased diffusion
Herpes virus encephalitis	Necrotizing meningoencephalitis with cytotoxic edema
Creutzfeldt–Jakob disease	Spongiform change with myelin vacuolization
Diffuse axonal injury	Cytotoxic edema or axonal retraction balls
Hypoglycemia	Cytotoxic edema
Lymphoma, medulloblastoma	High tumor cellularity
Bacterial abscess	Viscous pus
Hemorrhage – oxyhemoglobin and extracellular methemoglobin	Oxyhemoglobin – cell membranes intact Extracellular methemoglobin – undetermined
Acute multiple sclerosis or acute disseminated encephalomyelitis	Increased inflammatory infiltrate, myelin vacuolization
Epidermoid tumors	Tumor cellularity
Venous sinus thrombosis[a]	Cytotoxic edema
Transient global amnesia[a]	Cytotoxic edema or spreading depression
Seizure[a]	Cytotoxic edema
Hemiplegic migraine[a]	Cytotoxic edema or spreading depression

[a] May be reversible

acute infarctions, the lesions have elevated diffusion (Fig. 7.20). Also, there may be increased rather than diminished flow-related enhancement in the ipsilateral MCA. It is thought that, similar to PRES, increased pressure damages endothelial tight junctions, leading to a capillary leak syndrome and development of vasogenic edema.

7.14.3 Other Syndromes

Rarely, other disease entities such as human immunodeficiency virus (HIV) or other viral encephalopathies, tumor, and acute demyelination can present with acute neurologic deficits and patterns of edema on conventional images suggestive of stroke. Similar to PRES and hyperperfusion syndrome following carotid endarterectomy, DWI show increased diffusion.

7.15 Other Entities with Decreased Diffusion

A number of other entities have decreased diffusion [37] (Table 7.8). These include acute demyelinative lesions with decreased diffusion due to myelin vacuolization; some products of hemorrhage (oxyhemoglobin and extracellular methemoglobin); herpes encephalitis with decreased diffusion due to cytotoxic edema from cell necrosis; diffuse axonal injury with decreased diffusion due to cytotoxic edema or axotomy with retraction ball formation; abscess with decreased diffusion due to the high viscosity of pus; tumors such as lymphoma and small round cell tumors with decreased diffusion due to dense cell packing; and Creutzfeldt–Jakob disease with decreased diffusion from myelin vacuolization. When these lesions are reviewed in combination with routine T1-, FLAIR-, T2- and gadolinium-enhanced T1-weighted images, they are usually readily differentiated from acute infarctions. However, occasionally diffusion and conventional imaging cannot distinguish between a single demyelinative lesion or nonenhancing tumor and an acute stroke. In these situations, spectroscopy may be helpful.

7.16 Venous Infarction

Cerebral venous sinus thrombosis (CVT) is a rare condition that affects fewer than 1 in 10,000 people (Table 7.9). The most common presenting signs and symptoms are headache, seizures, vomiting, and papilledema. Visual changes, altered consciousness, cranial nerve palsies, nystagmus, and focal neurologic deficits are also relatively common. Predisposing factors are protein C and S deficiencies; malignancies; pregnancy; medications such as oral contraceptives, steroids, and hormone replacement therapy; collagen vascular diseases; infection; trauma; surgery; and immobilization [122].

The pathophysiology of CVT is not completely clear [123–134]. Venous obstruction results in increased venous pressure, increased intracranial pressure, decreased perfusion pressure, and decreased cerebral blood flow. Increased venous pressure may result in vasogenic edema from breakdown of the blood–brain barrier and extravasation of fluid into the extracellular space. Blood may also extravasate into the extracellular space. Severely decreased blood flow may also result in cytotoxic edema associated with infarction. Increases in CSF production and resorption have also been reported.

Parenchymal findings on imaging correlate with the degree of venous pressure elevation [135]. With mild to moderate pressure elevations, there is parenchymal swelling with sulcal effacement but without signal abnormality. As pressure elevations become more severe, there is increasing edema and development of intraparenchymal hemorrhage. Superior sagittal sinus thrombosis is characterized by bilateral parasagittal T2-hyperintense lesions involving cortex and subcortical white matter. Transverse sinus thrombosis results in T2-hyperintense signal abnormality involving temporal cortex and subcortical white matter. Deep venous thrombosis is characterized by T2-hyperintense signal abnormalities in the bilateral thalami and sometimes the basal gan-

Table 7.9. Cerebral venous sinus thrombosis

Clinical

Headache
Seizure
Vomiting
Papilledema

Pathophysiology

Increased venous pressure leads to vasogenic edema from blood–brain barrier breakdown and fluid extravasation into the extracellular space

Increased venous pressure leads to increased intracranial pressure, decreased perfusion pressure, decreased cerebral blood flow, and cytotoxic edema

Conventional MR imaging

Hydrocephalus
Parenchymal swelling with sulcal effacement
Intraparenchymal edema
Intraparenchymal hemorrhage
Venous clot

Diffusion MR imaging of T2-hyperintense parenchymal lesions

Lesions with elevated diffusion due to vasogenic edema resolve

Lesions with decreased diffusion due to cytotoxic dema that resolve – resolution may be related to early drainage of blood through collateral pathways or to seizure activity

Lesions with decreased diffusion due to cytotoxic edema that persists

Heterogeneous lesions due to combination of vasogenic and cytotoxic edema

Treatment

Heparin

Intravascular thrombolysis for patients with rapidly progressive brain swelling

glia. Hemorrhage is seen in up to 40% of patients with CVT [136, 137] and is usually located at gray white matter junctions or within the white matter.

DWI has proven helpful in the differentiation of venous from arterial infarction and in the prediction of tissue outcome (Figs. 7.11, 7.21). T2-hyperintense

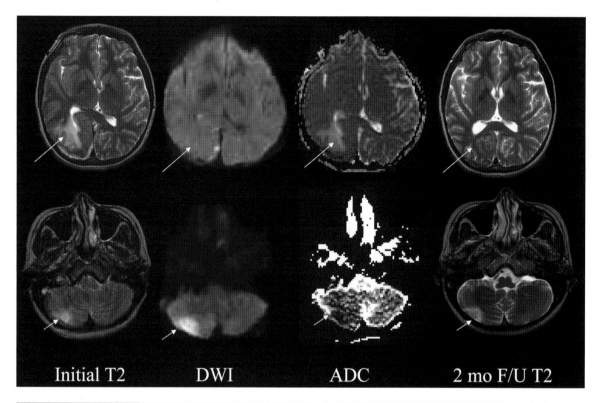

Initial T2   DWI   ADC   2 mo F/U T2

Figure 7.21

Superior sagittal, right transverse, and right sigmoid sinus thrombosis with parenchymal lesions characterized by vasogenic and cytotoxic edema. Patient is 31-year-old male with severe headache and vomiting. MR venogram (not shown) demonstrated thrombosis of the superior sagittal, right transverse, and right sigmoid sinuses. The T2-hyperintense right cerebellar lesion has decreased diffusion (DWI hyperintense and ADC hypointense), consistent with cytotoxic edema (*short white arrow*). The lesion is present at follow-up. The T2-hyperintense right occipital parietal lesion has elevated diffusion (DWI isointense, ADC hyperintense), consistent with vasogenic edema (*long white arrow*). It is no longer present at follow-up

lesions may have decreased diffusion, elevated diffusion or a mixed pattern. Lesions with elevated diffusion are thought to represent vasogenic edema and usually resolve. Lesions with decreased diffusion are thought to represent cytotoxic edema. Unlike arterial stroke, some of these lesions resolve and some persist. Resolution of lesions with decreased diffusion may be related to better drainage of blood through collateral pathways in some patients. In one paper, lesions with decreased diffusion that resolved were only seen in patients with seizure activity [138].

7.17 Conclusion

Diffusion MR imaging has vastly improved evaluation of acute ischemic stroke. It is highly sensitive and specific in the detection of acute ischemic stroke at early time points when CT and conventional MR sequences are unreliable. The initial DWI lesion is thought to represent infarct core and usually progresses to infarction unless there is early reperfusion. The initial DWI lesion volume and ADC ratios correlate highly with final infarct volume as well as with acute and chronic neurologic assessment tests. ADC values may be useful in differentiating tissue destined to infarct from tissue that is ischemic but potentially salvageable with reperfusion therapy. ADC values may also be useful in determining tissue at risk of undergoing hemorrhagic transformation following reperfusion therapy. Diffusion tensor imaging can delineate the differences in responses of gray versus white matter to ischemia. Fractional anisotropy may be important in determining stroke onset time and tractography provides early detection of Wallerian degeneration that may be important in determining prognosis. Finally, diffusion MR imaging can determine which patients with transient ischemic attack are at risk for subsequent large vessel infarction and can reliably differentiate stroke from stroke mimics. With improvements in MR software and hardware, diffusion MR will undoubtedly continue to improve our management and treatment of acute stroke patients.

References

1. Cooper R et al (1974) Restricted diffusion in biophysical systems. Exp Biophys J 14(3):161–177
2. Stejskal E, Tanner J (1965) Spin diffusion measurements: spin echos in the presence of time-dependent field gradient. J Chem Phys 42:288–292
3. Basser PJ, Pierpaoli C (1996) Microstructural and physiological features of tissues elucidated by quantitative-diffusion-tensor MRI. J Magn Reson B 111(3):209–219
4. Sevick RJ et al (1992) Cytotoxic brain edema: assessment with diffusion-weighted MR imaging. Radiology 185(3): 687–690
5. Mintorovitch J et al (1994) Diffusion-weighted magnetic resonance imaging of acute focal cerebral ischemia: comparison of signal intensity with changes in brain water and Na$^+$,K(+)-ATPase activity. J Cereb Blood Flow Metab 14(2):332–336
6. Benveniste H, Hedlund LW, Johnson GA (1992) Mechanism of detection of acute cerebral ischemia in rats by diffusion-weighted magnetic resonance microscopy. Stroke 23(5): 746–754
7. Niendorf T et al (1996) Biexponential diffusion attenuation in various states of brain tissue: implications for diffusion-weighted imaging. Magn Reson Med 36(6):847–857
8. Sykova E et al (1994) Extracellular volume fraction and diffusion characteristics during progressive ischemia and terminal anoxia in the spinal cord of the rat. J Cereb Blood Flow Metab 14(2):301–311
9. Wick M et al (1995) Alteration of intracellular metabolite diffusion in rat brain in vivo during ischemia and reperfusion. Stroke 26(10):1930–1933; discussion 1934
10. Van der Toorn A et al (1996) Diffusion of metabolites in normal and ischemic rat brain measured by localized 1H MRS. Magn Reson Med 36(6):914–922
11. Duong TQ et al (1998) Evaluation of extra- and intracellular apparent diffusion in normal and globally ischemic rat brain via 19F NMR. Magn Reson Med 40(1):1–13
12. Morikawa E et al (1992) The significance of brain temperature in focal cerebral ischemia: histopathological consequences of middle cerebral artery occlusion in the rat. J Cereb Blood Flow Metab 12(3):380–389
13. Le Bihan DJ, Delannoy, Levin RL (1989) Temperature mapping with MR imaging of molecular diffusion: application to hyperthermia. Radiology 171(3):853–857
14. Szafer A, Zhong J, Gore JC (1995) Theoretical model for water diffusion in tissues. Magn Reson Med 33(5):697–712
15. Helpern J, Ordidige R, Knight R (1992) The effect of cell membrane water permeability on the apparent diffusion of water. Society of Magnetic Resonance in Medicine, Berlin
16. Kucharczyk J et al (1993) Echo-planar perfusion-sensitive MR imaging of acute cerebral ischemia. Radiology 188(3): 711–717
17. Matsumoto K et al (1995) Role of vasogenic edema and tissue cavitation in ischemic evolution on diffusion-weighted imaging: comparison with multiparameter MR and immunohistochemistry. Am J Neuroradiol 16(5):1107–1115
18. Kucharczyk J et al (1991) Diffusion/perfusion MR imaging of acute cerebral ischemia. Magn Reson Med 19(2):311–315
19. Moseley ME et al (1990) Early detection of regional cerebral ischemia in cats: comparison of diffusion- and T2-weighted MRI and spectroscopy. Magn Reson Med 14(2): 330–346
20. Moseley ME et al (1990) Diffusion-weighted MR imaging of acute stroke: correlation with T2-weighted and magnetic susceptibility-enhanced MR imaging in cats. Am J Neuroradiol 11(3):423–429
21. Mintorovitch J et al (1991) Comparison of diffusion- and T2-weighted MRI for the early detection of cerebral ischemia and reperfusion in rats. Magn Reson Med 18(1):39–50
22. Moonen CT et al (1991) Restricted and anisotropic displacement of water in healthy cat brain and in stroke studied by NMR diffusion imaging. Magn Reson Med 19(2): 327–332
23. Warach S et al (1995) Acute human stroke studied by whole brain echo planar diffusion-weighted magnetic resonance imaging. Ann Neurol 37(2):231–241
24. Schlaug G et al (1997) Time course of the apparent diffusion coefficient (ADC) abnormality in human stroke. Neurology 49(1):113–119
25. Lutsep HL et al (1997) Clinical utility of diffusion-weighted magnetic resonance imaging in the assessment of ischemic stroke. Ann Neurol 41(5):574–580

26. Schwamm LH et al (1998) Time course of lesion development in patients with acute stroke: serial diffusion- and hemodynamic-weighted magnetic resonance imaging. Stroke 29(11):2268–2276

27. Copen WA et al (2001) Ischemic stroke: effects of etiology and patient age on the time course of the core apparent diffusion coefficient. Radiology 221(1):27–34

28. Marks MP et al (1999) Evaluation of early reperfusion and i.v. tPA therapy using diffusion- and perfusion-weighted MRI. Neurology 52(9):1792–1798

29. Nagesh V et al (1998) Time course of ADCw changes in ischemic stroke: beyond the human eye! Stroke 29(9):1778–1782

30. Gonzalez RG et al (1999) Diffusion-weighted MR imaging: diagnostic accuracy in patients imaged within 6 hours of stroke symptom onset. Radiology 210(1):155–162

31. Mohr J et al (1995) Magnetic resonance versus computed tomographic imaging in acute stroke. Stroke 26:807–812

32. Bryan R et al (1991) Diagnosis of acute cerebral infarction: comparison of CT and MR imaging. Am J Neuroradiol 12:611–620

33. Lovblad KO et al (1998) Clinical experience with diffusion-weighted MR in patients with acute stroke. Am J Neuroradiol 19(6):1061–1066

34. Mullins ME et al (2002) CT and conventional and diffusion-weighted MR imaging in acute stroke: study in 691 patients at presentation to the emergency department. Radiology 224(2):353–360

35. Marks MP et al (1996) Acute and chronic stroke: navigated spin-echo diffusion-weighted MR imaging. Radiology 199(2):403–408

36. Ay H et al (1999) Normal diffusion-weighted MRI during stroke-like deficits. Neurology 52(9):1784–1792

37. Schaefer PW, Grant PE, Gonzalez RG (2000) Diffusion-weighted MR imaging of the brain. Radiology 217(2):331–345

38. Singer MB et al (1998) Diffusion-weighted MRI in acute subcortical infarction. Stroke 29(1):133–136

39. Grant PE et al (2001) Frequency and clinical context of decreased apparent diffusion coefficient reversal in the human brain. Radiology 221(1):43–50

40. Kidwell CS et al (2002) Late secondary ischemic injury in patients receiving intraarterial thrombolysis. Ann Neurol 52(6):698–703

41. Schaefer PW et al (2002) Predicting cerebral ischemic infarct volume with diffusion and perfusion MR imaging. Am J Neuroradiol 23(10):1785–1794

42. Fiehler J et al (2002) Severe ADC decreases do not predict irreversible tissue damage in humans. Stroke 33(1):79–86

43. Fiehler J et al (2001) Apparent diffusion coefficient decreases and magnetic resonance imaging perfusion parameters are associated in ischemic tissue of acute stroke patients. J Cereb Blood Flow Metab 21(5):577–584

44. Jones TH et al (1981) Thresholds of focal cerebral ischemia in awake monkeys. J Neurosurg 54(6):773–782

45. Horowitz SH et al (1991) Computed tomographic-angiographic findings within the first five hours of cerebral infarction. Stroke 22(10):1245–1253

46. Hornig CR, Dorndorf W, Agnoli AL (1986) Hemorrhagic cerebral infarction – a prospective study. Stroke 17(2):179–185

47. Hakim AM, Ryder-Cooke A, Melanson D (1983) Sequential computerized tomographic appearance of strokes. Stroke 14(6):893–897

48. Calandre L, Ortega LF, Bermejo F (1984) Anticoagulation and hemorrhagic infarction in cerebral embolism secondary to rheumatic heart disease. Arch Neurol 41(11):1152–1154

49. Kidwell CS et al (2002) Predictors of hemorrhagic transformation in patients receiving intra-arterial thrombolysis. Stroke 33(3):717–724

50. Ogata J et al (1989) Hemorrhagic infarct of the brain without a reopening of the occluded arteries in cardioembolic stroke. Stroke 20(7):876–883

51. Lijnen HR et al (1998) Regulation of gelatinase activity in mice with targeted inactivation of components of the plasminogen/plasmin system. Thromb Haemost 79(6):1171–1176

52. Liotta LA et al (1981) Effect of plasminogen activator (urokinase), plasmin, and thrombin on glycoprotein and collagenous components of basement membrane. Cancer Res 41(11 Pt 1):4629–4636

53. Carmeliet P et al (1997) Urokinase-generated plasmin activates matrix metalloproteinases during aneurysm formation. Nat Genet 17(4):439–444

54. Selim M et al (2002) Predictors of hemorrhagic transformation after intravenous recombinant tissue plasminogen activator: prognostic value of the initial apparent diffusion coefficient and diffusion-weighted lesion volume. Stroke 33(8):2047–2052

55. Tong DC et al (2001) Prediction of hemorrhagic transformation following acute stroke: role of diffusion- and perfusion-weighted magnetic resonance imaging. Arch Neurol 58(4):587–593

56. Oppenheim C et al (2002) DWI prediction of symptomatic hemorrhagic transformation in acute MCA infarct. J Neuroradiol 29(1):6–13

57. Von Kummer R et al (1997) Acute stroke: usefulness of early CT findings before thrombolytic therapy. Radiology 205(2):327–333

58. Vo KD et al (2003) MR imaging enhancement patterns as predictors of hemorrhagic transformation in acute ischemic stroke. Am J Neuroradiol 24(4):674–679

59. Ueda T et al (1994) Evaluation of risk of hemorrhagic transformation in local intra-arterial thrombolysis in acute ischemic stroke by initial SPECT. Stroke 25(2):298–303

60. Schaefer PW, Roccatagliata L, Schwamm L, Gonzalez RG (2003) Assessing hemorrhagic transformation with diffusion and perfusion MR imaging. In: Book of abstracts of the 41st annual meeting of the American Society of Neuroradiology, Washington DC, 28 April – 2 May 2003

61. Kidwell CS et al (2002) Magnetic resonance imaging detection of microbleeds before thrombolysis: an emerging application. Stroke 33(1):95–98

62. Le Bihan D et al (2001) Diffusion tensor imaging: concepts and applications. J Magn Reson Imaging 13(4):534–546

63. Shimony JS et al (1999) Quantitative diffusion-tensor anisotropy brain MR imaging: normative human data and anatomic analysis. Radiology 212(3):770–784

64. Bammer R, Acar B, Moseley ME (2003) In vivo MR tractography using diffusion imaging. Eur J Radiol 45(3):223–234

65. Conturo TE et al (1999) Tracking neuronal fiber pathways in the living human brain. Proc Natl Acad Sci USA 96(18):10422–10427

66. Makris N et al (1997) Morphometry of in vivo human white matter association pathways with diffusion-weighted magnetic resonance imaging. Ann Neurol 42(6):951–962

67. Mukherjee P et al (2000) Differences between gray matter and white matter water diffusion in stroke: diffusion-tensor MR imaging in 12 patients. Radiology 215(1):211–220

68. Sorensen AG et al (1999) Human acute cerebral ischemia: detection of changes in water diffusion anisotropy by using MR imaging. Radiology 212(3):785–792

69. Pierpaoli C et al (1996) Diffusion tensor MR imaging of the human brain. Radiology 201(3):637–648

70. Reese TG et al (1995) Imaging myocardial fiber architecture in vivo with magnetic resonance. Magn Reson Med 34(6):786–791

71. Moseley ME et al (1990) Diffusion-weighted MR imaging of anisotropic water diffusion in cat central nervous system. Radiology 176(2):439–445

72. Moseley ME et al (1991) Anisotropy in diffusion-weighted MRI. Magn Reson Med 19(2):321–326

73. Le Bihan D, van Zijl P (2002) From the diffusion coefficient to the diffusion tensor. NMR Biomed 15(7–8):431–434

74. Beaulieu C (2002) The basis of anisotropic water diffusion in the nervous system – a technical review. NMR Biomed 15(7–8):435–455

75. Zelaya F et al (1999) An evaluation of the time dependence of the anisotropy of the water diffusion tensor in acute human ischemia. Magn Reson Imaging 17(3):331–348

76. Yang Q et al (1999) Serial study of apparent diffusion coefficient and anisotropy in patients with acute stroke. Stroke 30(11):2382–2390

77. Ozsunar Y et al (2004) Evolution of water diffusion and anisotropy in hyperacute stroke: significant correlation between fractional anisotropy and T2. Am J Neuroradiol 25(5):699–705

78. Higano S et al (2001) Diffusion anisotropy of the internal capsule and the corona radiata in association with stroke and tumors as measured by diffusion-weighted MR imaging. Am J Neuroradiol 22(3):456–463

79. Watanabe T et al (2001) Three-dimensional anisotropy contrast magnetic resonance axonography to predict the prognosis for motor function in patients suffering from stroke. J Neurosurg 94(6):955–960

80. Werring DJ et al (2000) Diffusion tensor imaging can detect and quantify corticospinal tract degeneration after stroke. J Neurol Neurosurg Psychiatry 69(2):269–272

81. Van Everdingen KJ et al (1998) Diffusion-weighted magnetic resonance imaging in acute stroke. Stroke 29(9):1783–1790

82. Tong DC et al (1998) Correlation of perfusion- and diffusion-weighted MRI with NIHSS score in acute (<6.5 hour) ischemic stroke. Neurology 50(4):864–870

83. Lovblad KO et al (1997) Ischemic lesion volumes in acute stroke by diffusion-weighted magnetic resonance imaging correlate with clinical outcome. Ann Neurol 42(2):164–170

84. Engelter S et al (2003) Infarct volume on apparent diffusion coefficient maps correlates with length of stay and outcome after middle cerebral artery stroke. Cerebrovasc Dis 15(3):188–191

85. Nighoghossian N et al (2003) Baseline magnetic resonance imaging parameters and stroke outcome in patients treated by intravenous tissue plasminogen activator. Stroke 34(2):458–463

86. Rohl L et al (2001) Correlation between diffusion- and perfusion-weighted MRI and neurological deficit measured by the Scandinavian Stroke Scale and Barthel Index in hyperacute subcortical stroke (≤6 hours). Cerebrovasc Dis 12(3):203–213

87. Thijs V et al (2000) Is early ischemic lesion volume on diffusion-weighted imaging an independent predictor of stroke outcome? A multivariable analysis. Stroke 31(11):2597–2602

88. Engelter S et al (2004) The clinical significance of diffusion-weighted MR imaging in infratentorial strokes. Neurology 62(4):474–480

89. Davalos A et al (2004) The clinical-DWI mismatch: a new diagnostic approach to the brain tissue at risk of infarction. Neurology 62(12):2187–2192

90. Arenillas J et al (2002) Prediction of early neurologic deterioration using diffusion- and perfusion-weighted imaging in hyperacute middle cerebral artery stroke. Stroke 33(9):2197–2203

91. Ay H et al (2002) "Footprints" of transient ischemic attacks: a diffusion-weighted MRI study. Cerebrovasc Dis 14(3–4):177–186

92. Kidwell CS et al (1999) Diffusion MRI in patients with transient ischemic attacks. Stroke 30(6):1174–1180

93. Purroy F et al (2004) Higher risk of further vascular events among transient ischemic attack patients with diffusion-weighted imaging acute lesions. Stroke 35(10):2313–2319

94. Crisostomo R, Garcia M, Tong D (2003) Detection of diffusion-weighted MRI abnormalities in patients with transient ischemic attack: correlation with clinical characteristics. Stroke 34(4):932–937

95. Inatomi Y et al (2004) DWI abnormalities and clinical characteristics in TIA patients. Neurology 62(3):376–380

96. Huber R et al (2002) Transient global amnesia. Evidence against vascular ischemic etiology from diffusion weighted imaging. J Neurol 249(11):1520–1524

97. Saito K et al (2003) Transient global amnesia associated with an acute infarction in the retrosplenium of the corpus callosum. J Neurol Sci 210(1–2):95–97

98. Matsui M et al (2002) Transient global amnesia: increased signal intensity in the right hippocampus on diffusion-weighted magnetic resonance imaging. Neuroradiology 44(3):235–238

99. Ay H et al (1998) Diffusion-weighted MRI characterizes the ischemic lesion in transient global amnesia. Neurology 51(3):901–903

100. Greer DM, Schaefer PW, Schwamm LH (2001) Unilateral temporal lobe stroke causing ischemic transient global amnesia: role for diffusion-weighted imaging in the initial evaluation. J Neuroimaging 11(3):317–319

101. Woolfenden AR et al (1997) Diffusion-weighted MRI in transient global amnesia precipitated by cerebral angiography. Stroke 28(11):2311–2314

102. Sedlaczek O et al (2004) Detection of delayed focal MR changes in the lateral hippocampus in transient global amnesia. Neurology 62(12):2165–2170

103. Ebisu T et al (1993) Discrimination between different types of white matter edema with diffusion-weighted MR imaging. J Magn Reson Imaging 3(6):863–868

104. Schaefer PW et al (1997) Diffusion-weighted imaging discriminates between cytotoxic and vasogenic edema in a patient with eclampsia. Stroke 28(5):1082–1085

105. Schwartz RB et al (1998) Diffusion-weighted MR imaging in hypertensive encephalopathy: clues to pathogenesis. Am J Neuroradiol 19(5):859–862

106. Hinchey J et al (1996) A reversible posterior leukoencephalopathy syndrome. N Engl J Med 334(8):494–500

107. Nakazato T et al (2003) Reversible posterior leukoencephalopathy syndrome associated with tacrolimus therapy. Intern Med 42(7):624–625

108. Henderson RD et al (2003) Posterior leukoencephalopathy following intrathecal chemotherapy with MRA-documented vasospasm. Neurology 60(2):326–328

109. Sylvester SL et al (2002) Reversible posterior leukoencephalopathy in an HIV-infected patient with thrombotic thrombocytopenic purpura. Scand J Infect Dis 34(9): 706–709

110. Utz N et al (2001) MR imaging of acute intermittent porphyria mimicking reversible posterior leukoencephalopathy syndrome. Neuroradiology 43(12):1059–1062

111. Edwards MJ et al (2001) Reversible posterior leukoencephalopathy syndrome following CHOP chemotherapy for diffuse large B-cell lymphoma. Ann Oncol 12(9): 1327–1329

112. Soylu A et al (2001) Posterior leukoencephalopathy syndrome in poststreptococcal acute glomerulonephritis. Pediatr Nephrol 16(7):601–603

113. Ikeda M et al (2001) Reversible posterior leukoencephalopathy in a patient with minimal-change nephrotic syndrome. Am J Kidney Dis 37(4):E30

114. Kamar N et al (2001) Reversible posterior leukoencephalopathy syndrome in hepatitis C virus-positive long-term hemodialysis patients. Am J Kidney Dis 37(4): E29

115. Honkaniemi J et al (2000) Reversible posterior leukoencephalopathy after combination chemotherapy. Neuroradiology 42(12):895–899

116. Taylor MB, Jackson A, Weller JM (2000) Dynamic susceptibility contrast enhanced MRI in reversible posterior leukoencephalopathy syndrome associated with haemolytic uraemic syndrome. Br J Radiol 73(868):438–442

117. Lewis MB (1999) Cyclosporin neurotoxicity after chemotherapy. Cyclosporin causes reversible posterior leukoencephalopathy syndrome. Br Med J 319(7201):54–55

118. Ito Y et al (1998) Cisplatin neurotoxicity presenting as reversible posterior leukoencephalopathy syndrome. Am J Neuroradiol 19(3):415–417

119. Covarrubias DJ, Luetmer PH, Campeau NG (2002) Posterior reversible encephalopathy syndrome: prognostic utility of quantitative diffusion-weighted MR images. Am J Neuroradiol 23(6):1038–1048

120. Ay H et al (1998) Posterior leukoencephalopathy without severe hypertension: utility of diffusion-weighted MRI. Neurology 51(5):1369–1376

121. Breen JC et al (1996) Brain edema after carotid surgery. Neurology 46(1):175–181

122. Smith WH, Easton DJ (2001) Cerebrovascular disease. In: Braunwald E, Kasper DL, Hauser SL, Longo DL, Jameson JL (eds) Harrison's principles of internal medicine. McGraw-Hill, New York, pp 2369–2391

123. Ameri A, Bousser MG (1992) Cerebral venous thrombosis. Neurol Clin 10(1):87–111

124. Daif A et al (1995) Cerebral venous thrombosis in adults. A study of 40 cases from Saudi Arabia. Stroke 26(7): 1193–1195

125. Hickey WF et al (1982) Primary cerebral venous thrombosis in patients with cancer – a rarely diagnosed paraneoplastic syndrome. Report of three cases and review of the literature. Am J Med 73(5):740–750

126. Crawford SC et al (1995) Thrombosis of the deep venous drainage of the brain in adults. Analysis of seven cases with review of the literature. Arch Neurol 52(11):1101–1108

127. Villringer A, Einhaupl KM (1997) Dural sinus and cerebral venous thrombosis. New Horiz 5(4):332–341

128. Lefebvre P et al (1998) Cerebral venous thrombosis and procoagulant factors – a case study. Angiology 49(7): 563–571

129. Ito K et al (1997) Cerebral hemodynamics and histological changes following acute cerebral venous occlusion in cats. Tokai J Exp Clin Med 22(3):83–93

130. Nagai S et al (1998) Superior sagittal sinus thrombosis associated with primary antiphospholipid syndrome – case report. Neurol Med Chir (Tokyo) 38(1):34–39

131. Vielhaber H et al (1998) Cerebral venous sinus thrombosis in infancy and childhood: role of genetic and acquired risk factors of thrombophilia. Eur J Pediatr 157(7):555–560

132. Van den Berg JS et al (1999) Cerebral venous thrombosis: recurrence with fatal course. J Neurol 246(2):144–146

133. Forbes KP, Pipe JG, Heiserman JE (2001) Evidence for cytotoxic edema in the pathogenesis of cerebral venous infarction. Am J Neuroradiol 22(3):450–455

134. Allroggen H, Abbott RJ (2000) Cerebral venous sinus thrombosis. Postgrad Med J 76(891):12–15

135. Tsai FY et al (1995) MR staging of acute dural sinus thrombosis: correlation with venous pressure measurements and implications for treatment and prognosis. Am J Neuroradiol 16(5):1021–1029

136. Yuh WT et al (1994) Venous sinus occlusive disease: MR findings. Am J Neuroradiol 15(2):309–316

137. Dormont D et al (1994) MRI in cerebral venous thrombosis. J Neuroradiol 21(2):81–99

138. Kassem-Moussa H et al (2000) Early diffusion-weighted MR imaging abnormalities in sustained seizure activity. Am J Roentgenol 174(5):1304–1306

Perfusion MRI of Acute Stroke

Pamela W. Schaefer, William A. Copen,
R. Gilberto González

8.1 Introduction

Perfusion describes the circulation of blood through a vascular bed within living tissue, so that oxygen, nutrients, and waste products may be exchanged via capillary walls. Accordingly, perfusion-weighted magnetic resonance imaging (PWI) describes techniques that study perfusion by visually depicting hemodynamic conditions at the microvascular level. This is in contrast to other vascular MR imaging techniques, notably magnetic resonance angiography (MRA), that depict the flow of blood in larger, macroscopically visible vessels. Ischemic damage to brain tissue is caused most directly by impairments in microvascular perfusion, rather than by events occurring in large vessels. Therefore, PWI uniquely offers the ability to guide acute stroke therapy by identifying regions of brain tissue that are threatened by impaired perfusion, though not yet irreversibly damaged, and that consequently may be rescued by timely initiation of thrombolytic or neuroprotective therapy.

The first portion of this chapter reviews techniques that are currently used for performing PWI in the clinical setting, including applicable pulse sequences, contrast agents, and post-processing techniques. Subsequently, we discuss strategies for incorporating the information provided by PWI into clinical decision-making.

8.2 Dynamic Susceptibility Contrast Imaging

PWI studies blood flow within vessels that are orders of magnitude smaller than image voxels; therefore, all PWI techniques rely on measurement of the concentration within each voxel of a contrast agent that is dissolved in the blood. In current clinical practice, the great majority of PWI studies are performed using contrast agents based upon the gadolinium ion. Images are acquired dynamically before, during, and after the injection of a bolus of a gadolinium-based contrast agent, and these images are used to track the bolus, and therefore the blood in which it is dissolved, as it passes through the microvasculature of the brain.

The free gadolinium ion is toxic, and it is therefore tightly chelated to a relatively large molecule in all available gadolinium-based contrast agents. When injected intravenously, these gadolinium chelates can exit the bloodstream and enter the interstitial space within most body tissues. However, they are too large and polarized to cross the blood–brain barrier. This fact is exploited by conventional gadolinium-enhanced MR imaging, in which T1-weighted images are acquired several minutes after injection of the contrast agent. Disruptions of the blood–brain barrier due to conditions such as inflammation or neoplasm result in persistence of gadolinium in the interstitial space, with resultant shortening of T1 relaxation, and hyperintensity on post-contrast T1-weighted images.

The T1 relaxivity effect of gadolinium operates over extremely short distances, and water spins must approach within a few micrometers of a gadolinium ion in order to experience a significant change in T1 relaxation. Such close approximation of water spins and gadolinium is frequent when gadolinium is present in the interstitial space, but is much more rare when an intact blood–brain barrier confines gadolinium to the intravascular compartment, which occupies approximately 4% of tissue volume in gray matter, and 2% in white matter. If the T1 relaxivity effect were used to provide the basis for image contrast in PWI, at most only 4% of spins would exhibit any difference in signal intensity, and the ability of PWI to measure differences in perfusion would be limited.

In order to provide improved ability to measure changes in the concentration of gadolinium as it passes through the cerebral vasculature, most PWI techniques in current clinical use rely on dynamic susceptibility contrast (DSC) imaging, in which image contrast is based on gadolinium's magnetic susceptibility effect, rather than its T1 relaxivity effect [1]. Magnetic susceptibility refers to the propensity of some species with a magnetic moment to align with an externally applied magnetic field, resulting in small, nonuniform local intensifications of the magnetic field. When present in high enough concentrations, gadolinium ions confined within a cerebral blood vessel create a magnetic susceptibility effect that results in substantial loss of signal on T2*-weighted images, which extends over a distance comparable in magnitude to the diameter of the blood vessel.

Acquisition of high-quality DSC data requires rapid injection of a gadolinium-based contrast agent, usually using a mechanical power injector. It also requires a pulse sequence capable of repeatedly acquiring T2*-weighted images rapidly enough that the concentration of gadolinium within each tissue voxel can be sampled with sufficient temporal resolution, typically every 1–2 s. This can be accomplished for a single image slice by most medium-field or high-field MRI scanners. However, in order to perform multi-slice PWI, it is necessary to use a fast imaging technique such as echo planar imaging (EPI), with which interleaved images of many tissue slices can be obtained within a single repetition time (TR).

Both EPI spin-echo and EPI gradient-echo sequences have been used successfully for PWI. Gradient-echo images have the disadvantage of disproportionately weighting the contribution of gadolinium in relatively large vessels, whereas spin-echo images provide a more accurate assessment of blood flow through vessels of all sizes. Therefore, spin-echo imaging allows for more accurate assessment of hemodynamic conditions in the capillary bed, which is theoretically of greatest interest in stroke imaging [2]. However, the 180° radiofrequency pulse in spin-echo sequences renders spin-echo images less sensitive to

Table 8.1. Gradient echo-planar perfusion-weighted imaging parameters. (*TE* Echo time, *TR* repetition time)

Sequence	Single-shot echo-planar gradient echo
TR	1500 ms
TE	40 ms
Flip angle	60°
Field of view	22 cm
Matrix	128×128
Slice thickness	5 mm
Interslice gap	1 mm
Number of slices	16
Number of time points	46
Contrast material gadopentetate dimeglumine	20 ml
Injection rate	5 ml/s
Injection delay	Injection begins 10 s after imaging begins

susceptibility effects, resulting in a reduction in contrast-to-noise ratio [3]. For this reason, most institutions use an EPI gradient-echo sequence for PWI. Our PWI sequence is described in detail in Table 8.1, and enables imaging of virtually the entire brain every 1.5 s. Our sequence requires 69 s of imaging time, and uses a standard dose of 20 ml of contrast material injected at 5 ml/s.

8.3 PWI Using Endogenous Contrast Agents

MRI is unlike x-ray computed tomography or radionuclide imaging, in that, theoretically, MRI can be used for totally noninvasive perfusion imaging using endogenous contrast agents that are already present within the blood. Two such approaches have been successful in the laboratory. In the first, the endogenous contrast agent is deoxyhemoglobin, which, like gadolinium, is paramagnetic, and therefore has similar effects on MR images. Deoxyhemoglobin-based techniques such as BOLD (blood oxygen level dependent) have been shown to be a reliable method of perfusion imaging in numerous experimental brain activation studies [4]. However, variations in signal resulting from changes in local deoxyhemoglobin concentrations are small, approximately 1 % at usual field strengths. As a result, these techniques generally require very long imaging times that would be impractical for clinical imaging, especially in the setting of acute stroke. Furthermore, they rely upon extraction of oxygen by brain tissue to produce deoxyhemoglobin, a process which may not reliably remain intact under ischemic conditions.

A second approach to noninvasive PWI utilizes the protons within blood as an endogenous contrast agent. In this approach, called arterial spin labeling (ASL), a pre-imaging radiofrequency pulse is used to invert the spins within blood before it flows into the imaged portion of the brain [5,6]. Because it does not require an exogenous contrast agent, ASL offers several potential advantages over DSC in the clinical setting. These include lower cost, lack of adverse reactions to injected contrast material, and the ability to perform a perfusion examination repeatedly during a short time, in order to assess the effects of thrombolytic drugs, induced changes in blood pressure, or other therapeutic interventions. However, ASL suffers from an intrinsic technical limitation, in that the change in spin orientation produced by the inversion pulse decays quickly as a result of T1 relaxation. Because T1 relaxation is very rapid in comparison to the time it takes for blood to flow from an inverted slice to an imaged slice of the brain, the signal changes produced by labeled blood are small in magnitude. Furthermore, because many ASL pulse sequences are relatively time-consuming, they can be very susceptible to artifacts related to patient motion, and multislice imaging can be especially challenging. These limitations are being addressed by ongoing advances in pulse sequence design [7,8], and by the increasing availability of high-field magnets, which increase the T1 of blood and therefore increase the detectable signal change resulting from spin inversion.

At the present time, DSC remains the preferred PWI method at nearly all clinical centers, and subsequent discussion of PWI post-processing methods will refer solely to those used for DSC imaging.

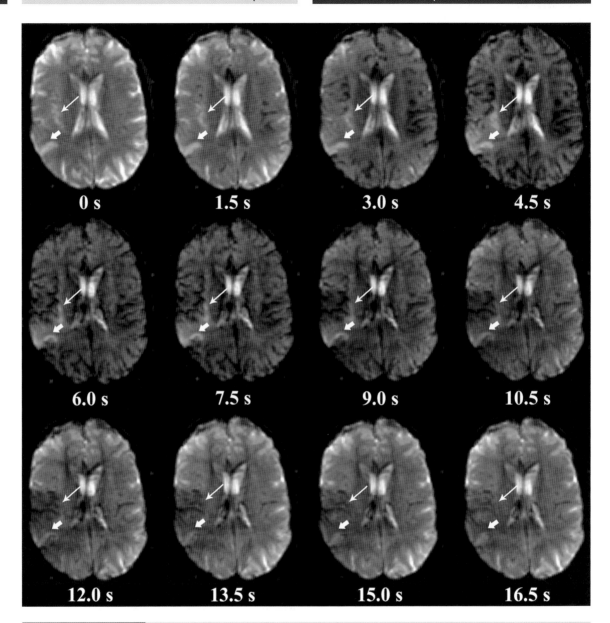

Figure 8.1

Dynamic susceptibility contrast images. These images were acquired during the injection of a bolus of gadolinium. Parenchymal signal intensity decreases as the bolus passes through the microvasculature, then increases again as the bolus washes out. Note that there is an area of severely diminished cerebral blood flow (*thick arrows*), which demonstrates virtually no decrease in signal until the 10.5 s image. Adjacent to this, there is a region of moderately diminished cerebral blood flow (*thin arrows*), in which signal loss occurs more slowly than in normally perfused tissue and persists for a greater time, due to increased intravascular transit time

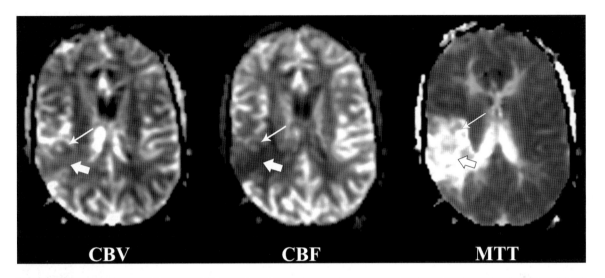

Figure 8.2

Perfusion-weighted image maps. These images were generated from the dynamic susceptibility contrast images shown in Fig. 8.1, using the post-processing method summarized in Fig. 8.3. In the region of severely impaired perfusion (*thick arrows*), abnormally low cerebral blood volume (*CBV*) and flow (*CBF*) are represented by *darker shades* of *gray* on the corresponding perfusion maps. In a region of only moderately impaired perfusion (*thin arrows*), CBV appears normal but CBF is abnormally low (this is appreciated most easily by comparing the ipsilateral to the contralateral cortical gray matter on the CBF map). Mean transit time (*MTT*) is abnormally elevated in both regions, resulting in increased signal intensity on the MTT map

8.4 Post-Processing of Dynamic Susceptibility Contrast Images

Although some information about regional perfusion differences may be gleaned by direct interpretation of raw DSC images as a cine loop or a mosaic (Fig. 8.1), the large number of images at each slice (typically 40–50) make review of individual images impractical. Far more straightforward and thorough interpretation of the images can be performed if one of various post-processing algorithms is used to convert the sequence of individual, dynamically acquired images into synthetic maps that depict any of several perfusion parameters for each brain voxel (Fig. 8.2).

This process may be understood by considering the raw DSC images in Fig. 8.1. The image labeled "0 s" was acquired before the arrival into the brain of an intravenously injected bolus of contrast material.

Several other baseline images were also acquired prior to this one, in order to allow more precise calculation of baseline signal intensity by the averaging of multiple images. Images acquired after the "0 s" image depict the arrival of the contrast bolus, with a resultant drop in signal intensity, followed by washout of the contrast material from the brain, which is manifested by a rebound of signal intensity to a level close to the baseline signal intensity at 0 s.

All of these images are T2*-weighted. In the "0 s" baseline image, as well as the other baseline images acquired before bolus arrival, signal intensities are related only to time-invariant properties of brain tissue and the scanner. However, in each subsequent image, signal intensity in each pixel has been decreased by an amount proportional to the concentration of gadolinium in the corresponding voxel. The concentration of gadolinium in each voxel is linearly related to ΔR_2^*, the change in the rate of T2* relaxation in comparison to the baseline, according to:

$$C_{Gd} = k\Delta R_2^*$$

where C_{Gd} is the concentration of gadolinium in the voxel, ΔR_2^* is the change in the rate of T2* relaxation relative to the baseline image(s), and k is a constant whose value depends on factors that are not usually measured clinically. T2* relaxation is an exponential process, so the concentration of gadolinium is related to change in signal intensity by the equation:

$$C_{Gd}(t) = -k' \ln\left(\frac{S_t}{S_0}\right)$$

where $C_{Gd}(t)$ is the concentration of gadolinium at time t after bolus arrival, S_t is the signal intensity at that time, S_0 is the signal intensity at time 0 or earlier, before the arrival of the bolus, and k' is a new constant.

Because it may be assumed that the gadolinium concentration in blood is uniform at any particular instant in time, the concentration of gadolinium within each tissue voxel is proportional to the volume of blood within that voxel, and regional cerebral blood volume (rCBV) in each volume may be calculated by averaging the gadolinium concentration measured at every time point after bolus arrival:

$$rCBV \approx \frac{\sum_{t=1}^{n} C_{Gd}(t)}{n}$$

assuming that measurements are obtained at n time points after bolus arrival. Cerebral blood volume is one of the simplest hemodynamic parameters to measure with DSC, and its calculation requires relatively little post-processing time. Because rCBV is preserved under all but the most severe ischemic conditions, tissue demonstrating abnormally diminished rCBV is usually suffering from severe ischemia, and has a low likelihood of viability regardless of therapeutic intervention.

Regional cerebral blood flow (rCBF) is a more sensitive indicator of tissue ischemia. Decrements in rCBF are seen in tissue experiencing even mild degrees of ischemia, and therefore such tissue may be amenable to therapeutic rescue if reperfusion can be achieved in a timely manner. The magnitude of rCBF in each voxel is reflected roughly by the slope of the concentration-versus-time curve representing the arrival of the gadolinium bolus. In general, a steeper slope reflects more rapid arrival of gadolinium in the voxel, and therefore greater rCBF. However, calculation of rCBF is made more complicated by the fact that the slope of the concentration-versus-time function is influenced not only by rCBF, but also by the rapidity with which gadolinium is delivered to the voxel by the feeding artery or arteries (Fig. 8.3). Mathematically, the concentration-versus-time function is the convolution of an arterial input function (AIF), which represents the delivery of gadolinium to the voxel by the feeding artery or arteries, and a residue function, which represents the proportion of gadolinium remaining in the voxel at each instant after bolus arrival, and whose height numerically represents the rCBF in that voxel. Therefore, calculation of rCBF requires estimation of an AIF, which is then used for deconvolution and calculation of the residue function (and therefore rCBF).

Once calculated, rCBF can be used to calculate the mean transit time (MTT) of blood through the tissue voxel, according to the central volume theorem:

$$MTT = \frac{CBV}{CBF}.$$

MTT is abnormally elevated in ischemic brain tissue, and synthetic images depicting regional differences in MTT, like rCBF maps, can be used to identify tissue experiencing even mild degrees of ischemia. MTT maps are often easier to interpret than rCBF maps, because the large differences that exist between rCBF in normal gray matter and normal white matter sometimes make visual detection of an ischemic lesion difficult (Fig. 8.2). The process for producing CBV, CBF, and MTT maps is summarized in Fig. 8.4.

AIF computation may be accomplished by a technologist, physician, or other trained person, often using a workstation separate from the MR scanner's main console. This process takes a few minutes to complete, and involves review of the raw DSC images in order to identify a few pixels that are close to a large artery of interest, and therefore can be used to represent the concentration of gadolinium within that artery. After the AIF has been selected, it is

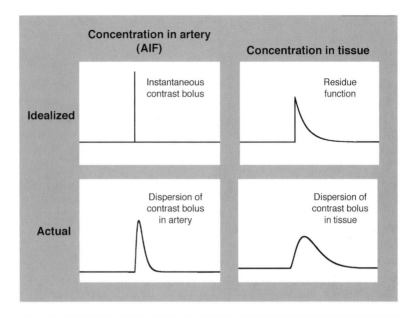

Concentration in artery
(AIF)

Concentration in tissue

Idealized

Instantaneous
contrast bolus

Residue
function

Actual

Dispersion of
contrast bolus
in artery

Dispersion of
contrast bolus
in tissue

Figure 8.3

Idealized and actual perfusion experiments. In all of the above graphs, time is depicted on the *x* axis and concentration of contrast material on the *y* axis. In an idealized perfusion experiment, the entirety of a bolus of contrast material would be delivered instantaneously to brain tissue via a feeding artery. This is depicted in the arterial input function in the *upper left hand corner*. In this case, the tissue concentration-versus-time curve (*upper right*) is a "residue function," reflecting the proportion of the contrast bolus remaining in the tissue at each moment in time. In the actual case, contrast is injected intravenously over a finite period of time, and the bolus is further dispersed as it travels through the circulatory system before reaching the brain. This results in an arterial input function (*AIF*) that is not instantaneous (*lower left*). As a result, there is also dispersion of the contrast bolus as it passes through the parenchymal microvasculature (*lower right*). If the actual AIF and tissue concentration curve are both known, the residue function can be computed by deconvolution

then used by a computer to perform deconvolution for each pixel, a process that usually consumes approximately 5–10 min for a typical multi-slice DSC sequence.

At our institution, we use singular value decomposition (SVD), a deconvolution algorithm that is relatively robust, in that it performs well in a wide variety of ischemic conditions [9, 10]. Because of its robustness, SVD is used at the majority of centers where PWI is performed. However, the SVD algorithm does have some limitations. In particular, its measurements of rCBF are artifactually influenced by differences that may exist between the AIF that is chosen, and the unmeasured AIF that corresponds to the actual arterial supply of each voxel (Table 8.2). SVD underestimates rCBF when arrival of the contrast bolus

Table 8.2. Pitfalls in dynamic susceptibility contrast perfusion-weighted imaging

Patient motion
Delay of contrast bolus
Dispersion of contrast bolus
Susceptibility artifact due to air or metallic objects
Unreliable for calculating absolute values of perfusion parameters

to tissue is delayed, relative to its arrival in the large artery used for calculation of the AIF. For this reason, the AIF is typically chosen from the proximal vessel supplying the ischemic territory [e.g., ipsilateral

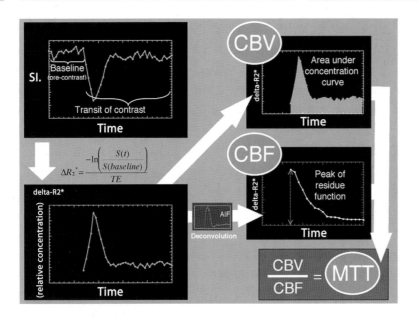

Figure 8.4

Post-processing of dynamic susceptibility images using deconvolution. For each pixel in each image slice, a graph of signal intensity (*S.I.*) as a function of time is converted into one of R_2^* as a function of time. R_2^*, the change in the rate of T2* relaxation due to the presence of gadolinium, is proportional to the concentration of gadolinium present. The R_2^*-versus-time curve is then used to compute three hemodynamic measurements. CBV (whose calculation does not require deconvolution) is proportional to the area under the curve. Deconvolution using a separately measured arterial input function (*AIF*) allows computation of a residue function, which describes the fraction of a hypothetical instantaneous contrast bolus that would remain at each time after injection. The peak of the residue function is proportional to CBF. CBV is divided by CBF to yield MTT

middle cerebral artery (MCA) stem for MCA infarction]. An AIF chosen from a more remote vessel allows an increase in the time delay between contrast reaching the AIF and the tissue. This causes underestimation of blood flow and overestimation of tissue at risk of infarction (Fig. 8.5). This is especially problematic when there is an ipsilateral carotid stenosis or occlusion and blood reaches the tissue through collateral circulation [11]. SVD also underestimates rCBF when the quantity of gadolinium that arrives in the voxel is dispersed over a longer time period [12–14]. When interpreting images of rCBF or MTT that are prepared by SVD deconvolution, it is important to keep in mind these potential causes of underestimation of rCBF, and therefore overestimation of the quantity of tissue placed at risk by ischemia. Recent efforts to develop deconvolution methods that are not artifactually influenced by delay or dispersion of the contrast bolus may reduce these concerns in the near future [15].

The AIF selection and deconvolution processes required for calculation of rCBF and MTT require some human intervention, computing resources, and time to complete; therefore, it is often useful to measure other hemodynamic parameters that can serve as more easily computed, though less physiologically precise measurements of regional perfusion. For example, many centers compute "time to peak" (TTP)

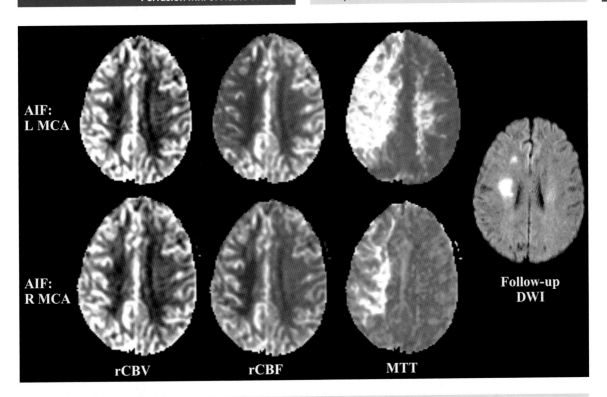

AIF:
L MCA

AIF:
R MCA

Follow-up
DWI

rCBV   rCBF   MTT

Figure 8.5

Choice of different arterial input functions. Patient is 39-year-old female with a history of right internal carotid artery dissection and left sided weakness, who was imaged at 8 h after symptom onset. When the left middle cerebral artery (*MCA*) stem is chosen as the arterial input function (*AIF*), there is longer delay between the AIF and the tissue sampling versus when the right MCA stem is chosen as the AIF. This results in underestimation of CBF and the corresponding maps demonstrate larger areas with low CBF and elevated MTT. The patient was started on heparin and hypertensive therapy. The final infarct is much more closely approximated by the CBF and MTT maps constructed with the right MCA AIF

maps, in which each pixel is assigned a number representing the amount of time it took for the contrast bolus to reach maximum concentration in the corresponding tissue voxel. TTP is a parameter whose exact physiological correlates are difficult to determine in any particular case, as it can become elevated as a result of reduced rCBF, prolonged MTT, delayed contrast arrival, dispersion of the bolus, or any combination of these factors. Therefore, TTP maps suffer from even greater technical limitations than maps of rCBF and MTT produced by deconvolution [11]. However, they can be produced extremely rapidly, and with a minimum of technical expertise and computing power.

At our institution, PWI data from acute stroke patients are used to compute maps of rCBV, TTP, and the maximum decrease in signal intensity over any two images, which serves as a rough estimation of rCBF. These synthetic images can be derived from raw DSC data in less than 1 min, and can therefore provide clinically important information to the physicians caring for the patient before he or she has left the MR scanner. Subsequently, we transfer the raw DSC images to another workstation and use deconvolution to produce maps of rCBF and MTT that can be available within 20–30 min, and used to further guide clinical decision-making. Absolute quantification of CBV, CBF, and MTT values can sometimes

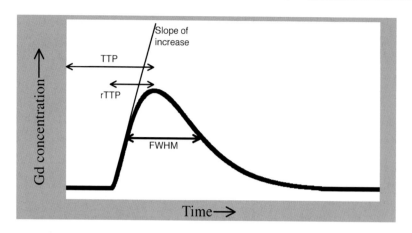

Figure 8.6

Post-processing of dynamic susceptibility images without deconvolution. Because of the extra time and human intervention required to calculate CBF and MTT with deconvolution techniques, alternative metrics that approximate CBF and MTT without deconvolution have been used. Measurement of the slope of increase of gadolinium concentration is an approximation of CBF, whereas the full width of the concentration curve at half of the maximum value (*FWHM*) is an approximation of MTT. Relative time to peak (*rTTP*) is influenced by both CBF and MTT. Time to peak (*TTP*) is influenced by CBF and MTT as well as any delay in the arrival of the contrast bolus

be obtained with the deconvolution method, although this is not routinely done clinically [9, 10]. Other post-processing techniques allow calculation of different transit time parameters such as first moment, ratio of area to peak, relative TTP, arrival time, and full-width at half-maximum (Fig. 8.6). However, deconvolution techniques that calculate MTT have proven superior to these parameters [11].

8.5 Reliability

In general, perfusion images are less sensitive than DWI images in the detection of acute stroke, with sensitivities for rCBV, rCBF, and MTT ranging from 74% to 84%. Lesions missed on perfusion images include: (1) lesions with small abnormalities on DWI that are not detected because of the lower resolution of MR perfusion images, and (2) lesions with early reperfusion. Specificities for perfusion images range from 96% to 100%. Occasional false-positive scans occur when there is an ischemic, but viable hypoperfused region that recovers [16].

8.6 Diffusion in Combination with Perfusion MRI in the Evaluation of Acute Stroke

8.6.1 Diffusion and Perfusion MRI in Predicting Tissue Viability

The clinical role of PWI in conjunction with DWI has not been completely defined (Tables 8.3, 8.4). The most important potential clinical impact may result from defining the ischemic penumbra, a region that is ischemic but still viable and that may infarct if not treated. Therefore, most investigation is focused on strokes with a diffusion–perfusion mismatch or strokes with a perfusion lesion larger than the diffusion lesion. Proximal occlusions are much more likely to result in a diffusion–perfusion mismatch than distal or lacunar infarctions. Operationally, the diffusion abnormality is thought to represent the ischemic core and the region characterized by normal diffusion but abnormal perfusion is thought to represent the ischemic penumbra [1, 17–22]. Definition of the penumbra is complicated because of the multiple

Table 8.3. Lesion volumes of diffusion and perfusion. (*DWI* Diffusion-weighted imaging, *PWI* perfusion-weighted imaging)

Pattern	Cause	Comment
PWI but no DWI	Proximal occlusion or critical stenosis with penumbra perfused via collaterals	DWI abnormalities may develop depending on collateralization and timing of reperfusion. Good candidate for reperfusion therapy
PWI>DWI	Proximal occlusion or critical stenosis with penumbra partially perfused via collaterals	DWI may expand into part or all of the PWI abnormality depending on collateralization and timing of reperfusion. Good candidate for reperfusion therapy
PWI=DWI	Usually lacunes or distal occlusion, but can be proximal occlusion	Entire territory has infarcted. No tissue at risk
PWI<DWI	Proximal, distal or lacunar infarct	Ischemic tissue has reperfused. No tissue at risk
DWI but no PWI	Proximal, distal or lacunar infarct	Ischemic tissue has reperfused. No tissue at risk. Also, tiny infarctions not seen on PWI due to lower resolution

hemodynamic parameters that may be calculated from the perfusion MRI data.

A number of papers have focused on volumetric data. With arterial occlusion, brain regions with decreased diffusion and decreased perfusion are thought to represent nonviable tissue or the core of an infarction. The majority of strokes increase in volume on DWI with the peak volumetric measurements achieved at 2–3 days postictus. The initial DWI lesion volume correlates highly with final infarct volume with reported correlation coefficients (r^2) ranging from 0.69 to 0.98 [16, 23–26]. The initial CBV lesion volume is usually similar to the DWI lesion volume, and CBV also correlates highly with final infarct volume, with reported correlation coefficients (r^2) ranging from 0.79 to 0.81 [16, 25, 27]. In one large series, predicted lesion growth from the initial DWI to the follow-up lesion size was 24% and from the initial CBV to the follow-up lesion size was 22%. When there is a rare DWI–CBV mismatch, the DWI lesion volume still correlates highly with final infarct volume, but the predicted lesion growth increases to approximately 60% [16]. The CBV, in this setting, also correlates highly with final infarct volume with no predicted lesion growth. In other words, when there is a DWI–CBV mismatch, the DWI abnormality grows into the size of the CBV abnormality (Fig. 8.7).

Many more strokes are characterized by a DWI–CBF or a DWI–MTT mismatch (Figs. 8.7–8.10). In general, initial CBF and MTT volumes correlate less well with final infarct volume than CBV, and on average greatly overestimate final infarct volume. Reported correlation coefficients (r^2) range from 0.3 to 0.67 for CBF and from 0.3 to 0.69 for MTT [16, 25, 27–29]. Predicted final infarct volume was 44% of the initial CBF abnormality, and 32% of the initial MTT abnormality in one study [16]. Another study demonstrated that size of the DWI–CBF and DWI–MTT mismatches correlates with final infarct volume. The correlation coefficients for DWI–CBF and DWI–MTT mismatch volume versus final infarct volume were 0.657 and 0.561 respectively [27].

In small-vessel infarctions (perforator infarctions and distal embolic infarctions) and in whole territory large-vessel infarctions, the initial perfusion (CBV, CBF, and MTT) and diffusion lesion volumes are usually similar and there is little to no lesion growth (Fig. 8.11). A diffusion lesion larger than the perfusion lesion or a diffusion lesion without a perfusion abnormality usually occurs with early reperfusion (Fig. 8.12). Similarly, in this situation, there is usually no significant lesion growth.

Table 8.4. Diffusion and perfusion MRI in predicting tissue viability. (*ADC* Apparent diffusion coefficient, *CBF* cerebral blood flow, *CBV* cerebral blood volume, *MTT* mean transit time, *TTP* time to peak)

DWI

Represents ischemic infarct core, is in general irreversible and is highly predictive of final infarct volume with strokes on average growing 20%

With thrombolysis, a portion of the DWI abnormality may be reversible, especially in white matter

ADC ratios and values may be important in predicting reversibility, hemorrhagic transformation and tissue viability. ? Threshold ADC ratio of ~ 0.8

CBV

Usually matched with DWI

Represents ischemic infarct core, is in general irreversible and is highly predictive of final infarct volume with strokes on average growing 20%

When CBV>DWI, the infarct usually grows into the CBV abnormality

Low CBV (<50% of normal) is predictive of tissue infarction

Elevated CBV is an unstable state – tissue may or may not infarct

CBF

With proximal occlusions, is usually larger than DWI

Usually overestimates final infarct size

Best parameter for distinguishing between penumbra likely to infarct from penumbra likely to survive in spite of intervention. ? Threshold CBV ratio of ~0.35

Best parameter for predicting hemorrhagic transformation

MTT

With proximal occlusions, is usually larger than DWI and yields the largest operational penumbra

Usually overestimates final infarct size

Controversy as to whether or not MTT is useful for distinguishing between penumbra likely to infarct and that likely to survive

TTP

With proximal occlusions, is usually larger than DWI

TTP of 6–8 s correlates well with final infarct size

Factors affecting calculations of thresholds for tissue viability

Timing of reperfusion

Gray versus white matter

Timing of initial scan

Timing of follow-up scan

Variability in post ischemic tissue responses

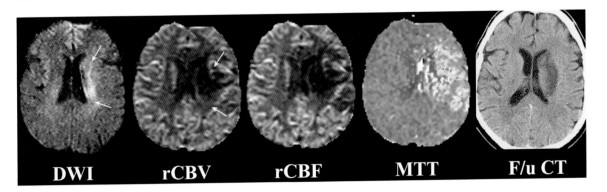

Figure 8.7

Diffusion–perfusion mismatch where there is a DWI–CBV mismatch and the stroke grows into the DWI–CBV but not the DWI–CBF or MTT mismatch region. Patient is 55-year-old male with right hemiparesis due to left MCA stem embolus. The DWI image demonstrates a small region of hyperintensity, consistent with acute infarction, in the left corona radiata (*white arrows*). The CBV map demonstrates a larger, hypointense abnormality involving more of the corona radiata as well as the caudate nucleus (*black arrows*). The CBF and MTT maps show larger abnormalities (CBF hypointense and MTT hyperintense) involving the left frontal and parietal lobes as well as the corona radiata and caudate nucleus. Follow-up CT (*F/u CT*) demonstrates growth of the infarct into the CBV abnormality but not into the CBF or MTT abnormalities

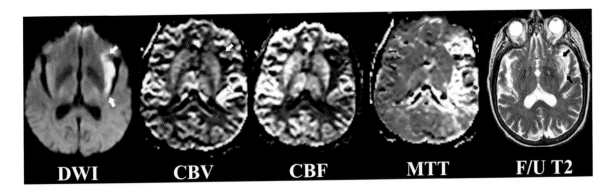

Figure 8.8

Diffusion–perfusion mismatch with the entire penumbra recovering. Patient is 80-year-old female with mild right hemiparesis, right facial droop with left MCA stem embolus, imaged at 4 h. There is hyperintensity on the DWI images and hypointensity on the CBV maps in the left insula (*arrow*). This region is thought to represent the core of ischemic tissue and was abnormal on follow-up T2-weighted images (*F/U T2*). The CBF and MTT images show larger abnormalities involving most of the visualized left MCA territory. The DWI- and CBV-normal but CBF- and MTT-abnormal tissue is thought to represent the ischemic penumbra. The patient was started on heparin and hypertensive therapy. None of the ischemic penumbra progressed to infarction

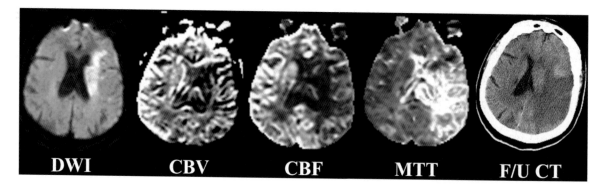

Figure 8.9

Diffusion–perfusion mismatch with infarct growing into nearly all of the tissue at risk of infarction. Patient is 70-year-old female with aphasia and right-sided weakness due to a left MCA stem embolus, imaged at 4 h. The DWI image demonstrates hyperintensity, consistent with acute infarction, in the left corona radiata and caudate nucleus. The CBV map demonstrates a hypointense lesion similar in size to the DWI abnormality. CBF and MTT images demonstrate much larger abnormal regions (CBF hypointense and MTT hyperintense) involving the left frontal and parietal lobes. The CBF- and MTT-abnormal but DWI-normal tissue reflects the operational ischemic penumbra. In spite of heparin and hypertensive therapy, follow-up CT (*F/U CT*) demonstrates growth of the infarct into most of the ischemic penumbra

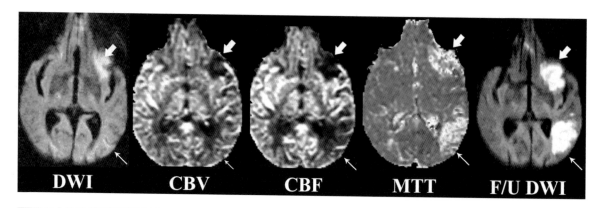

Figure 8.10

Diffusion–perfusion mismatch where there is DWI- and CBV-normal but CBF- and MTT-abnormal tissue that infarcts. Patient is 78-year-old female with aphasia during cardiac catheterization. There is a CBF-hypointense and MTT-hyperintense region (*thin arrow*) in the posterior left temporal lobe that appears normal on the DWI and CBV images. This entire region appears infarcted on follow-up DWI images (*F/U DWI*). In the inferior left frontal lobe, there is a lesion that is similar in size on all diffusion and perfusion images. There is no significant growth of this lesion on follow-up DWI

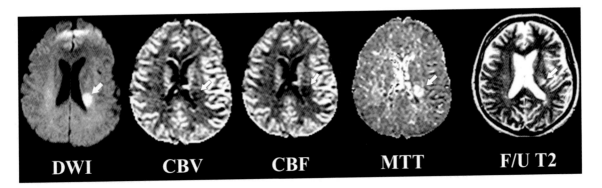

Figure 8.11

Lacunar infarct with matched diffusion and perfusion defects. Patient is 75-year-old male with right lower extremity weakness. The DWI image demonstrates an acute infarction in the left corona radiata (*arrow*). Defects similar in size are seen on the CBV, CBF, and MTT maps. There is no diffusion–perfusion mismatch. Follow-up T2-weighted image (*F/U T2*) demonstrates no significant lesion growth

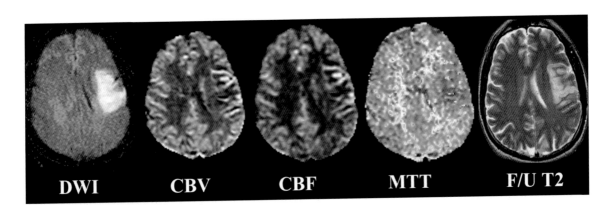

Figure 8.12

Diffusion abnormality without perfusion abnormality. Patient is 51-year-old male with right hemiparesis status post left carotid endarterectomy. DWI image demonstrates an acute left MCA infarction involving the left frontal and parietal lobes. The CBV, CBF, and MTT images demonstrate normal to elevated volume and flow and normal to decreased transit time in the corresponding region. This is consistent with early reperfusion. The follow-up T2-weighted image (*F/U T2*) demonstrates no significant infarct growth

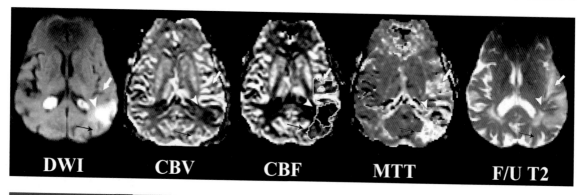

Figure 8.13

Diffusion–perfusion mismatch in a region with elevated CBV but low CBF that progresses to infarction. Patient is 83-year-old female with right hemiparesis and aphasia. Three regions are outlined on the CBF maps. The *white arrowhead* marks infarction core characterized by decreased diffusion, low CBV, low CBF, elevated MTT, and infarction on follow-up imaging. The *thick white arrow* marks penumbra that infarcts, which in this case is a DWI-normal region with elevated CBV, low CBF, elevated MTT, and follow-up infarction. The *thin black arrow* marks penumbra that remains viable which is a DWI- and CBV-normal region with low CBF, elevated MTT, and normal follow-up imaging

More recently, research has focused on differentiating diffusion and perfusion MR parameter lesion ratios or absolute values in infarct core, penumbra that progresses to infarction, and penumbra that remains viable. Most papers have demonstrated that rCBF is the most useful parameter in distinguishing hypoperfused tissue that will progress to infarction from hypoperfused tissue that will remain viable in patients not treated with thrombolysis. Reported rCBF values, expressed as a ratio or fraction of normal values, range from 0.12–0.44; for penumbra that progresses to infarction, 0.35–0.56; and for penumbra that remains viable, 0.58–0.78 [30–34]. Assuming a normal CBF of 50 ml · 100 g^{-1} · min^{-1} [35], these ratios translate to 6–22 ml · 100 g^{-1} · min^{-1} for core, 17.5–28 ml · 100 g^{-1} · min^{-1} for penumbra that progresses to infarction, and 29–39 ml · 100 g^{-1} · min^{-1} for penumbra that remains viable.

The variability in CBF ratios likely results from a number of different factors. Most importantly, the data obtained represent only a single time point in a dynamic process. One major factor is variability in timing of tissue reperfusion. Jones et al. [36] demonstrated that viability of ischemic tissue depends on both the severity and duration of CBF reduction in monkeys [36]. The CBF threshold for tissue infarction with reperfusion at 2–3 h was 10–12 ml · 100 g^{-1} · min^{-1} while the threshold for tissue infarction with permanent occlusion was 17–18 ml · 100 g^{-1} · min^{-1}. Ueda et al. [37], in a study of patients treated with thrombolysis, demonstrated that the duration of ischemia affected the CBF threshold for tissue viability for up to 5 h. Another factor is that normal average CBF in human parenchyma varies greatly, from 21.1 to 65.3 ml · 100 g^{-1} · min^{-1}, depending on age and location in gray matter versus white matter [35, 38–41]. Other factors affecting thresholds of tissue viability include variability methodologies, variability in initial and follow-up imaging times, and variability in post ischemic tissue responses.

Low rCBV ratios are highly predictive of infarction. However, elevated rCBV is not predictive of tissue viability, and rCBV ratios for penumbral regions that do and do not infarct may not be significantly different (Fig. 8.13). Lesion ratios range from 0.25 to 0.89 for lesion core, 0.69 to 1.44 for penumbra that progresses to infarction, and from 0.94 to 1.29 for penumbra that remains viable [30–34, 42]. The finding of elevated rCBV in the ischemic penumbra is in accordance with PET studies demonstrating that in the early stages of ischemia, decreased cerebral perfusion pressure produces vasodilatation and an increase in the CBV, which is associated with prolonged intravascular transit time, increased oxygen extraction fraction, and initially preserved oxygen delivery [43]. With further decreases in cerebral perfusion pressure, the compensatory vasodilatation reaches a maximum, and CBV initially continues to rise and then falls as capillary beds collapse. Thus, elevated rCBV is not necessarily sustainable over time and may represent a very unstable situation.

Some studies have demonstrated no statistically significant differences in MTT between infarct core and the two (viable and nonviable) penumbral regions, while others have demonstrated differences between all three regions or between the viable and nonviable penumbral regions [30–34, 42]. Reported MTT ratios for core range 1. 70–2.53; for penumbra that progresses to infarction, 1.74–2.19; and for hypoperfused tissue that remains viable, 1.65–1.66 [30–34, 42]. A number of studies have demonstrated that only patients with a TTP≥6 s are at risk of significant lesion enlargement and that tissue with TTP>6–8 s correlates highly with final infarct volume [44, 45]. One study that evaluated the abilities of CBF, MTT, TTP, and relative peak height to predict infarct growth found that a combination of TTP and relative peak height provided the best prediction of infarct growth (peak height <54% and TTP>5.2 s had a sensitivity of 71% and a specificity of 98%) [46].

Some reports demonstrate significant differences between the ADC values for the core, penumbra that infarcts, and penumbra that does not infarct, while others have not found such differences. In one large study, absolute mean ADC values for infarct core, penumbra that progresses to infarction, and penumbra that remains viable were $661{\times}10^{-6}\,mm^2/s$, $782{\times}10^{-6}\,mm^2/s$ and $823{\times}10^{-6}\,mm^2/s$, respectively [47]. Other authors report ADC ratios for infarct core, penumbra that progresses to infarction and hypoperfused tissue that remains viable of 0.62–0.63, 0.89–0.90, and 0.93–0.96, respectively [30, 32].

The aforementioned approaches have focused on regions or volumes of tissue. Since there is heterogeneity in diffusion and perfusion parameters within ischemic tissue, Wu et al. [48] performed a voxel-by-voxel multi parametric analysis of abnormalities on six maps (T2, ADC, DWI, CBV, CBF, and MTT) compared with follow-up T2-weighted images and developed thresholding and generalized linear model algorithms to predict tissue outcome [48]. They found that, at their optimal operating points, thresholding algorithms combining DWI and PWI provided 66% sensitivity and 83% specificity, and that generalized linear model algorithms combining DWI and PWI provided 66% sensitivity and 84% specificity.

8.6.2 Perfusion MRI and Thrombolysis in Acute Ischemic Stroke

Recently, a number of investigators have evaluated perfusion in patients treated with intravenous (i.v.) or intra-arterial thrombolytic therapy. In one study it was reported that a greater proportion of severely hypoperfused (>6 s MTT) tissue recovered in stroke patients treated with i.v. tissue plasminogen activator (t-PA) versus stroke patients treated with conventional therapies [49]. In another report, the presence of a tissue volume of equal to or greater than 50 ml with a CBF equal to or less than $12\,ml{\cdot}100\,g^{-1}{\cdot}min^{-1}$ predicted lesion growth [50]. In spite of successful recanalization with intra-arterial thrombolysis, some strokes grow into the penumbral region. In one study of 14 patients who underwent successful intra-arterial recanalization, it was reported that the best threshold for identifying irreversibly infarcted tissue was a T_{max} (time to peak contrast concentration) of 6–8 s or more [51]. CBV, CBF, and MTT thresholds have not been evaluated in these patients to date. In another study, regions with initial hypoperfusion that subsequently had elevated CBF following intra-arterial thrombolysis had a higher incidence of infarction compared to regions with initial hypoperfusion that did not develop hyperperfusion [52]. Also, Derex et al. [53] demonstrated that the degree of TTP delay correlated with recanalization rate in acute stroke patients treated with i.v. t-PA.

8.6.3 Diffusion and Perfusion MRI in Predicting Hemorrhagic Transformation of Acute Stroke

Hemorrhagic transformation (HT) of brain infarction represents secondary bleeding into ischemic tissue, varying from small petechiae to parenchymal hematoma (Table 8.5). It has a natural incidence of 15% to 26% during the first 2 weeks and up to 43% over the first month after cerebral infarction [54–57]. Predisposing factors include stroke etiology (HT is more frequent with embolic strokes), reperfusion, good collateral circulation, hypertension, anticoagulant therapy, and thrombolytic therapy. In patients treated with intra-arterial (i.a.) thrombolytic therapy, higher National Institutes of Health Stroke Scale (NIHSS) score, longer time to recanalization, lower platelet count, and higher glucose level are associated with HT [58].

The most commonly proposed pathophysiological mechanism for HT is the following. Severe ischemia leads to greater disruption of the cerebral microvasculature and greater degradation of the blood–brain barrier. Reperfusion into the damaged capillaries following clot lysis leads to blood extravasation with the development of petechial hemorrhage or hematoma. Reopening of a proximal occluded artery is not a sine qua non condition for HT, as multiple studies describe HT in spite of persistent arterial occlusion [54, 59]. HT in this setting may result from preservation of collateral flow. rt-PA thrombolytic therapy may aggravate ischemia-induced microvascular damage by activation of the plasminogen-plasmin system with release and activation of metalloproteinases [60–62]. Metalloproteinases are thought to be important factors in the degradation of the basal lamina during an ischemic insult.

Table 8.5. Factors associated with hemorrhagic transformation. (*MCA* Middle cerebral artery, *NIHSS* National Institutes of Health Stroke Scale)

Imaging parameters
Very low CBF on MR perfusion or SPECT imaging
Higher percentage of pixels with ADC $<550\times10^{-6}$ mm^2/s
Larger volume of the initial DWI abnormality
Prior microbleeds detected on T2* gradient echo images
Hypodensity in greater than one-third of the MCA territory on CT
Early parenchymal enhancement
Clinical
High NIHSS
Low platelets
High glucose
Hypertension
Vascular
Good collateral vessels
Early reperfusion
Embolic stroke
Therapy
Anticoagulation
Thrombolytic therapy

Since ADC values and perfusion parameters can mark the severity and extent of ischemia, a number of investigators have assessed these parameters in predicting HT (Fig. 8.14). Selim et al. [63] demonstrated that the volume of the initial DWI lesion and the absolute number of voxels with ADC value of

Figure 8.14 ▶

Hemorrhagic transformation. Patient is 76-year-old male with left hemiparesis. DWI and ADC images demonstrate a relatively large area with very low ADC values in the right basal ganglia, internal capsule, and corona radiata (*short thick arrows*). This region also has very low CBF values. CBF images also demonstrate less reduced perfusion throughout most of the rest of the visualized right MCA territory. Follow-up CT images (*F/U CT*) demonstrate hemorrhage into the right basal ganglia and deep white matter as well as into the right parietal cortex

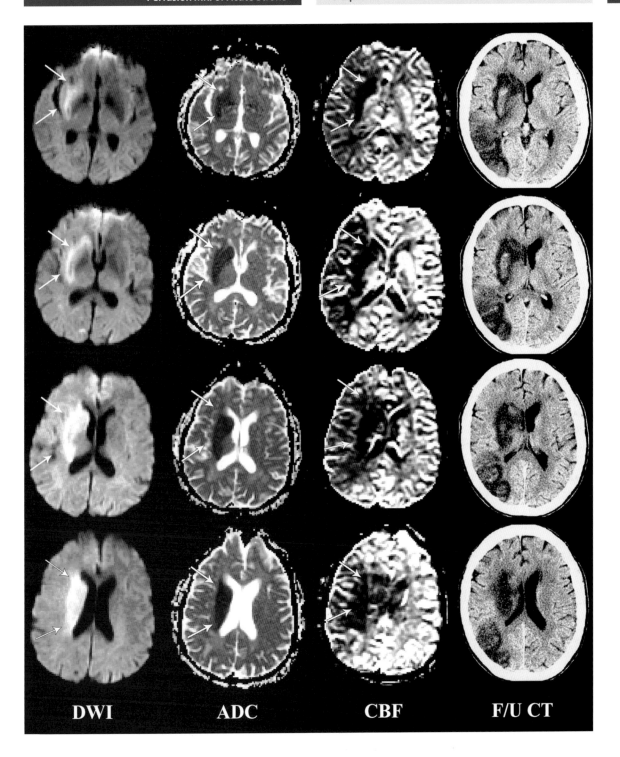

DWI   **ADC**   **CBF**   **F/U CT**

≤550 × 10^{-6}) mm^2/s correlated with HT of infarctions treated with i.v. t-PA [63], and Tong et al. [64] demonstrated that the mean ADC of ischemic regions that experienced HT was significantly lower than the overall mean ADC of all ischemic areas analyzed [(510±140)×10^{-6} mm^2/s vs. (623±113)×10^{-6} mm^2/s]. There was also a significant difference when comparing the HT-destined ischemic areas with non-HT-destined areas within the same ischemic lesion (P=0.02). Oppenheim et al. [65] demonstrated 100% sensitivity and 71% specificity for predicting HT when they divided infarcts into those with a mean ADC core of less than 300×10^{-6} mm^2/s compared to those with a mean ADC core of greater than 300×10^{-6} mm^2/s [65].

Cerebral blood flow may be the best perfusion parameter for identifying ischemic tissue that will undergo HT. With SPECT imaging, Ueda et al. [66] demonstrated an increased likelihood of HT in ischemic brain tissue with a CBF less than 35% of the normal cerebellar blood flow on SPECT imaging. It has also been demonstrated that CBF ratios are significantly lower in MCA infarctions that undergo HT than in those that do not. In one study, all ischemic tissue with a mean CBF ratio of less than 0.18 developed hemorrhage [67]. Other imaging parameters predictive of HT include:
1. Hypodensity in greater than one-third of the MCA territory on CT [68].
2. Early parenchymal enhancement on gadolinium-enhanced T1-weighted images [69].
3. Prior microbleeds detected on T2* gradient echo [70].

8.6.4 Correlation of Diffusion and Perfusion MRI with Clinical Outcome

A number of studies have shown how DWI can be used to predict clinical outcome (Table 8.6). Some studies have demonstrated statistically significant correlations between the acute anterior circulation DWI and ADC lesion volume and both acute and chronic neurological assessment tests including the NIHSS, the Canadian Neurological Scale, the Glasgow Outcome Score, the Barthel Index, and the Modified Rankin Scale [19, 26, 71–76]. Correlations between

Table 8.6. Diffusion and perfusion MRI in predicting clinical outcome

1. DWI, CBV, CBF, MTT, and TTP initial lesion volumes all correlate with acute and chronic neurologic assessment tests. It's unclear which parameter is best

2. DWI initial lesion volume correlation with outcome scales is higher for cortical than for penetrator artery strokes

3. Patients with a mismatch (proximal stroke) usually have worse clinical outcomes compared to patients without a mismatch (distal or lacunar stroke)

4. Size of the diffusion–perfusion mismatch volume correlates with clinical outcome

5. Amount of decrease in size of MTT abnormality volume following intravenous thrombolysis correlates with clinical outcome

DWI and ADC volume and clinical outcome, r, range from 0.65 to 0.78. In general, correlations are stronger for cortical strokes than for penetrator artery strokes [19, 72]. Lesion location may explain this difference. For example, a small ischemic lesion in the brainstem could produce a worse neurologic deficit than a cortical lesion of the same size. In fact, one study of posterior circulation strokes showed no correlation between initial DWI lesion volume and NIHSS [77]. A significant correlation has also been reported between the acute ADC ratio (ADC of lesion/ADC of normal contralateral brain) and chronic neurologic assessment scales [19, 71]. Furthermore, one study demonstrated that patients with a mismatch between the initial NIHSS score (>than 8) and the initial DWI lesion volume (<25 ml) had a higher probability of infarct growth and early neurologic deterioration [78]. Another demonstrated that for internal carotid artery (ICA) and middle cerebral artery (MCA) strokes, a DWI volume greater than 89 cm^3 was highly predictive (ROC curve with 85.7% sensitivity and 95.7% specificity) of early neurologic deterioration [79].

Initial CBV, CBF, MTT, and TTP lesion volumes also correlate with NIHSS, the Canadian Neurologic Scale, the Barthel Index, the Scandinavian Stroke Scale, and the modified Rankin Scale. Correlation coefficients, r, range from 0.71 to 0.96 [26, 29, 75, 80, 81].

Correlations are widely variable and it is unclear which initial perfusion map best predicts clinical outcome. In one study that compared initial CBV, CBF, and MTT volumes with modified Rankin scale, initial CBF volume had the highest correlation [81]. In another study that compared initial DWI, CBV, and MTT volumes with modified NIHSS, Rankin and Barthel Index, initial CBV had the highest correlation [82]. In general, patients who have perfusion lesion volumes larger than diffusion MR lesion volumes (perfusion–diffusion mismatches) have worse outcomes with larger final infarct volumes compared to patients without a diffusion–perfusion mismatch. Furthermore, the size of the diffusion–perfusion mismatch correlates with clinical outcome scales. In one study, patients with a DWI–MTT mismatch larger than 100 ml had a significantly larger lesion growth and a poorer outcome than patients with a smaller mismatch [75]. Thrombolytic therapy, due to early recanalization with reperfusion, can limit lesion growth and alter these correlations. In one study of patients treated with i.v. rt-PA, initial MTT volume correlated with the initial NIHSS but did not correlate with the NIHSS measured at 2–3 months [49]. In another study, the best independent predictor of excellent outcome in patients treated with i.v. t-PA was an MTT lesion volume decrease of more than 30 % 2 h after i.v. t-PA therapy [83].

8.6.5 Perfusion/Diffusion Mismatch in Patient Selection for Thrombolysis.

The Desmoteplase In Acute Ischemic Stroke trial (DIAS) [83] was a placebo-controlled, double-blind, randomized, dose-finding phase II trial designed to evaluate the safety and efficacy of intravenous desmoteplase administered within 3 to 9 hours of ischemic stroke onset in patients selected by the MRI criteria of a perfusion/diffusion mismatch on MRI. Patients with NIH Stroke Scale scores of 4 to 20 and MRI evidence of perfusion/diffusion mismatch were eligible. Reperfusion rates up to 71.4 % (P=0.0012) were observed with desmoteplase given at 125 mug/kg compared with 19.2 % with placebo. A favorable 90-day clinical outcome was found in 60.0of patients treated with desmoteplase % (125 mug/kg; P=0.0090)

compared to 22.2 % of placebo-treated patients. Further details are described in chapter 11. The imaging inclusion criteria included a DWI abnormality of less that 1/3 of the MCA territory, and a perfusion abnormality 20 % greater than the DWI abnormality. This was a multicenter trial and the specific perfusion analysis system varied among sites. The key requirement was that the perfusion data be immediately available. It appears that simple perfusion algorithms were primarily used such as time-to-peak (TTP) because these are easily generated at the MRI scanner console. A phase III trial of desmoteplase using the same imaging imaging criteria is currently underway.

8.7 Conclusion

Perfusion MRI allows evaluation of the hemodynamic status of acutely ischemic tissue and has greatly improved evaluation of acute stroke. The CBV abnormality correlates highly with the DWI abnormality, which is thought to represent the ischemic core. With proximal emboli, CBF and tissue transit time maps demonstrate the operational ischemic penumbra, additional tissue with altered perfusion that is at risk of progressing to infarction. Diffusion and perfusion MRI are useful in predicting tissue viability, and are also useful in predicting HT and clinical outcome. Most importantly, it has now been shown how DWI–PWI mismatch criteria may be used to successfully guide thrombolytic therapy.

References

1. Rosen BR, Belliveau JW, Vevea JM, Brady TJ (1990) Perfusion imaging with NMR contrast agents. Magn Reson Med 14:249–265
2. Speck O, Chang L, DeSilva N, Ernst T (2000) Perfusion MRI of the human brain with dynamic susceptibility contrast. Gradient-echo versus spin-echo techniques. J Magn Reson Imaging 12:381–387
3. Heiland S, Kreibich W, Benner T, Dorfler A, Forsting M, Sartor K (1998) Comparison of echo-planar sequences for perfusion weighted-MRI: which is best? Neuroradiology 40:216–221

4. Ogawa S, Lee T, Nayak A, Glynn P (1990) Oxygenation-sensitive contrast in magnetic resonance image of rodent brain at high magnetic fields. Magn Reson Med 14:68–78

5. Williams D, Detre J, Leigh L, Koretsky A (1992) Magnetic resonance imaging of perfusion using spin inversion of arterial water. Proc Natl Acad Sci USA 89:212–216

6. Edelman RR, Siewert B, Darby DG, Thangaraj V, Nobre A, Mesulam M, Warach S (1994) Qualitative mapping of cerebral blood flow and functional localization with echo-planar MR imaging and signal targeting with alternating radiofrequency. Radiology 192:513–520

7. Siewert B, Bly B, Schlaug G, Darby DG, Thangaraj V, Warach S, Edelman RR (1996) Comparison of the bold and epistar technique for functional brain imaging by using signal detection theory. Magn Reson Med 36:249–255

8. Ye F, Berman K, Ellmore T, Esposito G, van Horn J, Yang Y, Duyn J, Smith A, Frank J, Weinberger D, McLaughlin A (2000) H(2)(15)o PET validation of steady-state arterial spin tagging cerebral blood flow measurements in humans. Magn Reson Med 44:450–456

9. Ostergaard L, Weisskoff RM, Chesler DA, Gyldensted C, Rosen BR (1996) High resolution measurement of cerebral blood flow using intravascular tracer bolus passages, part 1. Mathematical approach and statistical analysis. Magn Reson Med 36:715–725

10. Ostergaard L, Sorensen AG, Kwong KK, Weisskoff RM, Gyldensted C, Rosen BR (1996) High resolution measurement of cerebral blood flow using intravascular tracer bolus passages, part 2. Experimental comparison and preliminary results. Magn Reson Med 36:726–736

11. Yamada K, Wu O, Gonzalez RG, Bakker D, Ostergaard L, Copen WA, Weisskoff RM, Rosen BR, Yagi K, Nishimura T, Sorensen AG (2002) Magnetic resonance perfusion-weighted imaging of acute cerebral infarction: effect of the calculation methods and underlying vasculopathy. Stroke 33:87–94

12. Calamante F, Gadian DG, Connelly A (2000) Delay and dispersion effects in dynamic susceptibility contrast MRI: simulations using singular value decomposition. Magn Reson Med 44:466–473

13. Wu O, Ostergaard L, Koroshetz WJ, Schwamm LH, O'Donnell J, Schaefer PW, Rosen BR, Weisskoff RM, Sorensen AG (2003) Effects of tracer arrival time on flow estimates in MR perfusion-weighted imaging. Magn Reson Med 50:856–864

14. Thijs V, Somford D, Bammer R, Robberecht W, Moseley ME, Albers GW (2004) Influence of arterial input function on hypoperfusion volumes measured with perfusion-weighted imaging. Stroke 35:94–98

15. Wu O, Ostergaard L, Weisskoff RM, Benner T, Rosen BR, Sorensen AG (2003) Tracer arrival timing-insensitive technique for estimating flow in MR perfusion-weighted imaging using singular value decomposition with a block-circulant deconvolution matrix. Magn Reson Med 50:164–174

16. Schaefer PW, Hunter GJ, He J, Hamberg LM, Sorensen AG, Schwamm LH, Koroshetz WJ, Gonzalez RG (2002) Predicting cerebral ischemic infarct volume with diffusion and perfusion MR imaging. Am J Neuroradiol 23:1785–1794

17. Kucharczyk J, Mintorovitch J, Asgari HS, Moseley M (1991) Diffusion/perfusion MR imaging of acute cerebral ischemia. Magn Reson Med 19:311–315

18. Mintorovitch J, Moseley ME, Chileuitt L, Shimizu H, Cohen Y, Weinstein PR (1991) Comparison of diffusion- and T2-weighted MRI for the early detection of cerebral ischemia and reperfusion in rats. Magn Reson Med 18:39–50

19. Schwamm LH, Koroshetz WJ, Sorensen AG, Wang B, Copen WA, Budzik R, Rordorf G, Buonanno FS, Schaefer PW, Gonzalez RG (1998) Time course of lesion development in patients with acute stroke: serial diffusion- and hemodynamic-weighted magnetic resonance imaging. Stroke 29:2268–2276

20. Moseley ME, Cohen Y, Mintorovitch J, Chileuitt L, Shimizu H, Kucharczyk J, Wendland MF, Weinstein PR (1990) Early detection of regional cerebral ischemia in cats: comparison of diffusion- and T2-weighted MRI and spectroscopy. Magn Reson Med 14:330–346

21. Rosen BR, Belliveau JW, Buchbinder BR et al (1991) Contrast agents and cerebral hemodynamics. Magn Reson Med 19:285–292

22. Baird AE, Benfield A, Schlaug G, Siewert B, Lovblad KO, Edelman RR, Warach S (1997) Enlargement of human cerebral ischemic lesion volumes measured by diffusion-weighted magnetic resonance imaging. Ann Neurol 41:581–589

23. Beaulieu C, de Crespigny A, Tong DC, Moseley ME, Albers GW, Marks MP (1999) Longitudinal magnetic resonance imaging study of perfusion and diffusion in stroke: evolution of lesion volume and correlation with clinical outcome. Ann Neurol 46:568–578

24. Rordorf G, Koroshetz WJ, Copen WA, Cramer SC, Schaefer PW, Budzik RF Jr., Schwamm LH, Buonanno F, Sorensen AG, Gonzalez G (1998) Regional ischemia and ischemic injury in patients with acute middle cerebral artery stroke as defined by early diffusion-weighted and perfusion-weighted MRI. Stroke 29:939–943

25. Sorensen AG, Copen WA, Ostergaard L, Buonanno FS, Gonzalez RG, Rordorf G, Rosen BR, Schwamm LH, Weisskoff RM, Koroshetz WJ (1999) Hyperacute stroke: simultaneous measurement of relative cerebral blood volume, relative cerebral blood flow, and mean tissue transit time. Radiology 210:519–527

26. Tong DC, Yenari MA, Albers GW, O'Brien M, Marks MP, Moseley ME (1998) Correlation of perfusion- and diffusion-weighted MRI with NIHSS score in acute (<6.5 hour) ischemic stroke. Neurology 50:864–870

27. Karonen JO, Liu Y, Vanninen RL, Ostergaard L, Kaarina Partanen PL, Vainio PA, Vanninen EJ, Nuutinen J, Roivainen R, Soimakallio S, Kuikka JT, Aronen HJ (2000) Combined perfusion- and diffusion-weighted MR imaging in acute ischemic stroke during the 1st week: a longitudinal study. Radiology 217:886–894

28. Karonen JO, Vanninen RL, Liu Y, Ostergaard L, Kuikka JT, Nuutinen J, Vanninen EJ, Partanen PL, Vainio PA, Korhonen K, Perkio J, Roivainen R, Sivenius J, Aronen HJ (1999) Combined diffusion and perfusion MRI with correlation to single-photon emission ct in acute ischemic stroke. Ischemic penumbra predicts infarct growth. Stroke 30:1583–1590

29. Barber PA, Darby DG, Desmond PM, Yang Q, Gerraty RP, Jolley D, Donnan GA, Tress BM, Davis SM (1998) Prediction of stroke outcome with echoplanar perfusion- and diffusion-weighted MRI. Neurology 51:418–426

30. Schaefer PW, Ozsunar Y, He J, Hamberg LM, Hunter GJ, Sorensen AG, Koroshetz WJ, Gonzalez RG (2003) Assessing tissue viability with MR diffusion and perfusion imaging. Am J Neuroradiol 24:436–443

31. Schlaug G, Benfield A, Baird AE, Siewert B, Lovblad KO, Parker RA, Edelman RR, Warach S (1999) The ischemic penumbra: operationally defined by diffusion and perfusion MRI. Neurology 53:1528–1537

32. Rohl L, Ostergaard L, Simonsen CZ, Vestergaard-Poulsen P, Andersen G, Sakoh M, Le Bihan D, Gyldensted C (2001) Viability thresholds of ischemic penumbra of hyperacute stroke defined by perfusion-weighted MRI and apparent diffusion coefficient. Stroke 32:1140–1146

33. Liu Y, Karonen JO, Vanninen RL, Ostergaard L, Roivainen R, Nuutinen J, Perkio J, Kononen M, Hamalainen A, Vanninen EJ, Soimakallio S, Kuikka JT, Aronen HJ (2000) Cerebral hemodynamics in human acute ischemic stroke: a study with diffusion- and perfusion-weighted magnetic resonance imaging and SPECT. J Cereb Blood Flow Metab 20:910–920

34. Grandin CB, Duprez TP, Smith AM, Mataigne F, Peeters A, Oppenheim C, Cosnard G (2001) Usefulness of magnetic resonance-derived quantitative measurements of cerebral blood flow and volume in prediction of infarct growth in hyperacute stroke. Stroke 32:1147–1153

35. Lassen NA (1985) Normal average value of cerebral blood flow in younger adults is 50 ml/100 g/min. J Cereb Blood Flow Metab 5:347–349

36. Jones TH, Morawetz RB, Crowell RM, Marcoux FW, FitzGibbon SJ, DeGirolami U, Ojemann RG (1981) Thresholds of focal cerebral ischemia in awake monkeys. J Neurosurg 54:773–782

37. Ueda T, Sakaki S, Yuh WT, Nochide I, Ohta S (1999) Outcome in acute stroke with successful intra-arterial thrombolysis and predictive value of initial single-photon emission-computed tomography. J Cereb Blood Flow Metab 19:99–108

38. Rempp KA, Brix G, Wenz F, Becker CR, Guckel F, Lorenz WJ (1994) Quantification of regional cerebral blood flow and volume with dynamic susceptibility contrast-enhanced MR imaging. Radiology 193:637–641

39. Frackowiak RS, Lenzi GL, Jones T, Heather JD (1980) Quantitative measurement of regional cerebral blood flow and oxygen metabolism in man using ^{15}O and positron emission tomography: theory, procedure, and normal values. J Comput Assist Tomogr 4:727–736

40. Furlan M, Marchal G, Viader F, Derlon JM, Baron JC (1996) Spontaneous neurological recovery after stroke and the fate of the ischemic penumbra. Ann Neurol 40:216–226

41. Marchal G, Beaudouin V, Rioux P, de la Sayette V, Le Doze F, Viader F, Derlon JM, Baron JC (1996) Prolonged persistence of substantial volumes of potentially viable brain tissue after stroke: a correlative PET-CT study with voxel-based data analysis. Stroke 27:599–606

42. Hatazawa J, Shimosegawa E, Toyoshima H, Ardekani BA, Suzuki A, Okudera T, Miura Y (1999) Cerebral blood volume in acute brain infarction: a combined study with dynamic susceptibility contrast MRI and 99mTc-HMPAO-SPECT. Stroke 30:800–806

43. Powers WJ (1991) Cerebral hemodynamics in ischemic cerebrovascular disease. Ann Neurol 29:231–240

44. Neumann-Haefelin T, Wittsack HJ, Wenserski F, Siebler M, Seitz RJ, Modder U, Freund HJ (1999) Diffusion and perfusion-weighted MRI. The DWI/PWI mismatch region in acute stroke. Stroke 8:1591–1597

45. Wittsack HJ, Ritzl A, Fink GR, Wenserski F, Siebler M, Seitz RJ, Modder U, Freund HJ (2002) MR imaging in acute stroke: diffusion-weighted and perfusion imaging parameters for predicting infarct size. Radiology 222:397–403

46. Grandin CB, Duprez TP, Smith AM, Oppenheim C, Peeters A, Robert AR, Cosnard G (2002) Which MR-derived perfusion parameters are the best predictors of infarct growth in hyperacute stroke? Comparative study between relative and quantitative measurements. Radiology 223:361–370

47. Oppenheim C, Grandin C, Samson Y, Smith A, Duprez T, Marsault C, Cosnard G (2001) Is there an apparent diffusion coefficient threshold in predicting tissue viability in hyperacute stroke? Stroke 32:2486–2491

48. Wu O, Koroshetz WJ, Ostergaard L, Buonanno FS, Copen WA, Gonzalez RG, Rordorf G, Rosen BR, Schwamm LH, Weisskoff RM, Sorensen AG (2001) Predicting tissue outcome in acute human cerebral ischemia using combined diffusion- and perfusion-weighted MR imaging. Stroke 32:933–942

49. Parsons MW, Barber PA, Chalk J, Darby DG, Rose S, Desmond PM, Gerraty RP, Tress BM, Wright PM, Donnan GA, Davis SM (2002) Diffusion- and perfusion-weighted MRI response to thrombolysis in stroke. Ann Neurol 51:28–37

50. Fiehler J, von Bezold M, Kucinski T, Knab R, Eckert B, Wittkugel O, Zeumer H, Rother J (2002) Cerebral blood flow predicts lesion growth in acute stroke patients. Stroke 33:2421–2425

51. Shih LC, Saver JL, Alger JR, Starkman S, Leary MC, Vinuela F, Duckwiler G, Gobin YP, Jahan R, Villablanca JP, Vespa PM, Kidwell CS (2003) Perfusion-weighted magnetic resonance imaging thresholds identifying core, irreversibly infarcted tissue. Stroke 34:1425–1430

52. Kidwell CS, Saver JL, Mattiello J, Starkman S, Vinuela F, Duckwiler G, Gobin YP, Jahan R, Vespa P, Villablanca JP, Liebeskind DS, Woods RP, Alger JR (2001) Diffusion-perfusion MRI characterization of post-recanalization hyperperfusion in humans. Neurology 57:2015–2021

53. Derex L, Nighoghossian N, Hermier M, Adeleine P, Berthezene Y, Philippeau F, Honnorat J, Froment JC, Trouillas P (2004) Influence of pretreatment MRI parameters on clinical outcome, recanalization and infarct size in 49 stroke patients treated by intravenous tissue plasminogen activator. J Neurol Sci 225:3–9

54. Horowitz SH, Zito JL, Donnarumma R, Patel M, Alvir J (1991) Computed tomographic-angiographic findings within the first five hours of cerebral infarction. Stroke 22:1245–1253

55. Hornig CR, Dorndorf W, Agnoli AL (1986) Hemorrhagic cerebral infarction – a prospective study. Stroke 17:179–185

56. Hakim AM, Ryder-Cooke A, Melanson D (1983) Sequential computerized tomographic appearance of strokes. Stroke 14:893–897

57. Calandre L, Ortega JF, Bermejo F (1984) Anticoagulation and hemorrhagic infarction in cerebral embolism secondary to rheumatic heart disease. Arch Neurol 41:1152–1154

58. Kidwell CS, Saver JL, Carneado J, Sayre J, Starkman S, Duckwiler G, Gobin YP, Jahan R, Vespa P, Villablanca JP, Liebeskind DS, Vinuela F (2002) Predictors of hemorrhagic transformation in patients receiving intra-arterial thrombolysis. Stroke 33:717–724

59. Ogata J, Yutani C, Imakita M, Ishibashi-Ueda H, Saku Y, Minematsu K, Sawada T, Yamaguchi T (1989) Hemorrhagic infarct of the brain without a reopening of the occluded arteries in cardioembolic stroke. Stroke 20:876–883

60. Lin DD, Filippi CG, Steever AB, Zimmerman RD (2001) Detection of intracranial hemorrhage: comparison between gradient-echo images and b(0) images obtained from diffusion-weighted echo-planar sequences. Am J Neuroradiol 22:1275–1281

61. Liotta LA, Goldfarb RH, Brundage R, Siegal GP, Terranova V, Garbisa S (1981) Effect of plasminogen activator (urokinase), plasmin, and thrombin on glycoprotein and collagenous components of basement membrane. Cancer Res 41:4629–4636

62. Carmeliet P, Moons L, Lijnen R, Baes M, Lemaitre V, Tipping P, Drew A, Eeckhout Y, Shapiro S, Lupu F, Collen D (1997) Urokinase-generated plasmin activates matrix metalloproteinases during aneurysm formation. Nat Genet 17:439–444

63. Selim M, Fink JN, Kumar S, Caplan LR, Horkan C, Chen Y, Linfante I, Schlaug G (2002) Predictors of hemorrhagic transformation after intravenous recombinant tissue plasminogen activator: prognostic value of the initial apparent diffusion coefficient and diffusion-weighted lesion volume. Stroke 33:2047–2052

64. Tong DC, Adami A, Moseley ME, Marks MP (2001) Prediction of hemorrhagic transformation following acute stroke: role of diffusion- and perfusion-weighted magnetic resonance imaging. Arch Neurol 58:587–593

65. Oppenheim C, Samson Y, Dormont D, Crozier S, Manai R, Rancurel G, Fredy D, Marsault C (2002) DWI prediction of symptomatic hemorrhagic transformation in acute MCA infarct. J Neuroradiol 29:6–13

66. Ueda T, Hatakeyama T, Kumon Y, Sakaki S, Uraoka T (1994) Evaluation of risk of hemorrhagic transformation in local intra-arterial thrombolysis in acute ischemic stroke by initial SPECT. Stroke 25:298–303

67. Schaefer PW, Roccatagliata L, Schwamm L, Gonzalez RG (2003) Assessing hemorrhagic transformation with diffusion and perfusion MR imaging. In: Book of abstracts of the 41st annual meeting of the American Society of Neuroradiology, Washington DC, 28 April – 2 May 2003

68. Von Kummer R, Allen KL, Holle R, Bozzao L, Bastianello S, Manelfe C, Bluhmki E, Ringleb P, Meier DH, Hacke W (1997) Acute stroke: usefulness of early ct findings before thrombolytic therapy. Radiology 205:327–333

69. Vo KD, Santiago F, Lin W, Hsu CY, Lee Y, Lee JM (2003) MR imaging enhancement patterns as predictors of hemorrhagic transformation in acute ischemic stroke. Am J Neuroradiol 24:674–679

70. Kidwell CS, Saver JL, Villablanca JP, Duckwiler G, Fredieu A, Gough K, Leary MC, Starkman S, Gobin YP, Jahan R, Vespa P, Liebeskind DS, Alger JR, Vinuela F (2002) Magnetic resonance imaging detection of microbleeds before thrombolysis: an emerging application. Stroke 33:95–98

71. Van Everdingen KJ, van der Grond J, Kappelle LJ, Ramos LM, Mali WP (1998) Diffusion-weighted magnetic resonance imaging in acute stroke. Stroke 29:1783–1790

72. Lovblad KO, Baird AE, Schlaug G, Benfield A, Siewert B, Voetsch B, Connor A, Burzynski C, Edelman RR, Warach S (1997) Ischemic lesion volumes in acute stroke by diffusion-weighted magnetic resonance imaging correlate with clinical outcome. Ann Neurol 42:164–170

73. Engelter S, Provenzale JM, Petrella JR, DeLong D, Alberts M (2003) Infarct volume on apparent diffusion coefficient maps correlates with length of stay and outcome after middle cerebral artery stroke. Cerebrovasc Dis 15:188–191

74. Nighoghossian N, Hermier M, Adeleine P, Derex L, Dugor J, Philippea F, Yimaz H, Honnorat J, Dardel P, Berthezene Y, Froment JC, Trouillas P (2003) Baseline magnetic resonance imaging parameters and stroke outcome in patients treated by intravenous tissue plasminogen activator. Stroke 34:458–463

75. Rohl L, Geday J, Ostergaard L, Simonsen CZ, Vestergaard-Poulsen P, Andersen G, Le Bihan D, Gyldensted C (2001) Correlation between diffusion- and perfusion-weighted MRI and neurological deficit measured by the Scandinavian stroke scale and Barthel index in hyperacute subcortical stroke (<or = 6 hours). Cerebrovasc Dis 12:203–213

76. Thijs V, Lansberg M, Beaulieu C, Marks MP, Moseley M, Albers GW (2000) Is early ischemic lesion volume on diffusion-weighted imaging an independent predictor of stroke outcome? A multivariable analysis. Stroke 31:2597–2602

77. Engelter S, Wetzel S, Radue E, Rausch M, Steck A, Lyrer P (2004) The clinical significance of diffusion-weighted MR imaging in infratentorial strokes. Neurology 62:474–480

78. Davalos A, Blanco M, Pedraza S, Leira R, Castellanos M, Pumar J, Silva Y, Serena J, Castillo J (2004) The clinical-DWI mismatch: a new diagnostic approach to the brain tissue at risk of infarction. Neurology 62:2187–2192

79. Arenillas J, Rovira A, Molina C, Grive E, Montaner J, Alvarez-Sabin J (2002) Prediction of early neurologic deterioration using diffusion- and perfusion- weighted imaging in hyperacute middle cerebral artery stroke. Stroke 33:2197–2203

80. Baird AE, Lovblad KO, Dashe JF, Connor A, Burzynski C, Schlaug G, Straroselskaya I, Edelman RR, Warach S (2000) Clinical correlations of diffusion and perfusion lesion volumes in acute ischemic stroke. Cerebrovasc Dis 10:441–448

81. Parsons MW, Yang Q, Barber PA, Darby DG, Desmond PM, Gerraty RP, Tress BM, Davis SM (2001) Perfusion magnetic resonance imaging maps in hyperacute stroke: relative cerebral blood flow most accurately identifies tissue destined to infarct. Stroke 32:1581–1587

82. Kluytmans M et al (2000) Prognostic value of perfusion- and diffusion-weighted MR imaging in first 3 days of stroke. Eur Radiol 10(9):1434–1441

83. Hacke W et al (2005) The Desmoteplase in Acute Ischemic Stroke Trial (DIAS): A Phase II MRI-Based 9-Hour Window Acute Stroke Thrombolysis Trial With Intravenous Desmoteplase. Stroke 36(1):66–73

Acute Stroke Imaging with SPECT, PET, Xenon-CT, and MR Spectroscopy

Mark E. Mullins

9.1 Introduction

This chapter briefly reviews current methods for diagnosing acute stroke other than the CT and MRI techniques described in the prior chapters. These include radionuclide perfusion imaging using the nuclear medicine techniques of single photon emission computed tomography (SPECT), perfusion and neurochemical imaging via positron emission tomography (PET), metabolic imaging through magnetic resonance spectroscopy (MRS), and inhalational-mediated xenon CT perfusion (Xe-CT). The intent of this chapter is to provide a brief overview of these techniques. The reader is directed to the Reference section for additional information. For a brief synopsis, please refer to Table 9.1.

9.2 SPECT

Technique and Theory. This modality uses a diffusible tracer. The active moiety is the "workhorse" of nuclear scintigraphy, technetium-99m ([Tc-99m]). [Tc-99m] is complexed with a carrier organic molecule that acts as an introducer into the neural axis, across the blood–brain barrier [1]. Most facilities use hexamethylpropyleneamine oxime (HMPAO) whereas others use ethylcysteine dimer (ECD) or DTPA (diethyleneamine pentaacetate) for the organic complex [1, 2]. Radiopharmaceutical administration is through the intravenous route and uptake within the neural tissue varies directly with blood flow, but the mechanism of stabilization within the tissues is unknown [1]. Alternatively, [Xe-133] (gas) may be inhaled and evaluated in the steady state, but

Table 9.1. Comparison and contrast of the modalities not in routine use for acute stroke evaluation. (*MRS* Magnetic resonance spectroscopy, *PET* positron emission tomography, *SPECT* single photon emission computed tomography, *Xe-CT* xenon computed tomography)

	PET	SPECT	Xe-CT	MR spectroscopy
Preparation time (approximate)	30 min	30 min	15 min	None
Scanning time (approximate)	30–60 min	5 min	15 min	5–30 min
Post-processing time (approximate)	15 min	15 min	5–15 min	0–15 min
Modality	Routine PET scanner	Routine 2- or 3-head SPECT camera	Multidetector CT scanner	MR scanner with MRS add-on
Administration	Intravenous	Intravenous	Inhalational	None
Tracer	[F-18]-Fluorodeoxy-glucose or [O-15]-O_2, -CO or -CO_2	[Tc-99m] HMPAO or [Tc-99m]-IMP	Xe-133	N/A
Tracer characteristic	Diffusible	Diffusible	Diffusible	N/A
Ionizing radiation	Yes	Yes	Yes	No
Radioactive tracer	Yes	Yes	No	N/A
Spatial resolution (relative)	Low	Low	High	Low
Portion of brain imaged	Entire	Entire	2-cm-thick slab in 4–6 slices	1 cm^3 (single voxel) or smaller (multiple voxel)
Contraindications (absolute)	Allergy	Allergy	Allergy	MR safety incompatibility
Sensitivity	N/A	61–74%	N/A	N/A
Specificity	N/A	88–98%	N/A	N/A
Primary references	[13]	[1]	[1]	[23, 24]

this type of imaging requires specialized equipment (ventilation) and is not in routine widespread use [3].

Product. Semi-quantitative manifestation of regional cerebral blood flow (rCBF) is typical [1]. Quantitative measurements of blood flow are possible via peripheral arterial blood sample evaluation in order to provide absolute counts of radioactivity in correlation to the imaging results [1]. However, because of the invasive nature of the quantitative measurements thus obtained, quantitative imaging is typically not invoked.

Availability. Excellent. Practically any Radiology Department with the capability to perform routine SPECT imaging is eligible. Requirements include routinely available gamma cameras with SPECT processing computers and the ability to make and administer the radionuclide.

Literature Review. Comparisons of the rCBF provided by [Tc-99m]-ECD SPECT have shown good correlation to results obtained using perfusion-weighted MR imaging (PWI) and PET [1, 4]. Comparisons of the rCBF provided by [Tc-99m]-HMPAO SPECT have shown good correlation with PWI [1, 5]. SPECT [6, 7] has been shown to have good/excellent sensitivity and outstanding specificity for detecting the presence and extent of acute stroke [1, 8]. Decisions regarding thrombolysis have been based upon SPECT thresholding as described by Ueda [9] and others [10] with good results [1]. The prediction of possible post-carotid endarterectomy hyperperfusion has been based upon SPECT results [11]. There are also data to support a good correlation with SPECT rCBF threshold values and severity and clinical outcome [12], including but not limited to development of intracranial hemorrhage [1, 3]. The conclusions of Ueda and colleagues are as follows [9]:

1. rCBF ratio >0.55 indicates possible reversibility, regardless of ictal onset time.
2. rCBF ratio <0.35 indicates increased risk of hemorrhage with therapy, regardless of ictal onset time.
3. rCBF ratio 0.35–0.55 indicates potential reversibility if treatment is instituted within the therapeutic window of <6 h.

9.2.1 Advantages

1. Most large departments contain the requisite materials and machinery to perform this technique.
2. Sedation issues and motion are typically not detrimental to imaging.
3. Imaging is quick, as are calculations and image production.
4. Literature-proven for very specific uses.
5. Could theoretically improve differentiation in specific situations where the differential diagnosis includes tumor.
6. Could potentially provide a surrogate marker for guiding stroke thrombolysis and treatment if threshold values are used despite placement within the 3- or 6-h therapeutic window.

9.2.2 Liabilities

1. Low spatial resolution.
2. Lack of fine anatomical detail/co-registration with anatomical imaging such as conventional MR imaging and/or CT scanning. Results must be corre-

lated with anatomical imaging to differentiate the simple absence of brain tissue from ischemic derangement of brain tissue; for example, an arachnoid cyst or surgical cavity may have the same appearance as infarct on SPECT scan and must be differentiated.
3. Ionizing radiation exposure, albeit minimal.
4. Patient remains at least somewhat radioactive after the procedure, thus bringing into play issues of protecting family and medical carers from additional exposure.
5. Not all medical facilities will be able to offer this service, especially at any time. For example, if radionuclide kits must be obtained from elsewhere, there is a great delay until imaging. Moreover, typical SPECT equipment is a necessity and not all facilities are set up for this, even if nuclear medicine facilities exist.
6. The technique is only semi-quantitative in its most typical use. Quantitative evaluation would require arterial access in an ongoing fashion (semi-invasive).
7. Internal comparison is utilized in the semi-quantitative approach; thus, the assumption is that the control regions have normal perfusion. This may be an erroneous assumption in certain patients and could result in misinterpretation.
8. White matter perfusion data thus obtained are apparently not reliable.

Summary. SPECT evaluation of stroke is a promising technique in that it images physiology and thus may eventually serve as a surrogate for the triage of stroke victims concerning treatment. Ueda's work suggests that this is possible with current technology. However, the need for specialized equipment and at least 30 min to evaluate the patient may be prohibitive in some settings. Moreover, additional anatomical imaging will be necessary, including at least noncontrast head CT. Thus, competition of this technique with CT and MR perfusion is likely to be limited, at least for the foreseeable future.

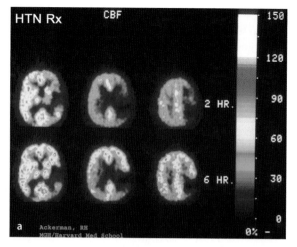

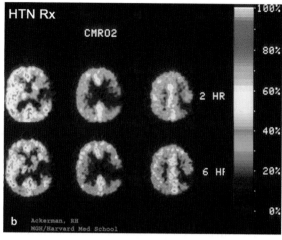

Figure 9.1 a–c

Patient with acute ischemic stroke treated with hypertensive therapy. a Positron emission tomography images of cerebral blood flow at 2 h (*top*) and 6 h (*bottom*) after the onset of symptoms. PET cerebral blood flow (*CBF*) images demonstrate a significant reduction in blood flow affecting a substantial portion of the left middle cerebral artery territory. b PET images of regional cerebral metabolic rate of oxygen at 2 h (*top*) and 6 h (*bottom*) after the onset of symptoms. Oxygen metabolism is abnormal in the left middle cerebral artery (*MCA*) territory, but in an area substantially smaller than the defect seen on the CBF images. This reduction in tissue at risk was presumably due to hypertensive therapy. c Follow-up CT scan of the head in the patient demonstrating that the ultimate cerebral infarct size most closely approximates the oxygen metabolism defect (b) than the CBF defect (a). (Images courtesy of Dr. Robert Ackerman, MD)

9.3 PET

Technique and Theory. This modality uses a diffusible tracer. The active moiety is either the "workhorse" of PET, [F-18]-fluorodeoxyglucose (FDG, half-life=110 min), or O_2, CO, or CO_2 labeled with [O-15] (half-life 2 min). Brain tissue typically takes up glucose as its primary energy substrate and is quite ac-

tively metabolic at baseline on PET scan. Decreased metabolism on PET scan indicates hypometabolism. Although there is a differential diagnosis for this appearance, once the clinical scenario and anatomic imaging are correlated to the PET scan findings, the PET results may predict infarction (Fig. 9.1). FDG imaging works on the basis of the glucose extraction fraction whereas [O-15] imaging works on the basis of the oxygen extraction fraction.

Product. Quantitative manifestation of cerebral blood flow (CBF), cerebral blood volume (CBV), mean transit time (MTT=CBV/CBF), cerebral perfusion pressure (CPP=1/MTT), cerebral metabolic rate of oxygen consumption (CMRO), oxygen extraction fraction (OEF), and cerebral glucose utilization is typical [1]. Normally, gray matter exceeds white matter extraction, and the supply of both glucose and oxygen to brain tissues exceeds its requirement by 2–3 times; derangement of this relationship is most common with ischemia/infarct. Quantitative measurements are possible using [O-15]-labeled substrates whereas nonquantitative measurements are typically used with FDG. Semi-quantitative measurements with FDG are possible with peripheral arterial blood sampling and comparison to internal standards (apparently unaffected brain). Specific uptake value (SUV) measurements are of limited utility in this clinical scenario.

Availability. Good. Practically any Radiology Department with the capability to perform routine PET imaging is eligible. However, due to the relatively short half-life of [O-15], use of this isotope requires specialized equipment and continuous flow-through devices for administration, as well as specialized ventilation. Requirements also include PET scanners and the ability to make or obtain and/or otherwise administer the radionuclide.

Literature Review. Reduced CPP induces changes in the remaining perfusion parameters [13]. Initially, however, a slight reduction in CPP has little effect on CBF whereas CBV may remain stable or increase slightly in relation to autoregulatory mechanisms (vasodilatation) [13]. Once the ability to vasodilate sufficiently to augment perfusion has been exhausted, CBF decreases at a rapid rate, CMRO declines slightly, and OEF increases at a rapid rate [13]. Regional OEF measurements thus represent an indicator of local autoregulatory failure, a direct manifestation of cerebrovascular disease [14, 15]. It is in this regard that PET [6, 7] exceeds provocative perfusion techniques such as cerebrovascular reserve measurements, which necessitate the administration of an additional medication and/or use of provocative maneuvers that may place the patient at additional risk. Increased OEF distal to known high-grade arterial disease in patients with no or reversible symptoms has been shown to be an independent predictor for stroke; moreover, this type of determination is not possible with any other current modality, and additionally it is relatively noninvasive and safe [13]. Studies evaluating the treatment of arterial disease have not shown statistically significant improvement in outcome when based on PET [13]. Moreover, although increased OEF suggests that brain tissue is still alive, studies indicate that, despite the plethora of measurements available with PET, determination of viability remains confounding [3, 13]. Prediction of clinical outcome based on PET thresholding has been controversial and variable [4, 13].

9.3.1 Advantages

1. Many large departments contain the baseline requisite materials and machinery to perform FDG-PET and some also can perform [O-15]-PET. Membership in this group is increasing all the time, as PET scanning becomes more popular.
2. Sedation issues and motion are typically not detriments to imaging, although the length of the examination may preclude acutely ill patients or those who are combative and cannot be sedated because of serial neurological testing.
3. This technique is quantitative.
4. OEF physiological measurements in relation to asymptomatic or TIA-related severe arterial disease have been statistically verified and are uniquely useful. Other uses, however, remain unproven in the literature.
5. The technique could theoretically improve differentiation in specific situations where the differential diagnosis includes tumor.
6. Could *potentially eventually* provide a surrogate marker for guiding stroke thrombolysis, and studies are underway to provide support for these applications. However, past studies have been unsuccessful in determining a significant benefit from its use in this regard.

9.3.2 Liabilities

1. Expensive.
2. This technique has low spatial resolution.
3. Lack of fine anatomical detail/co-registration with anatomical imaging such as conventional MR imaging and/or CT scanning. Results must be correlated with anatomical imaging to differentiate the simple absence of brain tissue from ischemic derangement of brain tissue; for example, an arachnoid cyst or surgical cavity may have the same appearance as infarct on PET scan and must be differentiated.
4. Ionizing radiation exposure.
5. Patient remains at least somewhat radioactive after the procedure, thus bringing into play issues of family and medical carer protection from additional exposure.
6. Not all medical facilities will be able to offer this service at any time. For example, if FDG must be obtained from elsewhere, there is a great delay until imaging. Moreover, typical PET equipment is a necessity and not all facilities are set up for this, even if nuclear medicine facilities exist.
7. Internal comparison is utilized in the semi-quantitative approach; thus, the assumption is that the control regions have normal perfusion. This may be an erroneous assumption in certain patients and could result in misinterpretation.

Summary. PET evaluation of stroke is a promising technique in that it images physiology such as OEF and thus may eventually serve as a surrogate for the triage of stroke victims concerning treatment. However, the need for specialized equipment and at least 75 min to evaluate the patient may be prohibitive in some settings. Its use in asymptomatic patients and/or those with TIA and severe arterial disease to predict increased risk of stroke has been validated, but studies concerning the ability of PET imaging to aid in the triage of acute stroke victims have not been corroborated. Moreover, additional anatomical imaging will remain necessary, including at least noncontrast head CT and likely both CT and MRI. Thus, competition of this technique with CT and MR perfusion is likely to remain limited until different methodologies for patient stratification emerge.

9.4 Xe-CT

Technique and Theory. A nonradioactive isotope of xenon gas (Xe, g) is a diffusible tracer and is utilized as a contrast material for CT based upon its density [1]. This inert gas is not metabolized and its concentration within the brain parenchyma is evidenced by increased density on CT and is a direct manifestation of perfusion in the steady state [1]. Xe is freely diffusible and thus its concentration depends on a steady state at the level of the lungs, which in turn produces a steady state in the bloodstream, which itself produces a steady state in the brain parenchyma – based on perfusion alone because Xe freely crosses the blood–brain barrier [1]. In contradistinction to PET and SPECT, the entire brain is not imaged; this is because of technical limitations. Multidetector CT techniques with current 32-slice scanners cannot yet cover the entire brain on perfusion CT scans; perhaps with 64-slice CT scanners this technical limitation will be removed. As opposed to PET and SPECT, Xe-CT is performed by initially carrying out a noncontrast baseline scan of several contiguous slices of brain (the number is determined by both the manufacturer and variations in slice thickness), then commencing the inhalation of Xe with subsequent serial CT scans at each individual slice level. These data are used, in turn, to form a graph and maps of cerebral perfusion parameters with respect to time; in this manner, Xe-CT's product(s) parallels that of CT perfusion using iodinated contrast material [1].

Product. Quantitative measurement via measurement of only CBF [1, 4, 16].

Availability. Moderate. Although equipment for Xe-CT is widely available (multidetector row CT scanner with 3D computer support) and software for data processing is available and partially automated, Xe (gas) storage and administration require specialized equipment and facilities that are not widely available. For example, specific ventilation is required in rooms where this technique is utilized, and most Radiology Departments are not equipped for this implementation.

Literature Review. Latchaw [1] reports that Xe-CT [6, 17–20] is able to well define the following clinically relevant categories:

1. CBF >20 ml/100 g tissue per minute: low flow without neurological dysfunction.
2. CBF 10–20 ml/100 g tissue per minute: possible reversible flow abnormality with neurological dysfunction. Best results were obtained with values in the 15–20 ml/100 g tissue per minute range with prompt thrombolysis.
3. CBF <10 ml/100 g tissue per minute: irreversible (has already or will infarct) flow abnormality with neurological dysfunction.
4. CBF <15 ml/100 g tissue per minute: increased risk of edema, hemorrhage, and, as a direct result, herniation with its associated morbidity and mortality. This risk is increased in large areas of abnormality.

9.4.1 Advantages

1. This technique is quantitative.
2. High spatial resolution.
3. May be easily combined with evaluation of the arteries on CT [CT angiography (CTA)]; the results of CTA and Xe-CT are complementary.
4. May be repeated (after a wash-out phase).
5. Could potentially provide a surrogate marker for guiding stroke thrombolysis and studies are apparently underway to provide support for these applications.

9.4.2 Liabilities

1. Motion artifact obviates quantitative, and severely degrades qualitative, interpretation.
2. Only CBF measurement is available.
3. Xenon gas has a mild sedative effect that mimics inebriation. As the typical stroke patient is both of increased age and frequently disoriented and/or combative because of neurological impairment, this sedative effect can be counterproductive.
4. Ionizing radiation exposure.
5. Referring physicians of patients with respiratory compromise may balk at the idea of Xe (g) ventilation due to its mild sedative effect and the reportedly occasional incidence of associated apnea.

6. Not all medical facilities will be able to offer this service, especially round the clock.
7. Typically, the entire brain is not imaged with current multidetector CT technology, although this may soon change.
8. Latchaw reports that although Xe (g) is commercially available, the performance of Xe-CT requires an investigational status and thus its use must be approved by the hospital human research committee. It is likely that this involvement would also necessitate written informed consent, thus potentially further delaying stroke diagnosis and treatment.

Summary. Xe-CT evaluation of stroke is a promising technique in that it images physiology such as CBF and thus may eventually serve as a surrogate for the triage of stroke victims concerning treatment. However, the need for specialized equipment, clinical limitations, and an investigational status have been prohibitive in most settings. Most centers utilize CTP (CT perfusion with iodinated contrast material) or PWI in lieu of this technique. Thus, competition of this technique with CT and MR perfusion is likely to remain limited until clinical parameters are enhanced and investment in the required facilities and equipment is mandated by improved study results in managing acute stroke patients.

9.5 MR Spectroscopy

Technique and Theory. MR spectroscopy (MRS) is essentially the application of one-dimensional nuclear magnetic resonance (NMR) techniques to clinical conventional MRI. A single or multiple voxels are defined based on a localizer or routine sequence set of images and currently available software upgrades are used to perform the pulse sequence and display the resultant one-dimensional MR spectrum. Water suppression and optimization of technical factors are critical because the clinically relevant peaks are very small compared to the water peak. Protons are by far the most commonly used nucleus in MRS but phosphorus has also been used experimentally [3].

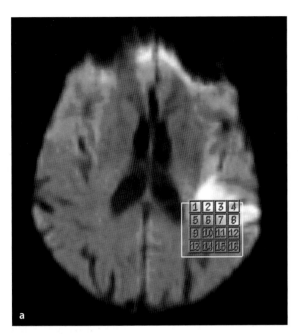
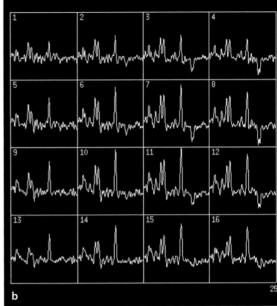

Figure 9.2

Proton MR spectroscopic imaging in a patient with acute stroke. Diffusion-weighted image (*left*) demonstrates an area of reduced diffusion in the left MCA territory. Overlaid are the voxel positions of the spectra shown on the *right*. The spectra in the *top row* are notable for decreases in N-acetyl-aspartate (*NAA*) resonance and the appearance of the inverted doublet of lactate. Going to *lower rows*, both of these resonances normalize

Product. Individual peaks are visualized including choline/phosphocholine (Cho, involved in cell membranes and energy transport), creatine/phosphocreatine (Cr, involved in energy transport), N-acetyl-aspartate (NAA, a neuronal marker) and lactate (Lac, a manifestation of anaerobic metabolism) [21–25]. The area under the curve may be calculated to give absolute spins if an external, known spin source is used prior to the patient's scan in order to calibrate the measurement. The internal comparison of peak heights within and among voxels is alternatively and almost exclusively used, especially for normal-appearing brain (internal standard for comparison). A word of caution regarding the literature and comparisons is advised. Peaks are not infinitely thin, therefore the area under the curve does not exactly equal peak height; however, because internal comparisons are used instead of absolute measurements, this in-

equality is assumed and obviated. Additionally, most software routinely re-scales the y axis (intensity) based on the largest value, and attention to the scale is recommended in order to compare separate spectral peaks.

Availability. Excellent. In general, all current MR scanners have MRS capability and upgrades are available for most recent MR scanner systems.

Literature Review. Saunders recently reviewed the MRS literature concerning stroke and summarized the data as follows [24]:

1. Lac is not visualized in the normal adult brain spectrum; its appearance is the "hallmark" of cerebral ischemia. Unfortunately, measurements within the core and penumbra of an infarct are not definitely different; moreover, the presence of Lac has

a differential diagnosis including abscess. Lac evolution and/or resolution may be observed with or without an associated infarct.

2. Decreased NAA is most consistent with neuronal degradation, may occur very early in ischemia, is likely irreversible (as opposed to disease processes such as demyelination), and may continue for days to weeks even after the cessation of ischemia. Correlation of NAA concentration to infarct size (volume) allows a better prediction of morbidity/outcome than does either NAA concentration or infarct volume alone (Fig. 9.2).

3. Changes in the Cho peak have been shown to be widely variable.

4. Reductions in Cr have been described both initially and progressively after ischemia/infarct but the degree of change is much less than that of NAA.

5. Amino acid, lipid, and other peak variations are not well defined. It is unlikely that these peaks will be of clinical diagnostic assistance for stroke in the near future.

9.5.1 Advantages

1. Potentially quantitative if external standards are used in addition to measurements on the patient (however, this may increase the time of the examination and further delay diagnosis and treatment of stroke – a liability).

2. May be easily combined with conventional MR imaging, MR angiography, PWI and diffusion-weighted imaging; these techniques are complementary.

3. May be repeated immediately.

4. No ionizing radiation exposure.

5. Could theoretically improve differentiation in specific situations where the differential diagnosis includes tumor.

6. Could potentially provide a surrogate marker for guiding stroke thrombolysis.

9.5.2 Liabilities

1. The patient must have MR compatibility (that is, no pacemaker, cochlear implant, neurostimulator, etc.).

2. Motion artifact obviates interpretation.

3. Low spatial resolution.

4. Perfusion data are unavailable.

5. Typically, the entire brain is not imaged.

6. Not all sites will have MR scanners readily available; furthermore, not all medical facilities will be able to offer this service round the clock.

Summary. MRS evaluation of stroke is a promising technique in that it images intracellular metabolites and thus may eventually serve as a surrogate for the triage of stroke victims concerning treatment. Despite its newfound speed of performance, constantly improving availability and lack of ionizing radiation, several problems persist and dominate its sparing use. Its manifestation of metabolites is relatively unique but apparently not yet distinctive or clinically relevant for most clinical stroke scenarios. At present, MRS should not be used alone but rather in combination with conventional, diffusion-weighted and perfusion-weighted MR imaging for optimal effect in the management of acute stroke patients.

References

1. Latchaw RE (2004) Cerebral perfusion imaging in acute stroke. J Vasc Interv Radiol 15:S29–S46

2. Lorberboym M, Lampl Y, Sadeh M (2003) Correlation of 99mTc-DTPA SPECT of the blood–brain barrier with neurologic outcome after acute stroke. J Nucl Med 44:1898–1904

3. Mountz JM, Liu HG, Deutsch G (2003) Neuroimaging in cerebrovascular disorders: measurement of cerebral physiology after stroke and assessment of stroke recovery. Semin Nucl Med 33:56–76

4. Vo KD, Lin W, Lee JM (2003) Evidence-based neuroimaging in acute ischemic stroke. Neuroimaging Clin North Am 13:167–183

5. Kim JH, Lee EJ, Lee SJ, Choi NC, Lim BH, Shin T (2002) Comparative evaluation of cerebral blood volume and cerebral blood flow in acute ischemic stroke by using perfusion-weighted MR imaging and SPECT. Acta Radiol 43:365–370

6. Bonaffini N, Altieri M, Rocco A, di Piero V (2002) Functional neuroimaging in acute stroke. Clin Exp Hypertens 24:647–657

7. Blake P, Johnson B, VanMeter JW (2003) Positron emission tomography (PET) and single photon emission computed tomography (SPECT): clinical applications. J Neuroophthalmol 23:34–41

8. Igarashi H, Hamamoto M, Yamaguchi H et al (2003) Cerebral blood flow index image as a simple indicator for the fate of acute ischemic lesion. Acta Neurochir [Suppl] 86:241–246

9. Ueda T, Sakaki S, Yuh WT, Nochide I, Ohta S (1999) Outcome in acute stroke with successful intra-arterial thrombolysis and predictive value of initial single-photon emission-computed tomography. J Cereb Blood Flow Metab 19:99–108

10. Heiss WD, Forsting M, Diener HC (2001) Imaging in cerebrovascular disease. Curr Opin Neurol 14:67–75

11. Hosoda K, Kawaguchi T, Ishii K et al (2003) Prediction of hyperperfusion after carotid endarterectomy by brain SPECT analysis with semiquantitative statistical mapping method. Stroke 34:1187–1193

12. Ogasawara K, Ogawa A, Terasaki K, Shimizu H, Tominaga T, Yoshimoto T (2002) Use of cerebrovascular reactivity in patients with symptomatic major cerebral artery occlusion to predict 5-year outcome: comparison of xenon-133 and iodine-123-IMP single-photon emission computed tomography. J Cereb Blood Flow Metab 22:1142–1148

13. Powers WJ, Zazulia AR (2003) The use of positron emission tomography in cerebrovascular disease. Neuroimaging Clin North Am 13:741–758

14. Okazawa H, Yamauchi H, Sugimoto K, Takahashi M (2003) Differences in vasodilatory capacity and changes in cerebral blood flow induced by acetazolamide in patients with cerebrovascular disease. J Nucl Med 44:1371–1378

15. Yamauchi H, Okazawa H, Kishibe Y, Sugimoto K, Takahashi M (2004) Oxygen extraction fraction and acetazolamide reactivity in symptomatic carotid artery disease. J Neurol Neurosurg Psychiatry 75:33–37

16. Wintermark M, Thiran JP, Maeder P, Schnyder P, Meuli R (2001) Simultaneous measurement of regional cerebral blood flow by perfusion CT and stable xenon CT: a validation study. Am J Neuroradiol 22:905–914

17. Jager HR (2000) Diagnosis of stroke with advanced CT and MR imaging. Br Med Bull 56:318–333

18. Pindzola RR, Balzer JR, Nemoto EM, Goldstein S, Yonas H (2001) Cerebrovascular reserve in patients with carotid occlusive disease assessed by stable xenon-enhanced ct cerebral blood flow and transcranial Doppler. Stroke 32:1811–1817

19. Kilpatrick MM, Yonas H, Goldstein S et al (2001) CT-based assessment of acute stroke: CT, CT angiography, and xenon-enhanced CT cerebral blood flow. Stroke 32:2543–2549

20. Meuli RA (2004) Imaging viable brain tissue with CT scan during acute stroke. Cerebrovasc Dis 17 [Suppl 3]:28–34

21. Beauchamp NJ Jr., Barker PB, Wang PY, van Zijl PC (1999) Imaging of acute cerebral ischemia. Radiology 212:307–324

22. Bonavita S, Di Salle F, Tedeschi G (1999) Proton MRS in neurological disorders. Eur J Radiol 30:125–131

23. Yoshiura T, Wu O, Sorensen AG (1999) Advanced MR techniques: diffusion MR imaging, perfusion MR imaging, and spectroscopy. Neuroimaging Clin North Am 9:439–453

24. Saunders DE (2000) MR spectroscopy in stroke. Br Med Bull 56:334–345

25. Chu WJ, Mason GF, Pan JW et al (2002) Regional cerebral blood flow and magnetic resonance spectroscopic imaging findings in diaschisis from stroke. Stroke 33:1243–1248

PART III
Intervention in Acute Ischemic Stroke

Clinical Management of Acute Stroke

W.J. Koroshetz, R.G. González

Contents

10.1 Introduction

The first minutes to hours after the onset of neurologic dysfunction in stroke patients frequently hold the only opportunity to prevent death or serious permanent disability. The goal in the first hours after the onset of acute stroke is to prevent infarction or minimize the degree of permanent brain injury. A system that ensures rapid and precise assessment of the variety of stroke patients is necessary to optimize acute stroke treatment. Consensus guidelines for acute stroke management have set the following goals for hospitals: (1) triage of the stroke patient to medical attention within 10 min, (2) history, physical examination, and blood tests as soon as possible, (3) brain imaging within 30 min, (4) CT interpretation within 20 min of scan completion, (5) treatment decisions within 60 min of presentation [National Institute of Neurological Disorders and Stroke (NINDS) consensus conference]. Local clinical pathways that are continually refined are necessary to coordinate the multidisciplinary effort.

10.2 History of Stroke Onset

It is important to know as precisely as possible the time of symptom onset and the characteristics of the initial symptoms. The patient may not be able to provide an accurate history due to their neurologic deficits; therefore, phone interviews with emergency medical technicians, family members or other eyewitnesses before, or at the time of, the patient's arrival can be invaluable.

The eyewitnesses to the event should be queried about:

- when the affected individual was last at neurologic baseline; an exact time of onset can be critical in treatment decisions
- whether there were clonic movements or other behaviors to suggest seizure at onset
- whether there is a history of previous seizure, diabetes, warfarin use, prior stroke, prior transient ischemic attack (TIA), prior myocardial infarction (MI), drug abuse, trauma, head or neck pain
- other relevant past medical history, such as recent surgery, angina, hypertension, bleeding disorder, clotting disorder, atrial fibrillation, overdose, febrile illness, and medication allergies.

Upon notification that a potential acute stroke case is on the way to the hospital the computed tomography (CT) technician and stroke physician should be paged.

The acute ischemic stroke patient may not be competent to make medical decisions. Because emergency treatments (i.e., decompressive surgery, hemorrhage evacuation, thrombolytic drug administration, intra-arterial clot removal, emergency endarterectomy) carry risk, it is advisable to discuss possible interventions with the patient's family members when they first call the hospital. If the noncompetent patient is unaccompanied by a responsible family member, then the treating physician should establish a means of remaining in contact. Cell phones allow communication with the family member who is in transit to the hospital, but in their absence it may be prudent for the responsible family member to delay travel until treatment decisions are made.

10.3 Clinical Presentation

The acute stroke evaluation should be made available for all patients with a sudden-onset neurologic deficit, the basis of the stroke syndrome. Though focal neurologic deficits are common in stroke patients they may not be present in some conditions,

for example subarachnoid hemorrhage, or they may require specific stroke expertise to be elicited, for example top of basilar artery embolus. The most difficult diagnostic problems usually occur in patients with an altered level of consciousness, especially if there are other potential causes of encephalopathy, such as alcohol intoxication, a fall, etc. There is tremendous variation in the presentation of acute stroke patients. This variation depends on whether the stroke is ischemic or hemorrhagic, which brain areas are affected, and underlying medical illnesses. In addition, the physician must also be able to identify stroke among other conditions that mimic stroke syndromes. The most common mimics of stroke include seizure, hypoglycemia, migrainous accompaniment, drug overdose, thiamine deficiency (Wernicke's syndrome), and other causes of encephalopathy. Tumor occasionally causes stroke-like symptoms due to intra-tumor hemorrhage or the epileptic or migrainous activity associated with tumor. (See Table 10.1 for conditions that mimic ischemic stroke.)

In the initial evaluation of a patient with an acute-onset neurologic deficit, the stroke physician needs to rapidly determine the cause of the neurologic disturbance in order to provide appropriate treatment. The usual sequence is: (1) stabilize the patient's medical condition, (2) treat if any suspicion of hypoglycemia, narcotic overdose, thiamine deficiency, (3) determine if there is intracranial hemorrhage, and (4) decide whether evidence is consistent with acute brain ischemia. If the stroke syndrome is thought likely due to ischemia and the patient is within 3 h of onset, then thrombolytic treatment with intravenous tissue plasminogen activator (i.v. t-PA) needs to be considered. To determine the cerebral localization of the deficits and the vascular mechanism responsible, the stroke physician depends upon knowledge of the vascular syndromes, the localization of neurologic function in the brain, and the forms of ischemia known to cause particular neurologic syndromes. In ischemic stroke, emergency brain imaging is essential in establishing the responsible vascular lesion and mapping the regional damage that is essential in offering prognostic

Table 10.1. Common conditions that may mimic acute ischemic stroke

Condition	Symptoms	Comments
Hypoglycemia	Encephalopathy and focal neurologic deficit, especially aphasia	Insulin or oral hypoglycemic use
		Blood sugar less than 40 mg/dl
		Rapid resolution of symptoms with glucose infusion
Seizure	Focal neurologic deficit often with post-ictal encephalopathy, i.e., post-ictus	History of witnessed seizure activity with onset of deficit. Can be very difficult to distinguish if there is a nonconvulsive seizure with focal cortical post-ictus deficit, such as aphasia or neglect
		May be an underlying lesion seen on noncontrast CT scan or contrast CT
Migraine	Focal neurologic deficits often with mild encephalopathy	History of migraine complicated by hemiparesis, hemisensory loss, aphasia, etc.
		Build up of symptoms over time with typical headache, photophobia, sonophobia
		Sometimes a diagnosis of exclusion
Drug overdose	Coma, may be associated with absent eye movements simulating basilar thrombosis	Toxic screen positive for narcotics, or barbiturates
Intracerebral hematoma	Focal neurologic deficit	Blood on CT scan
Subdural hematoma or empyema	Focal neurologic deficit	CT scan with subdural collection, that may be quite thin

information. In hemorrhagic stroke, brain imaging is critical in establishing the location and size of the hemorrhage, advisability of clot evacuation, the presence of mass effect, identification of hydrocephalus, and the presence of an underlying vascular lesion.

10.4 Emergency Management

Simultaneous execution of specific tasks by all members of the emergency stroke team permits efficient progression to diagnosis and treatment. There should be a plan of action and all members of the team should be familiar with it. Table 10.2 delineates the tasks of each member of a hypothetical acute stroke team.

10.5 General Medical Support

10.5.1 ABCs of Emergency Medical Management

Though poor outcome may occur due to delays in stroke evaluation, it is equally important that rapid triage to neurologic evaluation and brain imaging occur in a medically safe manner. The patient needs to be assessed for hemodynamic and respiratory stability as well as for signs or history of trauma, especially neck injury. The neck should be evaluated and stabilized if there is question of injury, not an uncommon scenario in the stroke patient who falls. A history and physical examination should be performed by a qualified physician. The identification of critical medical conditions is often made on the initial history and examination, and errors made if this is delayed until after the stroke evaluation.

Table 10.2. The schedule of tasks for each member of an acute stroke team. (*ASA* Acetylsalicylic acid, *AVM* arteriovenous malformations, *BP* blood pressure, *CTA* CT angiography, *D50* 50% dextrose, *EKG* electrocardiogram, *i.a.* intra-arterial, *ICH* intracranial hemorrhage, *i.v.* intravenous, *MI* myocardial infarction, *NS* normal saline, *PCP* primary care physician, *PT* prothrombin time, *PTT* partial thromboplastin time, *rt-PA* recombinant tissue plasminogen activator, *SAH* subarachnoid hemorrhage)

Acute stroke team member	Time (min)			
	0–15	15–30	30–45	45–60
Emergency nurse	1. Obtain vital signs	1. Infuse fast-acting agents to maintain blood pressure within the set range	1. Monitor patient in neuroimaging suite	1. If indicated, mix rt-PA, treat with fast-acting agents to maintain BP goals for t-PA, administer t-PA
	2. Start 18-gauge i.v. line and begin infusion of 0.9 NS	2. Use acetaminophen or cooling blanket to prevent hyperthermia		2. Ready fresh frozen plasma if needed to treat hemorrhage
	3. Administer D50, thiamine, naloxone in the appropriate setting	3. Prepare patient for transport to neuroimaging		
	4. Send blood including PT, PTT, platelet count, glucose, hematocrit, toxicology, type and cross for fresh frozen plasma for patients taking warfarin			
	5. Obtain EKG and monitor rhythm			
	6. Administer oxygen to maintain O$_2$ saturation >95%			
Emergency physician	1. Obtain medical history			
	2. Assess airway, blood pressure, breathing, cardiovascular state			
	3. Physical examination for signs of head trauma, seizure, bleeding, aortic dissection			
	4. Evaluate EKG for evidence of acute MI			

Table 10.2. (continued)

Acute stroke team member	Time (min) 0–15	15–30	30–45	45–60
Stroke physician	1. Obtain history of the event from patient and family 2. Neurologic examination to correlate neurologic symptoms and signs with ischemia in a particular vascular territory	1. Discuss findings with family and open discussion of risk and benefits of thrombolysis 2. Obtain detailed history of the event and the past medical history	1. Review the CT scan 2. Decide on whether to perform CTA 3. Consult PCP 4. Check platelet count, PT, PTT, hematocrit, blood glucose 5. Notify interventional team if i.a. therapy appropriate 6. Notify neurosurgery if intracranial hemorrhage	1. If ischemic stroke then decide on treatment plan: i.v. or i.a. thrombolytic, heparin or ASA 2. If hemorrhagic stroke then correct coagulation abnormalities and decide on need for intraventricular drain
CT technician	1. Prepare scanner to accept patient	1. Perform CT scan	1. CTA if needed	
Radiologist	1. Prepare injector for CTA	1. Evaluate CT images for evidence of SAH, ICH, early signs of stroke, bright artery sign. Notify interventional team if appropriate	1. Reconstruct CTA to identify aneurysm or AVM in hemorrhagic stroke, major vessel occlusion in ischemic stroke 2. Chest radiograph	1. Neuro-interventional team prepare for i.a. thrombolysis if indicated. This may include arranging anesthesia, consent from family or patient

Airway. Airway protection in stroke patients may require immediate intervention. An impaired level of consciousness combined with emesis can occur in patients with increased intracranial pressure and posterior circulation stroke. Vertebrobasilar ischemia may affect medullary respiratory centers and cause apnea, or more commonly paralysis of pharyngeal and tongue musculature with obstruction of the airway. The patient may require gastric suction and intubation to protect the airway from aspiration of gastric contents. An oral airway or nasal trumpet can be helpful if the patient has an upper airway obstruction.

Breathing. Consensus guidelines call for monitoring O_2 saturation and maintaining it above 95%. If needed, oxygen is usually administered by nasal cannula. Aspiration may have occurred prior to hospital arrival, which can lead to impaired oxygenation. Hypercarbia will further increase intracranial pressure (ICP) in patients with high ICP due to intracranial hemorrhage, hydrocephalus or brain swelling. It is sometimes necessary to ventilate the stroke patient who has an impaired respiratory drive or increased ICP.

Cardiovascular. As stroke is a cerebrovascular event the cardiovascular management and assessment are especially important. Patients at highest risk for stroke have coexisting cardiovascular disease. It is important to obtain an electrocardiogram (EKG) to evaluate the patient for evidence of acute cardiac ischemia and atrial fibrillation. Hypotension is uniformly bad. Most patients with acute stroke have elevated blood pressure even without pre-existing hypertension. Although chronic hypertension is the major risk factor for stroke, acute elevation of blood pressure may be protective in ischemic stroke. For example, elevated blood pressure can help augment the delivery of blood to ischemic areas via collateral circulation. Ischemic symptoms in patients who receive oral anti-hypertensive agents can worsen as blood pressure falls, and improve as blood pressure increases. Most consensus-based guidelines recommend that blood pressure be left untreated unless the systolic pressure is above 200 mmHg or the diastolic

above 120 mmHg. At these very high levels, malignant hypertension can occur with neurologic deficits simulating stroke but with papilledema, proteinuria, seizures, and encephalopathy. The pathologic process in hypertensive encephalopathy is impaired vasoregulation and vasogenic edema that responds to the lowering of blood pressure. In contrast, the use of intravenous t-PA has been pioneered with strict blood pressure control below a systolic blood pressure of 180 mmHg. In patients undergoing intra-arterial lysis, vessel recanalization may mark the time at which blood pressure needs to be lowered to prevent reperfusion hemorrhage. Blood pressure lowering may also be appropriate in acute ischemic stroke patients with concurrent acute myocardial ischemia or aortic dissection.

Rapid Reversal of Conditions Mimicking Stroke. Immediately after rapid assessment of the patient's circulatory and respiratory status (ABCs), the medical team should consider the possibility of hypoglycemia, thiamine deficiency, and drug overdose as etiologies. If there is any reasonable suspicion of these reversible causes of focal neurologic symptoms, often accompanied by a depressed level of consciousness, the medical team should perform the appropriate blood sampling followed by infusion of glucose, naloxone, and/or thiamine.

Osmolarity. Hypo-osmolarity will promote brain swelling. Patients with ischemic stroke at risk of ischemic brain swelling are treated with isotonic fluids. Dehydration, however, should be avoided as it promotes coagulation and impairs cerebral blood flow (CBF). The objective is to make the patient euvolemic with fluids containing little or no free water.

Hyperglycemia. Elevated blood glucose has been found to increase ischemic injury in animal models of stroke. It has been shown to be associated with poor outcome in ischemic stroke. Hypoglycemia is clearly an added insult to the brain that is suffering from a lack of energy supply. Insulin is used to maintain normal blood sugar.

Vascular Obstruction. The risk of hemorrhage causing an infarction is thought to be increased when the vascular obstruction resolves and the injured vascular wall is stressed by the return of systemic blood pressure. The National Institute of Neurological Disorders and Stroke (NINDS) study of i.v. thrombolysis was careful to exclude patients with hypertension, defined as systolic pressure over 180 mmHg or diastolic pressure over 120 mmHg. After infusion of recombinant t-PA (rt-PA), patient's blood pressure was carefully controlled with i.v., rapidly titratable agents, labetalol and nitroprusside. This level of blood pressure control has been recommended for patients who receive rt-PA. In patients undergoing intra-arterial (i.a.) lysis of thrombus, we have maintained the patient relatively hypertensive, often with phenylephrine (neosynephrine). At the time of clot lysis, the blood pressure is reduced to protect against hemorrhage and because blood flow is no longer dependent upon collateral flow.

In patients who are to undergo thrombolysis, care must be taken with attempts at instrumentation. An arterial puncture from attempted catheterization in a noncompressible site (e.g., subclavian vein) is contraindicated in patients to be treated with thrombolytic agents.

10.6 Medical Evaluation

Medical evaluation of the patient presenting with acute stroke is important because patients with cerebrovascular disease frequently have other forms of cardiovascular or other systemic disease, which may complicate medical management. If the patient is undergoing thrombolysis, bleeding from sites of systemic illness may become clinically evident. For this reason, medical teams should perform a stepwise analysis of the patient's organ systems, giving special consideration to the conditions listed in Table 10.3.

10.7 Neurologic Assessment

The neurological evaluation of the acute stroke patient must be efficient because of critical time constraints. This introduces an increased potential for errors, especially if the patient has an altered level of consciousness and is therefore unable to provide a detailed history or perform certain parts of the neurologic examination.

The experienced stroke physician immediately observes the patient for signs of eye and head deviation to the side of the lesion, external rotation of the paretic lower limb, and decerebrate or decorticate posture. The stroke physician will also monitor the patient's breathing pattern for signs of airway obstruction or impaired ventilatory drive, air escaping from the side of the facial paresis, unequal palpebral fissure (as occurs with ptosis on the side of a Horner's), or impaired lid closure on the side of facial weakness.

The physician subsequently assesses the patient's level of consciousness by attempting to arouse the patient or engage the patient in conversation. If the patient does not respond to verbal stimuli, the physician will try to evoke a response through tactile stimuli, proceeding from gentle shaking to pinch, nail pressure, and sternal rub.

If the patient's eyes remain closed and the patient responds to noxious stimuli with only reflexive movements, then the patient is in a state of coma. Alertness with the inability to comprehend spoken language suggests aphasia or severe abulia. Dysnomia, paraphasic errors, and stuttering effortful speech all suggest aphasia. Inattention to stimuli on one side of the visual field and body part suggests neglect syndrome. A single finding such as the patient's inability to find or identify their own left hand is strong evidence for right parietal dysfunction.

Next, the physician monitors the patient's:

- visual function, by testing visual fields to finger counting or threat
- pupils and their response to light
- eye movements to command or to the doll's head maneuver (if no suspicion of neck injury)

Table 10.3. Medical evaluation. (*AR* Aortic regurgitation, *CCA* common carotid artery, *ECA* external carotid artery, *ICA* internal carotid artery, *GI* gastrointestinal, *LV* left ventricular, *MR* mitral regurgitation, *PMI* point of maximal impulse, *TR* tricuspid regurgitation)

Organ system	Physical finding	Potential relevant underlying pathophysiology
Head	Soft tissue injury	Head trauma
	Tender, thickened, or pulseless temporal artery	Temporal arteritis
	Obliteration of flow through the trochlear artery with compression of the pre-auricular or supra-orbital vessels	ICA occlusion or severe stenosis with retrograde ophthalmic flow
	Anhidrosis	CCA dissection with damage to sympathetic fibers or brainstem stroke with interruption of sympathetic tract
	Tongue laceration	Consider seizure as the cause of the neurologic deterioration
Ear	Hemotympanum	Basilar skull fracture
	Vesicles	Facial weakness due to zoster-associated VIIth nerve palsy
Nose	Blood	Potential site of bleeding after thrombolysis, Osler Weber Rendu syndrome
	Chronic ulceration	Occasionally secondary to dissecting carotid artery rupture
		Nasopharyngeal carcinoma, Wegener's, with cranial nerve involvement
Neck	Carotid or vertebral bruit	Carotid or vertebral stenosis
	Absent carotid pulse	CCA occlusion
	Nuchal rigidity	Meningeal irritation in SAH or infectious meningitis
Nodes	Enlarged hard nodes	Metastatic disease (brain metastasis as cause of neurologic deficit, may need contrast CT scan) or marantic endocarditis
Throat	Pharyngeal mass	Abscess that can encase the carotid artery
	Inflammatory exudate	Diphtheria as cause of rapid demyelination and bulbar then systemic weakness
Eyes	Erythematous, painful globe with dilated unreactive pupil (rubeosis iridis)	Ischemic eye due to combined ICA and ECA disease
	Papilledema	Increased intracranial pressure from intracranial mass, venous sinus thrombosis, hydrocephalus, chronic meningitis
	Roth spot	Bacterial endocarditis
	Cholesterol embolus	Cholesterol embolus from aorta or carotid
	Hypertensive or diabetic retinopathy	Hypertension and/or diabetes
	Subhyaloid hemorrhage	Subarachnoid hemorrhage

Table 10.3. (continued)

Organ system	Physical finding	Potential relevant underlying pathophysiology
Skin	Splinter hemorrhages in nailbed	Bacterial endocarditis
	Osler's nodes on palmar surface	Bacterial endocarditis
	Punctate hemorrhages in conjunctiva or mucosa	Bacterial endocarditis
	Livedo reticularis, ischemic infarcts in toes or fingers	Cholesterol emboli
	Livedo reticularis	Anti-cardiolipin Ab (Sneddon's syndrome)
	Purplish nodules with white centers	Kohlemeier–Degos disease (stroke, bowel infarction)
	Purplish papules	Fabry's disease
	Malar rash	Systemic lupus erythematosus
	Telangiectasia	Osler Weber Rendu as potential bleeding source
	Purpura	Coagulation disorder (TTP, ITP)
	Venipuncture site	Endocarditis due to i.v. drug abuse
Cardiovascular	Regurgitant murmur of TR, MR or AR	Endocarditis
	Diffuse PMI or paradoxical motion of the PMI	AR with type I aortic dissection
	Asymmetry of blood pressure in two arms	MR and TR with dilated atria
		Cardiomyopathy
		LV aneurysm
		Subclavian stenosis or occlusion. Athero common cause if chronic, aortic dissection if acute
Abdominal	Varices, spider telangiectasia, icterus	Liver disease with likely coagulation system abnormality
	Mass	Cancer (consider brain metastasis as cause of neurologic deficit, may need contrast CT scan)
	Abdominal pain, GI bleeding	Mesenteric embolus
Extremities	Ischemic limb	Systemic embolus

- sensation, by testing corneal and facial sensation to a pin
- facial movement to command or in response to noxious stimulus (nasal tickle)
- pharyngeal and lingual function, by listening and evaluating speech and examining the mouth
- motor function, by testing for pronator drift, power, tone, speed of finger or toe movements
- sensory function, by testing patient's ability to detect pin, touch, vibration, and position (a sensory level on the body suggests that the pathology is the spinal cord)
- cerebellar function, by asking the patient to walk, and to touch repetitively first their own nose and then the examiner's finger
- ataxia in the legs, by asking the patient to touch the examiner's finger with their toes
- asymmetry of reflexes
- Babinski reflex.

Table 10.4. NIHSS

1a.	Level of consciousness: SCORE ___	0 1 2 3	Alert Not alert, but arousable with minimal stimulation Not alert, requires repeated stimulation to attend Coma
1b.	Ask patient the month and their age: SCORE ___	0 1 2	Answers both correctly Answers one correctly Both incorrect
1c.	Ask patient to open and close eyes: SCORE ___	0 1 2	Obeys both correctly Obeys one correctly Both incorrect
2.	Best gaze (only horizontal eye movement): SCORE ___	0 1 2	Normal Partial gaze palsy Forced deviation
3.	Visual field testing: SCORE ___	0 1 2 3	No visual field loss Partial hemianopia Complete hemianopia Bilateral hemianopia (blind including cortical blindness)
4.	Facial paresis (ask patient to show teeth or raise eyebrows and close eyes tightly): SCORE ___	0 1 2 3	Normal symmetrical movement Minor paralysis (flattened nasolabial fold, asymmetry on smiling) Partial paralysis (total or near-total paralysis of lower face) Complete paralysis of one or both sides (absence of facial movement in the upper and lower face)
5.	Motor function – arm (right and left): Right arm ___ Left arm ___ SCORE ___	0 1 2 3 4 9	Normal [extends arms 90° (or 45°) for 10 s without drift] Drift Some effort against gravity No effort against gravity No movement Untestable (joint fused or limb amputated)
6.	Motor function – leg (right and left): Right leg ___ Left leg ___ SCORE ___	0 1 2 3 4 9	Normal (hold leg 30° position for 5 s) Drift Some effort against gravity No effort against gravity No movement Untestable (joint fused or limb amputated)
7.	Limb ataxia SCORE ___	0 1 2	No ataxia Present in one limb Present in two limbs
8.	Sensory (use pinprick to test arms, legs, trunk and face – compare side to side) SCORE ___	0 1 2	Normal Mild to moderate decrease in sensation Severe to total sensory loss
9.	Best language (describe picture, name items, read sentences) SCORE ___	0 1 2 3	No aphasia Mild to moderate aphasia Severe aphasia Mute

Table 10.4. (continued)

10. Dysarthria (read several words)	0	Normal articulation
	1	Mild to moderate slurring of words
	2	Near unintelligible or unable to speak
SCORE ___	9	Intubated or other physical barrier
11. Extinction and inattention	0	Normal
	1	Inattention or extinction to bilateral simultaneous stimulation in one of the sensory modalities
SCORE ___	2	Severe hemi-inattention or hemi-inattention to more than one modality
TOTAL SCORE ___		

The above examination can usually be performed within 10 min. The NIHSS (Table 10.4) is a standardized assessment of the above systems that has been used in clinical trials and can be helpful in stratifying patient deficits. From the above information the physician can usually make an informed assessment of the patient's neurological insult. The goal is to combine any abnormalities noted on the examination with the patient's history to determine whether stroke is the most probable diagnosis.

The medical team must perform the neurological examination repeatedly over time to determine if the patient's condition is deteriorating. The performance of some patients improves in the hours following the onset of acute neurological deficits. This improvement can be due to the resolution of abnormal electrical activity in patients with seizure who mimic stroke. In addition, improvement sometimes occurs due to spontaneous recanalization of the affected vessel. In the presence of a rapidly improving deficit, physicians may withhold thrombolytic treatment.

10.8 Intervention and Treatment

Ready availability of imaging is crucial for the proper management of acute stroke. The noncontrast, head CT is the minimal imaging study necessary for proper stroke management. The immediate availability of more informative imaging modalities such as CT angiography/perfusion and/or MR diffusion/perfusion imaging greatly increases the knowledge of the patient's present pathophysiologic condition. The use of these modalities in acute ischemic stroke is described in detail in other chapters. After the clinical evaluation and imaging, the stroke physician has the necessary information to make decisions with the consent of the patient and/or the patient's family as to the most appropriate treatment, whether it is for ischemic or hemorrhagic stroke.

10.9 Conclusion

A predetermined course of action for the rapid, precise evaluation of the acute stroke patient is essential. The goal is to prevent cerebral infarction or to minimize the degree of permanent cerebral injury. Precise information on the time of onset, as well as a rapid and accurate medical and neurological evaluation is extremely important. The acute stroke team should be able to perform multiple tasks in parallel. A thorough evaluation (with imaging) should be complete within an hour of presentation. The treatment plan should then be immediately implemented.

Suggested Reading

Aboderin I, Venables G (1996) Stroke management in Europe. Pan European Consensus Meeting on Stroke Management. J Intern Med 240:173–180

Adams HP Jr., Brott TG, Furlan AJ et al (1996) Guidelines for thrombolytic therapy for acute stroke. Stroke 27:1711–1718

Adams HP Jr., Adams RJ, Brott TG et al (2003) Guidelines for the early management of patients with acute ischemic stroke. Stroke 34:1056–1083

Alberts MJ, Hademoenos G, Latchaw RE et al (2000) Recommendations for the establishment of primary stroke centers. J Am Med Assoc 283:3102–3109

American College of Surgeons, Subcommittee on Advanced Trauma Life Support (1993) Advanced Trauma Life Support, Program for Physicians, 5th edn. 1st Impression, Chicago, Ill., pp 47–52

Bath PMW, Soo J, Butterworth RJ et al (1996) Do acute stroke units improve care? J Stroke Cerebrovasc Dis 6:346–349

Benavente O, Hart RG (1999) Stroke, part II. Management of acute ischemic stroke. Am Fam Physician 59:2828–2834

Brott T, Adams HP, Olinger CP et al (1989) Measurements of acute cerebral infarction. A clinical examination scale. Stroke 20:864–870

Cook DJ, Guyatt GH, Laupacis A et al (1995) Clinical recommendations using levels of evidence for antithrombotic agents. Chest 108 [Suppl]:227S–230S

Cummins RO (ed) (1994) Textbook of advanced cardiac life support, 3rd edn. American Heart Association, Dallas, Tex., Chap. 1, 2

Feinberg WM, Alkers GW, Barnett HJM et al (1994) Guidelines for management of transient ischemic attack. Stroke 25:1320–1335

Futrell N, Millikan CH (1996) Stroke is an emergency. Dis Mon 42:199–264

Gomez CR, Malkoff MD, Sauer CM et al (1994) Code stroke. Stroke 25:1920–1923

Indredavik B, Bakke F, Solberg R et al (1992) Benefit of a stroke unit. A randomized controlled trial. Stroke 22:1026–1031

Langhorne P, William BO, Gilchrist W, Howie K (1993) Do stroke units save lives? Lancet 342:395–398

Laupacis A, Alders GW, Dalen JE et al (1995) Antithrombotic therapy in atrial fibrillation. Chest 108 [Suppl]:352S–359S

Lyden PD, Rapp K, Babcock T et al (1994) Ultra-rapid identification, triage, and enrollment of stroke patients into clinical trials. J Stroke Cerebrovasc Dis 4:106–113

Marler J, Jones P, Emr M (eds) (1997) Proceedings of a national symposium on rapid identification and treatment of acute stroke. National Institute of Neurological Disorders and Stroke, Arlington, Va.

McDowell FH, Brott TG, Goldstein M et al (1993) Stroke the first six hours. J Stroke Cerebrovasc Dis 3:133–144

Morris AD, Grosset DG, Squire IB et al (1993) The experiences of an acute stroke unit: implications for multicentre acute stroke trials. J Neurol Neurosurg Psychiatry 56:352–355

Quality Standards Subcommittee of the American Academy of Neurology: practice advisory (1996) Thrombolytic therapy for acute ischemic stroke. Neurology 47:835–839

Sherman D, Gifford MD, Dyken ML Jr., Gent M et al (1995) Antithrombotic therapy for cerebrovascular disorders. An update. Chest 108 [Suppl]:444S–456S

Teasedale G, Jennett B (1974) Assessment of coma and impaired consciousness. A practical scale. Lancet 2:81–83

Intravenous Thrombolysis

Lee H. Schwamm

Contents

11.1 Introduction

This chapter will review the basic mechanisms of clot formation (thrombosis) and dissolution (thrombolysis or fibrinolysis), the mechanisms of the major drug classes used in treatment, and the results from major clinical trials. This chapter will also present evidence-based recommendations and protocols for applying thrombolytic therapy to individual patients.

11.2 Thrombosis and Fibrinolysis

In the absence of injury, the vascular endothelium has antithrombotic properties, making it resistant to platelet adherence and coagulation factor interactions. Exposure of the subendothelial extracellular matrix to the blood elements by either vascular perforation or dissection initiates the coagulation cascade [1, 2]. Platelets adhere to the exposed subendothelium and are activated, releasing a variety of cytokines and forming a surface for the complex molecular interactions of the coagulation cascade [3, 4]. Platelet membrane phospholipids react with factors VII and V, which promote activation and conversion of factor X to Xa, and prothrombin II to thrombin IIa, respectively. When fibrin is produced by thrombin-mediated cleavage of fibrinogen, the conglomeration of platelets, trapped red blood cells, and leukocytes bound by interlocking fibrin strands defines the architecture of the early thrombus. The clot growth or stabilization is determined by the balance between endogenous coagulation and thrombolysis. Over time, cellular elements are destroyed by autolysis and fibrin strands become increasingly stable through cross-linking, defining the architecture of the mature thrombus. These mature thrombi are increasingly resistant to endogenous or exogenous enzymatic degradation.

Thrombolysis is mediated by enzymatic disruption of the cross-linked fibrin by plasmin [2]. Plasminogen, the precursor of plasmin, is present in circulating blood and has no enzymatic activity. Plasminogen activators (PA) are required to convert inert plasminogen into active plasmin, and must overcome the effects of plasminogen-activating inhibitors. However, circulating blood contains alpha2-antiplasmin, a potent plasmin inhibitor, which quickly neutralizes newly formed plasmin. To achieve systemic fibrinolysis, the production of plasmin must overcome circulating plasmin inhibitors. Within a thrombus, plasminogen is bound to fibrin and platelets. This geometry interferes with the action of alpha2-antiplasmin and allows the relatively unopposed activation of the plasminogen by local t-PA [5,6]. The thrombus-specific initiation of t-PA represents the predominant source of intrinsic fibrinolytic activity and works in concert with the coagulation cascade to determine the extent of thrombosis propagation or remodeling.

11.3 Fibrinolytic Agents

All currently available thrombolytic agents act through the conversion of plasminogen to plasmin. Some agents such as ancrod (pit viper venom) deplete fibrinogen stores and block clot initiation, but do not act as fibrinolytic agents per se. Large doses of an exogenous tissue plasminogen activator [e.g., urokinase (UK), streptokinase (SK), rt-PA] overwhelm plasmin inhibitors and induce systemic fibrinolysis. To date, there is no convincing evidence that any one agent is more effective at cerebrovascular recanalization, through either intravenous (i.v.) or intra-arterial (i.a.) delivery. However, there may be differences in the degree of systemic fibrinolysis induced and hemorrhagic complications [7].

Streptokinase (SK). SK is a plasminogen activator produced by *Streptococcus haemolyticus* that is not specific for fibrin-bound plasminogen. To produce

systemic fibrinolysis it must first bind to plasmin. The resulting SK–plasmin complex can then cleave plasminogen to form plasmin. Anistreplase (APSAC) is an inert SK–plasmin complex that is activated in circulating blood [8]. As an exogenous protein, SK can elicit hypersensitivity reactions. Inactivation by circulating antistreptococcal antibodies (formed by prior exposure to the antigen) as well as complex pharmacokinetics produces variable dose–response curves. For these reasons, as well as higher than expected hemorrhagic complications in recent myocardial and cerebrovascular trials, it has largely been replaced by UK and newer agents.

Urokinase (UK). UK is a glycoprotein plasminogen activator that can be isolated from renal tissues or urine and, like SK, is not specific for fibrin-bound plasminogen [8]. It has a half-life of 9–12 min. Unlike SK, it is an endogenous compound that does not produce an immune reaction. Pro-urokinase is a recombinant single-chain form of UK that must be activated by plasmin hydrolysis of a specific peptide bond, rendering it more thrombus-specific with a positive feedback loop at active clotting sites. Because pro-urokinase preferentially activates fibrin-bound plasminogen, the plasmin that is produced locally can then activate more pro-urokinase. Because the interaction is best facilitated at the clot surface (highest source of fibrin-bound plasminogen), the effects are concentrated locally with a theoretical reduction in systemic fibrinolytic effects. The phase III clinical trial has been completed, and preliminary results suggest that it is effective and safe in treating acute ischemic stroke in the middle cerebral artery (MCA) territory if given within 6 h of symptom onset via i.a. delivery [9, 10].

Tissue Plasminogen Activator (t-PA). t-PA is synthesized by vascular endothelial cells and is found in low concentrations in circulating blood [1]. It has a plasma half-life of 3–8 min, is relatively fibrin specific, and undergoes 100-fold enhancement of activity at fibrin-bound plasminogen [11]. Because there are t-PA-specific binding sites on platelet membranes and because fibrin-degradation products can also activate plasminogen, the degree of fibrin specificity is limited. For i.v. thrombolysis, the only theoretical disadvantage of t-PA is its high cost relative to UK and SK. It is the only drug currently approved by the Food and Drug Administration (FDA) for treatment of acute ischemic stroke.

Desmoteplase [*Desmodus rotundus* Salivary Plasminogen Activator Alpha-1 (DSPA1)]. Highly potent plasminogen activators were discovered in the New World vampire bat (*Desmodus rotundus*), animals that feed exclusively on blood. Its saliva contains plasminogen activators first described by Hawkey [12] that result in rapid lysis of fresh blood clots. Of four *D. rotundus* salivary plasminogen activators (DSPAs) that were identified, the full-length plasminogen activator (DSPA1) variant is the most comprehensively studied [13, 14]. The DSPAs are single-chain molecules [13]. One characteristic that distinguishes this agent from other plasminogen activators is its high fibrin specificity [14]. It has been reported that the activity of DSPA1 is 105,000 times higher in the presence of fibrin than in its absence compared to 550 for t-PA [15]. Furthermore, fibrinogen is a potent cofactor of plasminogen activation by t-PA, but has little effect on DSPA1. In animal models of arterial thrombosis DSPA1 has been shown to have faster and more sustained reperfusion than human t-PA [16]. The DSPAs appear to cause less fibrinogenolysis [17] and antiplasmin consumption than t-PA. Finally, desmoteplase has been shown to have little neurotoxicity compared to t-PA in an animal model [18].

11.4 Intravenous Fibrinolysis

Background. For more than 30 years, patients with acute ischemic stroke have been treated with thrombolytic agents. Because these early studies predated the availability of CT, the differentiation of ischemic from hemorrhagic stroke or intracerebral hemorrhage was based on clinical history, neurologic examination, and lumbar puncture. In these earlier uncontrolled studies, most patients were treated more than 6 h after stroke onset; hemorrhagic complications overwhelmed any potential benefits associated with

this delayed recanalization. These earlier studies were performed using UK, SK, thrombolysin, and plasmin. Despite angiographically verified arterial recanalization with thrombolysin and SK, clinical outcomes were poor. By the late 1970s, acute revascularization in ischemic stroke was considered too dangerous [19].

Interest in thrombolytic therapy for acute ischemic stroke re-emerged with reports of successful thrombolysis for arterial thrombosis in the peripheral vascular system. Local i.a. infusion was found to have higher rates of recanalization compared with systemic i.v. delivery of thrombolytics without increased levels of hemorrhagic complications; i.v. use of UK and SK was found to provide clinical benefit in patients with pulmonary embolism [5, 6]. In the early 1980s i.a. infusion of UK or SK for acute myocardial infarction (MI) was shown to be highly effective [5, 6]. At the same time, technical advances in endovascular microcatheter and microguidewire design made access to the intracranial vessels safer and easier, and improvements in CT made detection of cerebral ischemia more reliable.

Clinical Trials. Intravenous thrombolytic therapies for stroke during the 1980s were carried out using UK [20, 21], SK [22], and t-PA [23]. In the studies using UK and SK, patients were often treated many hours to several days after stroke symptom onset, with predictably poor outcomes. However, subsequent studies recognized the critical importance of early therapy, and several i.v. rt-PA trials used treatment windows of less than 8 h and performed serial angiographic evaluations of recanalization [23]. Von Kummer and Hacke [24] found very similar results in a regimen using t-PA 100 mg i.v. in 32 patients with angiographic and ultrasound evidence of vascular occlusion. Several patients with proximal MCA stem (M1) occlusions or distal internal cerebral artery (ICA) occlusions died. The results suggested that: (1) i.v. t-PA was effective in distal MCA branch occlusions, (2) risk–benefit ratios were higher (i.e., poorer outcomes) in proximal MCA occlusions, and (3) i.a. approaches to thrombolysis of proximal MCA occlusions should be pursued.

Based on these pilot data, three large multicenter randomized trials were performed to evaluate the safety and efficacy of i.v. SK alone or in combination with aspirin or heparin: the Australian Streptokinase Trial (ASK) [25], the Multicenter Acute Stroke Trial – Europe (MAST–E) [26], and the Multicenter Acute Stroke Trial – Italy (MAST–I) [27]. ASK and MAST–E, the two double-blind randomized trials, were stopped prematurely because of excess mortality in the thrombolysis-treated group. MAST–I was stopped after randomizing only about a third of the intended number of participants due to similar safety concerns. Despite negative results, these trials contributed important information that was critical in the successful design of the later i.v. t-PA trials.

ECASS. The European Cooperative Acute Stroke Study enrolled 620 patients with acute ischemic stroke in whom treatment could be initiated within 6 h of stroke onset [28]. Patients were excluded if pre-treatment CT showed signs of hemorrhage or major early infarction involving more than one-third of the MCA territory (diffuse sulcal effacement, poor differentiation between gray and white matter, and diffuse hypodensity). In a randomized double-blind study, patients either received placebo or i.v. t-PA (1.1 mg/kg to a maximum dose 100 mg; 10% bolus followed by infusion over 1 h) and could not receive anticoagulants, antiplatelet, cerebroprotective, or volume-expanding agents during the first 24 h. Outcome was measured by two primary end points: the modified Rankin scale and the Barthel index at 90 days after stroke onset.

At 3 months, there was no significant difference in the primary end points between rt-PA-treated and placebo-treated patients. Mortality was higher in the t-PA group at 30 days (17.9% versus 12.7%, $P=0.08$) and statistically higher at 3 months (22.4% versus 15.8%, $P=0.04$). Hemorrhages were common in both groups (t-PA 42.8% versus placebo 36.8%); however, large parenchymal hemorrhages were significantly increased with t-PA (19.8% versus 6.5%, $P<0.001$) with a significant increase in hemorrhage-associated deaths (6.3% versus 2.4%, $P=0.02$). The t-PA-treated patients who survived had shorter hospital stays and a more rapid recovery than placebo-treated patients.

Review of the patients' records and imaging studies showed 109 patients (17%) were actually protocol violators, many due to unappreciated abnormalities on the acute pre-treatment CT scans. This included errors in interpretation at centers known for their expertise in acute stroke. Mortality in this group approached 50%. In a post-hoc subgroup analysis that excluded the protocol violators, there was a statistically significant improvement in outcome at 3 months by Rankin score but no significant difference by Barthel index. However, the rate of symptomatic hemorrhages was still three times greater in the t-PA group compared with placebo, reinforcing the point that treatment with i.v. t-PA, even in carefully selected patients, still carries a risk of symptomatic intracranial hemorrhage.

NINDS. The NINDS rt-PA Stroke Study [29] was a two-part randomized trial of i.v. t-PA (0.9 mg/kg; maximum 90 mg; 10% bolus and infusion over 60 min) versus placebo with treatment initiated within 90 or 180 min after witnessed stroke onset. Half of the patients in the study received drug within 90 min of symptom onset. Pre-treatment CT scans excluded patients with intracranial hemorrhage, but no attempt was made to exclude patients on the basis of specific CT findings of stroke. Co-administration of anticoagulants, antiplatelet agents or cerebroprotective agents was not allowed for 24 h. In the first study cohort, the primary outcome measure was a four-point improvement at 24 h on the NIHSS. An early analysis did not demonstrate a significant difference between the groups, and so the first trial was "ended" and a second study begun, now utilizing a global outcome score at 90 days as the primary endpoint. This new primary endpoint was then applied to the first cohort as part of a combined analysis.

In the 624 patients studied, there was a trend toward neurological recovery at 24 h as assessed by the NIHSS. At 3 months, 50% of t-PA-treated patients had excellent global outcomes (minimal or no deficit) compared with 38% of controls (12% absolute improvement or 30% relative improvement). Despite a higher rate of symptomatic hemorrhage in the t-PA group (6.4% versus 0.6%), the mortality at 3 months was lower in the t-PA group (17% versus 21%,

P=0.3). Subgroup analysis showed statistically robust benefit for all stroke subtypes, including presumed lacunar strokes. Though the numbers were too small to be statistically significant, older patients (age >75 years) and those with severe deficits (NIHSS >20) had higher hemorrhage rates and mortality. Current aspirin use was not an exclusion criterion in the NINDS study, and there was a trend toward increased hemorrhage in this group.

The initial data analysis suggested that time of treatment (early versus late) within the 180-min window had no impact on outcome. However, subsequent re-analysis, when controlled for severity of deficit (bad strokes come to hospital sooner), demonstrated that there is a rapid decay of the drug effect as the 180-min window is approached. This finding, together with the negative results of two trials looking at the treatment windows of 0–6 h (ECASS II [30]) and 3–5 h (ATLANTIS, prematurely halted [31]), strongly suggests that treatment with i.v. t-PA should be initiated as rapidly as possible, and certainly no later than 3 h.

On the basis of the NINDS trial and the previously reported i.v. rt-PA experience, rt-PA was approved in the United States and its use endorsed in consensus guidelines published by the American Heart Association Stroke Council [32, 33]and the American Academy of Neurology [34] for treatment of acute ischemic stroke.

Pooled Data Analysis and Meta-Analysis. A pooled analysis was performed by the investigators of the ATLANTIS, ECASS, and NINDS [35]. These included data that were collected in six randomized controlled trials in which i.v. t-PA was administered with a total, N, of 2775. This analysis demonstrated evidence of a substantial benefit of t-PA delivered within the first 3 h and some benefit for up to 270 min after the onset of symptoms.

The Cochran group performed a meta-analysis [36]. The analysis included those studies that used t-PA (NINDS, ECASS, and ECASS II), and also those studies that evaluated SK: MAST–I, MAST–E, and the Australian streptokinase study. The meta-analysis included patients who were treated within 3 h after symptom onset. In this analysis, there were 126 fewer dead or dependent stroke patients for every 1000 patients treated with thrombolytic agents.

Phase IV Studies and Studies Based on Routine Clinical Practice. The Standard Treatment with Alteplase to Reverse Stroke Study (STARS) [37] included 389 patients treated within 3 h of stroke onset. The Canadian Activase for Stroke Effectiveness Study (CASES) [38] included 1,132 patients from 60 centers in Canada. These two phase IV studies demonstrated outcomes and safety comparable to the NINDS trials.

Finally, a series of publications [39–49] have described the use of t-PA in routine clinical practice. The results in general have been favorable. However, strict adherence to protocols and the experience of the individuals providing thrombolytic care were clearly important. Indeed, an increased rate of symptomatic intracerebral hemorrhage (ICH) was documented with protocol violations by several groups [42, 46, 47, 49]. In a study of 29 Cleveland area hospitals, a 15.7% rate of symptomatic ICH was found [44]. However, 50% of these patients had protocol deviations from treatment guidelines.

DIAS. The Desmoteplase in Acute Ischemic Stroke trial (DIAS) [50] was a placebo-controlled, double-blind, randomized, dose-finding phase II trial designed to evaluate the safety and efficacy of i.v. desmoteplase administered within 3–9 h of ischemic stroke onset in patients selected by the MRI criteria of a perfusion–diffusion mismatch on MRI. Patients with NIHSS scores of 4–20 and MRI evidence of perfusion–diffusion mismatch were eligible. A total of 104 patients were studied in two parts. The first 47 patients were in part 1, and were randomized to fixed doses of desmoteplase (25 mg, 37.5 mg, or 50 mg) or placebo. Because of an excessive rate of symptomatic intracranial hemorrhage (26.7%), part 1 was halted.

Part 2 was then undertaken using lower weight-adjusted doses escalating through 62.5 µg/kg, 90 µg/kg, and 125 µg/kg in 57 patients. MRI criteria for part 2 included a diffusion abnormality greater 2 cm, but no greater than one-third the MCA territory, and a perfusion abnormality that was at least 20% larger than the diffusion abnormality. Reperfusion rates of up to 71.4% (P=0.0012) were observed with desmoteplase given at 125 µg/kg compared with 19.2% with placebo. A favorable 90-day clinical outcome was found between 13.3% (62.5 µg/kg; $P=0.757$) and 60.0% (125 µg/kg; $P=0.0090$) of patients treated with desmoteplase compared to 22.2% of placebo-treated patients. Symptomatic ICH in part 2 occurred in one patient (2.2%) who received a 90 µg/kg dose. The authors of this study concluded that i.v. desmoteplase administered 3–9 h after acute ischemic stroke in patients selected with perfusion–diffusion mismatch is associated with a higher rate of reperfusion and better clinical outcome compared with placebo.

The DIAS study, while only a phase II trial, raises hopes that safe and effective i.v. fibrinolysis can be employed in selected patients several hours after the rt-PA limit of 3 h. The reported reduced neurotoxicity of desmoteplase [18] adds to the potential utility of this new agent. The results of a planned phase III trial are eagerly awaited.

11.5 Evidence-Based Recommendations for Acute Ischemic Stroke Treatment with Intravenous Fibrinolysis

Evidence-Based Recommendations for Use of t-PA. At the Seventh American College of Chest Physician's Conference on Antithrombotic and Thrombolytic Therapy: Evidence-Based Guidelines, the following course of action was recommended [51]. For eligible patients i.v. t-PA should be administered intravenously with a dose of 0.9 mg/kg. (maximum of 90 mg), with 10% of the total dose administered as an initial bolus and the remainder infused over 60 min, provided that treatment is initiated within 3 h of clearly defined symptom onset. The recommendation assumed a higher value of long-term functional improvement relative to the value of minimizing the risk of intracerebral hemorrhage in the immediate peristroke period. This recommendation was based on the criteria shown in Tables 11.2 and 11.3 to determine eligibility for treatment.

It was stressed that physicians with experience and skill in stroke management and the interpretation of CT scans should supervise treatment. While some have advocated vascular imaging before thera-

py, these authors indicate that treatment should not be unduly delayed in order to facilitate vascular imaging. Blood pressure should be closely monitored and kept below 180/105 mmHg and antithrombotic agents should not be administered for 24 h.

Evidence-Based Guidelines for Large Strokes. Evidence-based guidelines were also given for patients with extensive (greater than one-third of the MCA territory) and clearly identifiable hypodensities on CT. The recommendation was against giving thrombolytics to patients with these criteria. They did note, however, that minor ischemic changes are commonly present, such as subtle or small areas of hypodensity, loss of grey–white distinction and other subtle signs. These signs are not a contraindication to treatment [51].

Evidence-Based Guidelines for Time of Stroke Onset Greater than 3 h. Finally reviewing the evidence available, it was recommended that t-PA should not be given to individuals beyond 3 h of symptom onset. Furthermore, they recommended against the use of SK as an i.v. thrombolytic agent in acute ischemic stroke [51].

Neurotoxicity of t-PA. It has been demonstrated that t-PA is expressed in central nervous system cells, including neurons, where it has several functions [52]. In a series of animal studies, evidence has been produced to suggest that t-PA may have a deleterious effect in ischemic stroke [53–56]. It is postulated that these effects are produced by mechanisms related to normal physiological functions within the brain [52]. Additionally, there are data to suggest that t-PA may enhance the probability of hemorrhage through its upregulation of matrix metalloproteinases (MMPs) [57, 58]. Indeed, the deleterious effect of t-PA in a stroke model has been shown to be ameliorated by the use of a MMP inhibitor [59], leading to the suggestion that such inhibitors may be usefully employed clinically in combination with t-PA [58]. Finally, it has been reported that t-PA potentiates apoptosis in ischemic human brain endothelium and in mouse cortical neurons treated with N-methyl-D-aspartate (NMDA) by shifting the apoptotic pathways from caspase-9 to caspase-8, which directly activates caspase-3 without amplification through the Bid-mediated mitochondrial pathway [60].

It must be stressed that these data arise from animal experiments, and that the clinical data strongly suggest that if t-PA is administered within 3 h of ischemic stroke onset, the benefits clearly outweigh any potential deleterious effects. Nonetheless, research is being conducted to develop methods to minimize the potential neurotoxicity of t-PA [58, 60], or to develop alternative plasminogen activators that do not possess some of these properties, such as desmoteplase [18].

11.6 Acute Ischemic Stroke Treatment with Intravenous t-PA

Time from symptom onset and imaging are surrogate markers for the degree of ischemic brain injury. Whatever the upper limits are for the safe use of t-PA, outcomes will be best when the drug is given as early as possible. "Time is brain" and the clock starts when the symptoms start. Thrombolytic agents have the potential to rescue regions of brain destined for infarction; rapid reperfusion can transform would-be-strokes into transient ischemic attacks (TIAs). Intravenous

Table 11.1. Massachusetts General Hospital acute stroke service. Protocol for intravenous (*i.v.*) recombinant tissue plasminogen activator (*rt-PA*) for acute stroke. (*CHF* Congestive heart failure, *CTA* CT angiography, *DWI* diffusion-weighted imaging)

Start supplementary oxygen   www.acutestroke.com
Treat any fever with acetaminophen for brain protection
Nil by mouth (NPO) except medications
To prevent bleeding complications after thrombolysis, do not place foley, nasogastric tube, arterial line or central venous line unless it is absolutely necessary for patient safety or unless requested by the Acute Stroke Staff. Do not place any femoral catheters (venous or arterial)
To maintain cerebral perfusion, do not lower blood pressure unless it is causing myocardial ischemia or exceeds 220/120 mmHg. Use labetolol i.v. (5–20 mg i.v. q 10–20 min) or, if necessary, sodium nitroprusside iv (0.5–10 µg/kg per min). Monitor with noninvasive cuff pressures every 15 min or continuous arterial pressure monitoring
Do not administer heparin unless recommended by the Acute Stroke Team
Arrange for emergent head CT/CTA and possible MRI with DWI/perfusion imaging if available
Page Neurology Acute Stroke Staff/Fellow if not already done
Alert Interventional Neuroradiology and Anesthesia about possible case
Alert Interventional Neuroradiology technologist and nursing
Alert Neuro ICU and check for bed availability
Call Respiratory Therapy for a ventilator to CT if accepting an intubated patient in transfer
Place and check patency of 16- to 18-gauge forearm i.v. access for potential CTA and general anesthesia
Consider chest radiograph to exclude acute CHF or aortic dissection
Can patient undergo MRI? (e.g., severe claustrophobia, implanted pacemaker, metal fragments, shrapnel)
Consider bypassing CTA if renal failure, diabetes, CHF
Hold metformin for 48 h after iodinated contrast
Transfer patient to imaging site as soon as possible
Review CT/CTA or MRI with Neuroradiology and Neurology Stroke Team on-line at scanner
If patient is eligible for IV tPA, start bolus after review of non-contrast CT.
If proximal vessel occlusion present on CTA and brain at risk detected based on mismatch between clinical and/or imaging parameters, consider catheter-based thrombolysis or mechanical clot disruption/extraction
Transfer patient immediately from scanner to neurointerventional suite if eligible for IA therapy
Obtain informed consent for procedure and general anesthesia in writing from patient or family

Table 11.2. Inclusion criteria for i.v. rt-PA for acute stroke

A significant neurologic deficit expected to result in long-term disability

Noncontrast CT scan showing no hemorrhage or well-established infarct

Acute ischemic stroke symptoms with time of onset or time last known well clearly defined,
less than 3 h before rt-PA will be given

Table 11.3. Exclusion criteria for i.v. rt-PA for acute stroke. (*DBP* Diastolic blood pressure, *PT* prothrombin time, *PTT* partial thromboplastin time, *SBP* systolic blood pressure)

Absolute exclusion criteria

Hemorrhage or well-established acute infarct on CT

CNS lesion with high likelihood of hemorrhage s/p i.v. t-PA (e.g., brain tumors, abscess, vascular malformation, aneurysm, contusion)

Established bacterial endocarditis

Relative contraindications

Mild or rapidly improving deficits

Significant trauma within 3 months

Cardiopulmonary resuscitation with chest compressions within past 10 days

Stroke within 3 months

History of intracranial hemorrhage; or symptoms suspicious of subarachnoid hemorrhage

Major surgery within past 14 days

Minor surgery within past 10 days, including liver and kidney biopsy, thoracocentesis, lumbar puncture

Arterial puncture at a noncompressible site within past 14 days (see below for femoral artery puncture)

Pregnant (up to 10 days postpartum) or nursing woman

Gastrointestinal, urologic, or respiratory hemorrhage within past 21 days

Known bleeding diathesis (includes renal and hepatic insufficiency)

Life expectancy <1 year from other causes

Peritoneal dialysis or hemodialysis

PTT>40 s; platelet count <100,000

INR>1.7 (PT>15 if no INR available) with or without chronic oral anticoagulant use

SBP>180 mmHg or DBP>110 mmHg, despite basic measures to lower it acutely
(see Table 11.8 for treatment recommendations)

Seizure at onset of stroke. (This relative contraindication is intended to prevent treatment of patients with a deficit due to post-ictal Todd's paralysis or with seizure due to some other CNS lesion that precludes rt-PA therapy. If rapid diagnosis of vascular occlusion can be made, treatment may be given in some cases)

Glucose <50 or >400 mmol/l. (This relative contraindication is intended to prevent treatment of patients with focal deficits due to hypo- or hyperglycemia. If the deficit persists after correction of the serum glucose, or if rapid diagnosis of vascular occlusion can be made, treatment may be given in some cases)

Consideration should be given to the increased risk of hemorrhage in patients with severe deficits (NIHSS >20), age >75 years or early edema with mass effect on CT

Table 11.4. Pre-treatment work-up. (*CBC* Complete blood count, *ESR* erythrocyte sedimentation rate, *hCG* human chorionic gonadotrophin)

Temperature, pulse, BP, respirations
Physical exam/neurologic exam
EKG (may be completed after start of i.v. t-PA)
CBC with platelets, basic metabolic and hepatic function panel, PT (INR), PTT, ESR, fibrinogen
Urine hCG in women of child-bearing potential
Consider hypercoagulable panel in young patients without apparent stroke risk factors
Blood for type and cross match

Table 11.5. rt-PA infusion

Dose: 0.9 mg/kg (maximum dose of 90 mg)
Give 10% as a bolus followed by the remaining 90% as a continuous infusion over 60 min

Table 11.6. Pre- and post-treatment management

ICU admission or equivalent setting for monitoring during first 24 h
Vital signs q 15 min for 2 h, then q 30 min for 6 h, then q 1 h for 16 h
Strict control of BP for 24 h as per protocol
Neuro checks q 1 h for 24 h
Pulse oximeter; oxygen cannula or mask to maintain O_2 saturations >95%
Acetaminophen 650 mg po/pr q 4 h p.r.n. T>37 °C (99.4 °F); cooling blanket p.r.n. T>39 °C (102 °F), set to avoid shivering
No antiplatelet agents or anticoagulants in first 24 h
No foley catheter, nasogastric tube, arterial catheter or central venous catheter for 24 h, unless absolutely necessary
STAT head CT for any worsening of neurologic condition

Table 11.7. Procedures for symptomatic hemorrhage after rt-PA has been given. (*FFP* Fresh frozen plasma, *ICH* intracranial hemorrhage, *ICP* intracranial pressure)

STAT head CT, if ICH suspected
Consult Neurosurgery for ICH
Check CBC, PT, PTT, platelets, fibrinogen and D-dimer. Repeat q 2 h until bleeding is controlled
Give FFP 2 units every 6 h for 24 h after dose
Give cryoprecipitate 20 units. If fibrinogen level <200 mg/dl at 1 h, repeat cryoprecipitate dose
Give platelets 4 units
Give protamine sulfate 1 mg/100 U heparin received in last 3 h (give initial 10 mg test dose slow i.v. over 10 min and observe for anaphylaxis; if stable give entire calculated dose slow IVP; maximum dose 100 mg)
Institute frequent neurochecks and therapy of acutely elevated ICP, as needed
May give aminocaproic acid (Amicar®) 5 g in 250 ml normal saline i.v. over 1 h as a last resort

Time is of the essence; therefore, it is best if a stroke team is formed that is trained specifically for the triage and treatment of acute stroke patients, and that appropriate protocols are established. The Massachusetts General Hospital (MGH) Acute Stroke Service protocols are listed in Tables 11.1–11.8. They include procedures to be implemented immediately in the emergency room (Table 11.1), inclusion (Table 11.2) and exclusion (Table 11.3) criteria for the use of i.v. t-PA, the pre-treatment work-up for such patients (Table 11.4), and details of rt-PA infusion (Table 11.5). Also listed are protocols for pre- and post-treatment management (Table 11.6), procedures for symptomatic hemorrhage after rt-PA has been given (Table 11.7), and for blood pressure control after i.v. rt-PA has been given (Table 11.8) www.acutestroke.com.

The objective, clinical assessment of the stroke patient is important for therapeutic decisions and prognosis. The most valuable instrument during the acute stroke period is the NIHSS, which is listed in Table 11.9. Two other commonly used clinical stroke scales include the Modified Rankin Scale (Table 11.10) and the Barthel Index (Table 11.11).

t-PA has a narrow therapeutic time window and reduced efficacy in patients with large proximal artery occlusions or with severe deficits. However, it can be given without special expertise, is clearly beneficial in acute ischemic stroke, and requires minimal technology for patient selection (CT scan, laboratory).

Table 11.8. Protocol for blood pressure control after i.v. rt-PA for acute stroke

Patients will be admitted to the ICU for hemodynamic monitoring for a minimum of 24 h. A noninvasive BP cuff is recommended unless sodium nitroprusside is required. BP will be strictly controlled according to the guidelines used in the NINDS trial as listed below. Clinical deterioration associated with acute reduction in BP should be evaluated immediately

Monitor arterial blood pressure during the first 24 h after starting treatment:
    Every 15 min for 2 h after starting the infusion, then
    Every 30 min for 6 h, then
    Every 60 min for 24 h after starting treatment

If systolic blood pressure is 180–230 mmHg or if diastolic blood pressure is 105–120 mmHg for two
or more readings 5–10 minutes apart:
    Give i.v. labetolol 10 mg over 1–2 min. The dose may be repeated or doubled every 10–20 min up to a total dose
    of 150 mg
    Monitor blood pressure every 15 min during labetolol treatment and observe for development of hypotension

If systolic blood pressure in >230 mmHg or if diastolic blood pressure is in the range 121–140 mmHg for two
or more readings 5–10 min apart:
    Give i.v. labetolol 10 mg over 1–2 min. The dose may be repeated or doubled every 10 min up to a total dose of 150 mg
    Monitor blood pressure every 15 min during the labetolol treatment and observe for development of hypotension
    If no satisfactory response, infuse sodium nitroprusside (0.5–10 µg/kg per min)

If diastolic blood pressure is >140 mmHg for two or more readings 5–10 min apart:
    Infuse sodium nitroprusside (0.5–10 µg/kg per min)
    Monitor blood pressure every 15 min during infusion of sodium nitroprusside[a] and observe for development
    of hypotension

[a] Continuous arterial monitoring is advised if sodium nitroprusside is used. The risk of bleeding secondary to an arterial puncture should be weighed against the possibility of missing dramatic changes in pressure during infusion

Table 11.9. NIHSS

1a.	Level of consciousness:	0	Alert
		1	Not alert, but arousable with minimal stimulation
		2	Not alert, requires repeated stimulation to attend
	SCORE ___	3	Coma
1b.	Ask patient the month and their age:	0	Answers both correctly
		1	Answers one correctly
	SCORE ___	2	Both incorrect
1c.	Ask patient to open and close eyes:	0	Obeys both correctly
		1	Obeys one correctly
	SCORE ___	2	Both incorrect
2.	Best gaze (only horizontal eye movement):	0	Normal
		1	Partial gaze palsy
	SCORE ___	2	Forced deviation
3.	Visual field testing:	0	No visual field loss
		1	Partial hemianopia
		2	Complete hemianopia
	SCORE ___	3	Bilateral hemianopia (blind including cortical blindness)
4.	Facial paresis (ask patient to show teeth or raise eyebrows and close eyes tightly):	0	Normal symmetrical movement
		1	Minor paralysis (flattened nasolabial fold, asymmetry on smiling)
		2	Partial paralysis (total or near-total paralysis of lower face)
	SCORE ___	3	Complete paralysis of one or both sides (absence of facial movement in the upper and lower face)

Table 11.9. (continued)

5.	Motor function – arm (right and left):	0	Normal [extends arms 90° (or 45°) for 10 s without drift]
	Right arm ___	1	Drift
	Left arm ___	2	Some effort against gravity
		3	No effort against gravity
		4	No movement
	SCORE ___	9	Untestable (joint fused or limb amputated)
6.	Motor function – leg (right and left):	0	Normal (hold leg 30° position for 5 s)
	Right leg ___	1	Drift
	Left leg ___	2	Some effort against gravity
		3	No effort against gravity
		4	No movement
	SCORE ___	9	Untestable (joint fused or limb amputated)
7.	Limb ataxia	0	No ataxia
		1	Present in one limb
	SCORE ___	2	Present in two limbs
8.	Sensory (use pinprick to test arms, legs,	0	Normal
	trunk and face – compare side to side)	1	Mild to moderate decrease in sensation
	SCORE ___	2	Severe to total sensory loss
9.	Best language	0	No aphasia
	(describe picture, name items,	1	Mild to moderate aphasia
	read sentences)	2	Severe aphasia
	SCORE ___	3	Mute
10.	Dysarthria (read several words)	0	Normal articulation
		1	Mild to moderate slurring of words
		2	Near unintelligible or unable to speak
	SCORE ___	9	Intubated or other physical barrier
11.	Extinction and inattention	0	Normal
		1	Inattention or extinction to bilateral simultaneous stimulation in one of the sensory modalities
	SCORE ___	2	Severe hemi-inattention or hemi-inattention to more than one modality

TOTAL SCORE ___

Table 11.10. Modified Rankin scale

0	No symptoms at all
1	No significant disability despite symptoms: able to carry out all usual duties and activities
2	Slight disability: unable to carry out all previous activities, but able to look after own affairs without assistance
3	Moderate disability: requiring some help, but able to walk without assistance
4	Moderate to severe disability: unable to walk without assistance, and unable to attend to own bodily needs without assistance
5	Severe disability: bedridden, incontinent, and requiring constant nursing care and attention
6	Death

Table 11.11. Barthel index [61–65] (http://www.neuro.mcg.edu/mcgstrok/Indices/Barthel_Ind.htm)

Activity		Score			
Feeding	0 = unable 5 = needs help cutting, spreading butter, etc., or requires modified diet 10 = independent	0	5	10	
Bathing	0 = dependent 5 = independent (or in shower)	0	5		
Grooming	0 = needs to help with personal care 5 = independent face/hair/teeth/shaving (implements provided)	0	5		
Dressing	0 = dependent 5 = needs help but can do about half unaided 10 = independent (including buttons, zips, laces, etc.)	0	5	10	
Bowels	0 = incontinent (or needs to be given enemas) 5 = occasional accident 10 = continent	0	5	10	
Bladder	0 = incontinent, or catheterized and unable to manage alone 5 = occasional accident 10 = continent	0	5	10	
Toilet use	0 = dependent 5 = needs some help, but can do something alone 10 = independent (on and off, dressing, wiping)	0	5	10	
Transfers (bed to chair and back)	0 = unable, no sitting balance 5 = major help (one or two people, physical), can sit 10 = minor help (verbal or physical) 15 = independent	0	5	10	15
Mobility (on level surfaces)	0 = immobile or <50 yards 5 = wheelchair independent, including corners, >50 yards 10 = walks with help of one person (verbal or physical) >50 yards 15 = independent (but may use any aid; for example, stick) >50 yards				
Stairs	0 = unable 5 = needs help (verbal, physical, carrying aid) 10 = independent	0	5	10	
TOTAL (0–100)		_____			
Patient name: _____ Rater: _____ Date: ____/____/____ :					

The Barthel ADL Index: guidelines
1. The index should be used as a record of what a patient does, not as a record of what a patient could do
2. The main aim is to establish degree of independence from any help, physical or verbal, however minor and for whatever reason
3. The need for supervision renders the patient not independent
4. A patient's performance should be established using the best available evidence. Asking the patient, friends/relatives and nurses are the usual sources, but direct observation and common sense are also important. However direct testing is not needed
5. Usually the patient's performance over the preceding 24–48 h is important, but occasionally longer periods will be relevant
6. Middle categories imply that the patient supplies over 50% of the effort
7. Use of aids to be independent is allowed

11.7 Conclusion

Based on the currently available data, three conclusions can be drawn: (1) time from symptom onset remains critical, (2) better patient selection and triage criteria can be used to reduce risk and increase efficacy, and (3) centers must develop an organized response to acute ischemic stroke with clinical protocols and quality of care assessment tools.

Future research should focus on reducing the risks of hemorrhage through better patient selection and developing individualized drug delivery and dosing strategies. Rapid diagnostic imaging tools that identify the site of vascular occlusion, exclude nonischemic etiologies that mimic acute stroke, and characterize the energy state and perfusion status of brain parenchyma will help to ensure appropriate patient selection. As demonstrated in other chapters in this book, CTA, CT perfusion, and diffusion and perfusion MRI may provide this detailed information in a clinically meaningful manner. MR imaging can also identify patients with occult hemorrhage due to diseases such as amyloid angiopathy, who may be at increased risk of intracerebral lobar hemorrhage when given thrombolytic therapy.

Alternatively, promising results of i.a. recanalization trials have demonstrated benefit up to and beyond 6 h after stroke onset. Unfortunately, special expertise and technology are needed to support i.a. recanalization, and this is unlikely to be available to most community hospitals. However, a regional approach to acute stroke care might connect community hospitals with tertiary centers that are equipped for i.a. thrombolysis. In this context, rapid noninvasive diagnostic testing would facilitate optimal patient selection and guide therapeutic decisions. Because of its ability to rapidly identify or exclude proximal vessel occlusion, CTA may facilitate patient selection for i.v. versus i.a. thrombolytic therapy and trigger a system for rapid evacuation of those patients requiring i.a. therapy to an affiliated institution. For centers that do not have ready access to neuroendovascular specialists, i.v. t-PA is still superior to conventional therapy (e.g., heparin or antiplatelet agents) and should be initiated immediately in appropriate cases.

References

1. Collen D (1987) Molecular mechanisms of fibrinolysis and their application to fibrin-specific thrombolytic therapy. J Cell Biochem 33(2):77–86
2. Collen D, Lijnen HR (1991) Basic and clinical aspects of fibrinolysis and thrombolysis. Blood 78(12):3114–3124
3. Freiman D (1987) The structure of thrombi. In: Colman RW, Hirsch J, Marder V et al (eds) Hemostasis and thrombosis. Lippincott, Philadelphia, Pa., pp 1123–1135
4. Ruggeri ZM (1997) Mechanisms initiating platelet thrombus formation. Thromb Haemost 78(1):611–616
5. Marder VJ, Sherry S (1988) Thrombolytic therapy: current status (1). N Engl J Med 318(23):1512–1520
6. Marder VJ, Sherry S (1988) Thrombolytic therapy: current status (2). N Engl J Med 318(24):1585–1595
7. Theron J et al (1989) Local intraarterial fibrinolysis in the carotid territory. Am J Neuroradiol 10(4):753–765
8. Pessin MS, del Zoppo GJ, Estol CJ (1990) Thrombolytic agents in the treatment of stroke. Clin Neuropharmacol 13(4):271–289
9. Del Zoppo GJ et al (1998) PROACT: a phase II randomized trial of recombinant pro-urokinase by direct arterial delivery in acute middle cerebral artery stroke. PROACT Investigators. Prolyse in acute cerebral thromboembolism. Stroke 29(1):4–11
10. Furlan A et al (1999) Intra-arterial prourokinase for acute ischemic stroke. The PROACT II study: a randomized controlled trial. Prolyse in acute cerebral thromboembolism. J Am Med Assoc 282(21):2003–2011
11. Hoylaerts M et al (1982) Kinetics of the activation of plasminogen by human tissue plasminogen activator. Role of fibrin. J Biol Chem 257(6):2912–2919
12. Hawkey C (1966) Plasminogen activator in saliva of the vampire bat *Desmodus rotundus*. Nature 211(47):434–435
13. Kratzschmar J et al (1991) The plasminogen activator family from the salivary gland of the vampire bat *Desmodus rotundus*: cloning and expression. Gene 105(2):229–237
14. Schleuning WD (2001) Vampire bat plasminogen activator DSPA-alpha-1 (desmoteplase): a thrombolytic drug optimized by natural selection. Haemostasis 31(3–6):118–122
15. Bringmann P et al (1995) Structural features mediating fibrin selectivity of vampire bat plasminogen activators. J Biol Chem 270(43):25596–25603
16. Mellott MJ et al (1992) Vampire bat salivary plasminogen activator promotes rapid and sustained reperfusion without concomitant systemic plasminogen activation in a canine model of arterial thrombosis. Arterioscler Thromb 12(2):212–221
17. Toschi L et al (1998) Fibrin selectivity of the isolated protease domains of tissue-type and vampire bat salivary gland plasminogen activators. Eur J Biochem 252(1):108–112

18. Liberatore GT et al (2003) Vampire bat salivary plasminogen activator (desmoteplase): a unique fibrinolytic enzyme that does not promote neurodegeneration. Stroke 34(2): 537–543

19. Hanaway J et al (1976) Intracranial bleeding associated with urokinase therapy for acute ischemic hemispheral stroke. Stroke 7(2):143–146

20. Fujishima M et al (1986) Controlled trial of combined urokinase and dextran sulfate therapy in patients with acute cerebral infarction. Angiology 37(7):487–498

21. Sato Y et al (1986) Anticoagulant and thrombolytic therapy for cerebral embolism of cardiac origin. Kurume Med J 33(2):89–95

22. Nenci GG et al (1983) Thrombolytic therapy for thromboembolism of vertebrobasilar artery. Angiology 34(9): 561–571

23. Del Zoppo GJ et al (1992) Recombinant tissue plasminogen activator in acute thrombotic and embolic stroke. Ann Neurol 32(1):78–86

24. Von Kummer R, Hacke W (1992) Safety and efficacy of intravenous tissue plasminogen activator and heparin in acute middle cerebral artery stroke. Stroke 23(5):646–652

25. Yasaka M et al (1998) Streptokinase in acute stroke: effect on reperfusion and recanalization. Australian Streptokinase Trial Study Group. Neurology 50(3):626–632

26. The Multicenter Acute Stroke Trial Europe Study Group (1996) Thrombolytic therapy with streptokinase in acute ischemic stroke. N Engl J Med 335(3):145–150

27. Multicentre Acute Stroke Trial Italy (MAST-I) Group (1995) Randomised controlled trial of streptokinase, aspirin, and combination of both in treatment of acute ischaemic stroke. Lancet 346(8989):1509–1514

28. Hacke W et al (1995) Intravenous thrombolysis with recombinant tissue plasminogen activator for acute hemispheric stroke. The European Cooperative Acute Stroke Study (ECASS). J Am Med Assoc 274(13):1017–1025

29. NINDS Group (1995) Tissue plasminogen activator for acute ischemic stroke. N Engl J Med 333:1581–1587

30. Hacke W et al (1998) Randomised double-blind placebo-controlled trial of thrombolytic therapy with intravenous alteplase in acute ischaemic stroke (ECASS II). Second European-Australasian Acute Stroke Study Investigators. Lancet 352(9136):1245–1251

31. Clark WM et al (1999) Recombinant tissue-type plasminogen activator (alteplase) for ischemic stroke 3 to 5 hours after symptom onset. The ATLANTIS Study: a randomized controlled trial. Alteplase thrombolysis for acute noninterventional therapy in ischemic stroke. J Am Med Assoc 282(21):2019–2026

32. Adams HP Jr et al (1996) Guidelines for thrombolytic therapy for acute stroke: a supplement to the guidelines for the management of patients with acute ischemic stroke. A statement for healthcare professionals from a Special Writing Group of the Stroke Council, American Heart Association. Circulation 94(5):1167–1174

33. Adams HP Jr et al (2003) Guidelines for the early management of patients with ischemic stroke: a scientific statement from the Stroke Council of the American Stroke Association. Stroke 34(4):1056–1083

34. Report of the Quality Standards Subcommittee of the American Academy of Neurology (1996) Practice advisory: thrombolytic therapy for acute ischemic stroke – summary statement. Neurology 47(3):835–839

35. Hacke W et al (2004) Association of outcome with early stroke treatment: pooled analysis of ATLANTIS, ECASS, and NINDS rt-PA stroke trials. Lancet 363(9411):768–774

36. Wardlaw JM (2001) Overview of Cochrane thrombolysis meta-analysis. Neurology 57 [5 Suppl 2]:S69–S76

37. Albers GW et al (2000) Intravenous tissue-type plasminogen activator for treatment of acute stroke: the Standard Treatment with Alteplase to Reverse Stroke (STARS) study. J Am Med Assoc 283(9):1145–1150

38. Hill MD, Buchan AM (2001) Methodology for the Canadian Activase for Stroke Effectiveness Study (CASES). CASES Investigators. Can J Neurol Sci 28(3):232–238

39. Grond M et al (1998) Early intravenous thrombolysis for acute ischemic stroke in a community-based approach. Stroke 29(8):1544–1549

40. Chiu D et al (1998) Intravenous tissue plasminogen activator for acute ischemic stroke: feasibility, safety, and efficacy in the first year of clinical practice. Stroke 29(1):18–22

41. Trouillas P et al (1998) Thrombolysis with intravenous rtPA in a series of 100 cases of acute carotid territory stroke: determination of etiological, topographic, and radiological outcome factors. Stroke 29(12):2529–2540

42. Tanne D et al (1999) Initial clinical experience with IV tissue plasminogen activator for acute ischemic stroke: a multicenter survey. The t-PA Stroke Survey Group. Neurology 53(2):424–427

43. Akins PT et al (2000) Can emergency department physicians safely and effectively initiate thrombolysis for acute ischemic stroke? Neurology 55(12):1801–1805

44. Katzan IL et al (2000) Use of tissue-type plasminogen activator for acute ischemic stroke: the Cleveland area experience. J Am Med Assoc 283(9):1151–1158

45. Wang DZ et al (2000) Treating acute stroke patients with intravenous tPA. The OSF stroke network experience. Stroke 31(1):77–81

46. Lopez-Yunez AM et al (2001) Protocol violations in community-based rTPA stroke treatment are associated with symptomatic intracerebral hemorrhage. Stroke 32(1): 12–16

47. Bravata DM et al (2002) Thrombolysis for acute stroke in routine clinical practice. Arch Intern Med 162(17):1994–2001

48. Merino JG et al (2002) Extending tissue plasminogen activator use to community and rural stroke patients. Stroke 33(1):141–146

49. Tanne D et al (2002) Markers of increased risk of intracerebral hemorrhage after intravenous recombinant tissue plasminogen activator therapy for acute ischemic stroke in clinical practice: the Multicenter rt-PA Stroke Survey. Circulation 105(14):1679–1685

50. Hacke W et al (2005) The Desmoteplase in Acute Ischemic Stroke Trial (DIAS): a phase II MRI-based 9-hour window acute stroke thrombolysis trial with intravenous desmoteplase. Stroke 36(1):66–73

51. Albers GW et al (2004) Antithrombotic and thrombolytic therapy for ischemic stroke: the Seventh ACCP Conference on Antithrombotic and Thrombolytic Therapy. Chest 126 [Suppl 3]:483S–512S

52. Benchenane K et al (2004) Equivocal roles of tissue-type plasminogen activator in stroke-induced injury. Trends Neurosci 27(3):155–160

53. Tsirka SE, Rogove AD, Strickland S (1996) Neuronal cell death and tPA. Nature 384(6605):123–124

54. Wang YF et al (1998) Tissue plasminogen activator (tPA) increases neuronal damage after focal cerebral ischemia in wild-type and tPA-deficient mice. Nat Med 4(2):228–231

55. Nagai N et al (1999) Role of plasminogen system components in focal cerebral ischemic infarction: a gene targeting and gene transfer study in mice. Circulation 99(18):2440–2444

56. Nicole O et al (2001) The proteolytic activity of tissue-plasminogen activator enhances NMDA receptor-mediated signaling. Nat Med 7(1):59–64

57. Wang X et al (2004) Mechanisms of hemorrhagic transformation after tissue plasminogen activator reperfusion therapy for ischemic stroke. Stroke 35 [11 Suppl 1]:2726–2730

58. Lo EH, Broderick JP, Moskowitz MA (2004) tPA and proteolysis in the neurovascular unit. Stroke 35(2):354–356

59. Pfefferkorn T, Rosenberg GA (2003) Closure of the blood–brain barrier by matrix metalloproteinase inhibition reduces rtPA-mediated mortality in cerebral ischemia with delayed reperfusion. Stroke 34(8):2025–2030

60. Liu D et al (2004) Tissue plasminogen activator neurovascular toxicity is controlled by activated protein C. Nat Med 10(12):1379–1383

61. Collin C, Wade DT, Davies S, Horne V (1988) The Barthel ADL Index: a reliability study. Int Disability Study 10:61–63

62. Gresham GE, Phillips TF, Labi ML (1980) ADL status in stroke: relative merits of three standard indexes. Arch Phys Med Rehabil 61:355–358

63. Loewen SC, Anderson BA (1990) Predictors of stroke outcome using objective measurement scales. Stroke 21:78–81

64. Mahoney FI, Barthel D (1965) Functional evaluation: the Barthel Index. Maryland State Med J 14:56–61

Endovascular Treatment of Acute Stroke

Raul G. Nogueira, Johnny C. Pryor,
James D. Rabinov, Albert Yoo,
Joshua A. Hirsch

Contents

12.1 Rationale

Stroke remains the third most common cause of death in the industrialized nations, after myocardial infarction and cancer, and the single most common reason for permanent disability [1]. In 1996, the Food and Drug Administration (FDA) approved intravenous (i.v.) thrombolysis with recombinant tissue plasminogen activator (rt-PA, alteplase) for the treatment of acute ischemic stroke after reviewing the results of the National Institute of Neurological Disorders and Stroke (NINDS) and rt-PA Stroke Study Group trial [2]. Intravenous rt-PA thrombolysis was the first approved treatment for acute stroke that effectively treats the causative vascular occlusion. This strategy has the advantage of being relatively easy and rapid to initiate, and does not require specialized equipment or highly technical expertise. Even though thrombolysis was initially a matter of relative controversy, its benefits are now unquestionable. A Cochrane Database Review included 18 trials (16 double-blind) with a total of 5727 patients who received thrombolytics [i.v. urokinase, streptokinase, rt-PA or recombinant intra-arterial (i.a.) pro-urokinase] up to 6 h after ischemic stroke. The review showed a significant reduction in the proportion of patients who were dead or dependent (modified Rankin 3–6) at the end of follow-up at 3–6 months [odds ratio (OR) 0.84, 95% confidence interval (CI) 0.75–0.95] despite a significant increase in the odds of death within the first 10 days (OR 1.81, 95% CI 1.46–2.24), most of which were related to symptomatic intracranial hemorrhage (OR 3.37, 95% CI 2.68–4.22) [3]. Moreover, a recent pooled analysis of six major randomized placebo-controlled i.v. rt-PA stroke trials (ATLANTIS I and II, ECASS I and II, and NINDS I and II), including 2775 patients who were treated with i.v. rt-PA or placebo within 360 min of stroke onset, suggested a potential benefit beyond 3 h, even though the chances of a favorable 3-month outcome decreases as the interval from stroke onset to start of treatment increases.

However, i.v. rt-PA is not a panacea for acute stroke treatment. Indeed, the recanalization of proximal arterial occlusion by i.v. rt-PA ranges from 10% for internal carotid artery (ICA) occlusion to 30% for proximal middle cerebral artery (MCA) occlusion [4]. Analysis of the NINDS data shows only a 12% absolute increase in good outcomes between the placebo and rt-PA group at 3 months [5]. In other words, eight stroke patients must be treated with rt-PA to achieve one additional good patient outcome. However, this analysis understates the impact of rt-PA on stroke patients because it fails to include the patients who partially improved [6]. Even when considering this argument, rates of improvement are far from ideal and, given the prevalence and impact of acute ischemic stroke, it is imperative to devise strategies that can be more effective.

Local i.a. thrombolysis (IAT) has several theoretical advantages over i.v. thrombolysis. For instance, by using coaxial microcatheter techniques, the occluded intracranial vessel is directly accessible and the fibrinolytic agent can be infused into the thrombus. This allows a smaller dose of fibrinolytic agent to reach a higher local concentration than that reached by systemic infusion. With the smaller dose, complications from systemic fibrinolytic effects, including intracranial hemorrhage, can theoretically be reduced.

Moreover, thrombolytics need only be given for as long as the vascular occlusion persists, avoiding exposure to unnecessary higher doses. For these reasons, the treatment window for endovascular lysis can be extended over the typical i.v. window of 3 h. Another major advantage is the combination of thrombolytic treatment with mechanical manipulation of the clot, which may improve recanalization rates [7]. Indeed, mechanical lysis with little or no thrombolytic agent has emerged as a key option for patients who either have a contraindication to thrombolytics (e.g., recent surgery) or are late in their presentation [8, 9]. Furthermore, adjunctive endovascular treatment may be essential for the accomplishment of a successful thrombolysis; for example, through stenting of a dissected vessel, or through angioplasty with or without stenting of an occlusive lesion [10–12].

The major disadvantages to the endovascular strategy include the delay in initiating treatment because of the logistics of doing an angiogram, the additional risks and expense of an invasive procedure, and the fact that this therapy is not available in many communities.

12.2 Technical Aspects

The Massachusetts General Hospital (MGH) protocol for IAT in acute stroke, including inclusion and absolute exclusion criteria, relative contraindications, pre- and post-thrombolysis work-up and management, and management of symptomatic intracranial hemorrhage (ICH) after thrombolysis, is described in the Appendix at the end of this chapter.

Fig. 12.1 a–i ▶

A 74-year-old female presenting with sudden onset of left hemiparesis, right gaze deviation and slurred speech. a Noncontrast head CT showed a "hyperdense MCA sign" on the right. b, c CTA demonstrated a proximal right MCA cut-off. d CT perfusion showed reduction in cerebral blood flow (*CBF*) with e prolongation of mean transit time (*MTT*) and f relative preservation of cerebral blood volume (*CBV*) in the right MCA territory consistent with a salvable ischemic penumbra (CBF/CBV "mismatch"). g Angiogram confirmed proximal MCA occlusion with good collateral flow. h Complete recanalization occurred post intra-arterial thrombolysis (*IAT*) with 2.6 mg of rt-PA and wire manipulation. i Follow-up MRI demonstrated a right MCA infarct involving the deep nuclei but sparing the cortex. This frequently happens with occlusions proximal to the lenticulostriate vessels, given the poor collateral flow to this territory

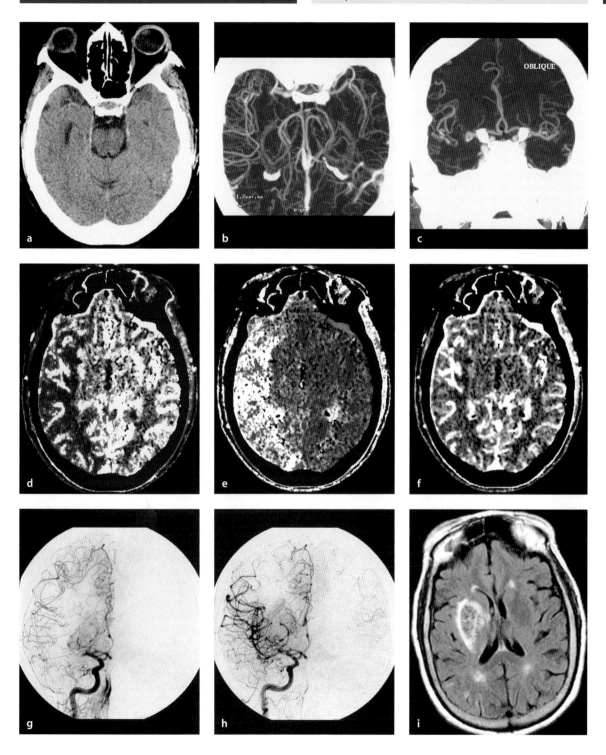

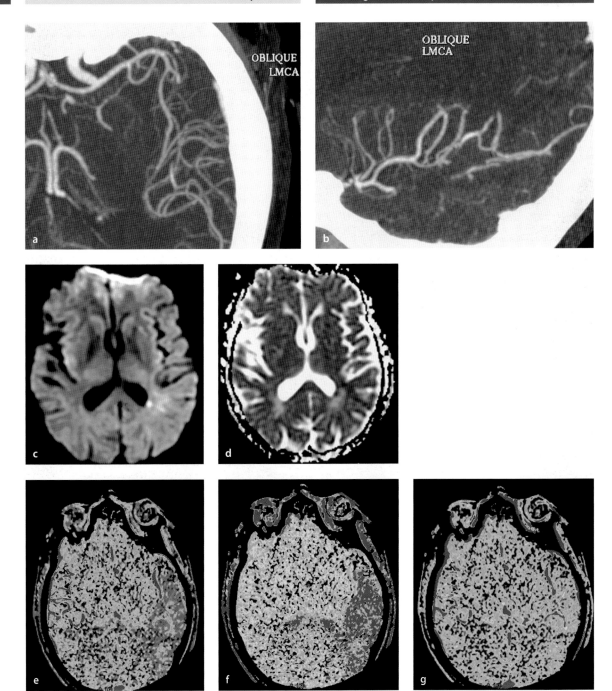

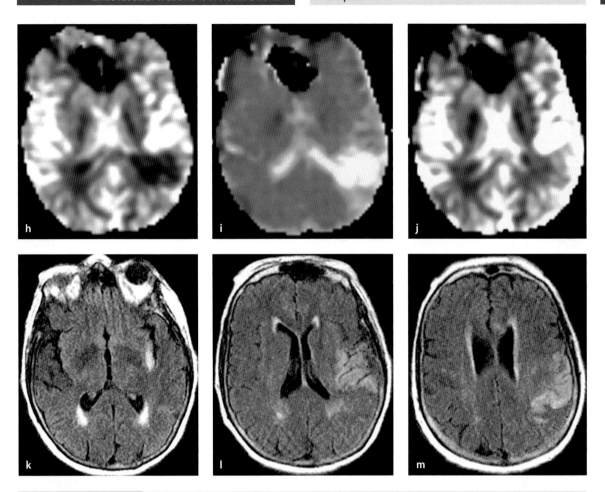

Fig. 12.2 a–m

A 69-year-old female presenting with sudden onset of right hemiparesis, left gaze deviation and aphasia. a, b CTA demonstrated a proximal cut-off in the inferior division of the left MCA. c, d Diffusion-weighted imaging (*DWI*) and apparent diffusion coefficient (*ADC*) maps showed a small focus of restricted diffusion in the left MCA territory. e–g CT perfusion and h–j MR perfusion showed reduction in CBF (e, h) with prolongation of MTT (f, i) and relative preservation of CBV (g, j) in the left MCA territory consistent with a salvageable ischemic penumbra (CBF/CBV or DWI/PWI "mismatch"). The patient could not undergo IAT given high INR on presentation. Follow-up MRI demonstrated growth of the left MCA infarct into the area of ischemic penumbra (k–m)

12.2.1 Pre-procedure Evaluation and Patient Monitoring

After clinical and imaging evaluation suggests the need for IAT, the anesthesia team is contacted and informed of the patient's estimated time of arrival at the interventional neuroradiology suite. Patients re-

ferred from other institutions who have had ICH and infarcts greater than one-third of the involved vascular territory excluded by outside CT may receive i.v. t-PA before transfer and while en route as part of a "bridging" approach [13]. When CT/CT angiography (CTA) confirms the presence of a large vessel occlusion, the patient is brought emergently to angiography. Soft-copy review of noncontrast CT with variable window width and center level settings to accentuate the contrast between normal and edematous tissue (e.g., width 30, level 30) may optimize the recognition of early ischemic changes [14]. We consider the presence of hypodensity involving greater than one-third of the affected vascular territory a contraindication for thrombolysis [15]. Review of post-contrast CTA source images provides a good estimative of whole-brain perfusion without the delay required to process the conventional CT perfusion images [16]. However, if time allows, CT perfusion maps can more accurately characterize the ischemic penumbra (Figs. 12.1, 12.2) [17]. Careful but expedited pre-procedural analysis of the CTA may be extremely helpful in establishing the presence of anatomic variants (e.g., bovine aortic arch) or pathological states (e.g., vessel origin or bifurcation disease) prior to the catheterization procedure. Concurrently, the team Neurologist and/or interventional Neuroradiologist obtain consent while other team members prepare the patient for the procedure.

MRI with MRA, as well as diffusion- and perfusion-weighted imaging (DWI/PWI), has the advantage of providing more complete information on brain parenchymal injury and penumbra at risk. However, it is important that the MRI is performed in a manner that does not significantly delay the endovascular therapy. Nonetheless, MRI can be particularly helpful in selected difficult cases. Patients who present with seizures at stroke onset, a contraindication to i.v. t-PA in the NINDS trial, may need to undergo MRI to exclude the possibility of post-ictal Todd's paralysis unless vascular occlusion is clearly seen on CTA [18]. Similarly, in other situations such as complex migraine, functional disorder, transient global amnesia, acute demyelination, amyloid angiopathy, and brain tumor, the diagnostic abilities of MR can be useful in distinguishing a stroke mimic from an acute ischemic stroke [19]. It should be noted, however, that prolonged seizures and acute demyelination can also cause restricted diffusion. We and others have found that DWI lesions can be partially reversed by IAT in as many as 19% of cases [20, 21]. The application of DWI and PWI in the extension of the therapeutic time window for acute stroke is currently under investigation [22, 23].

A sterile angiography equipment tray should always be prepared at the end of each workday for emergency use after hours to save time during set up. The patient is placed on a cooling blanket to induce moderate hypothermia for brain protection while on the angiography table. Stroke patients are often confused, uncooperative, and combative, which makes digital subtraction angiography and microcatheterization difficult. In addition, access to the patient is limited within the biplane angiographic unit making airway management problematic. The major disadvantage of general anesthesia is the inability to monitor neurological status during the procedure. In most cases the induction of general anesthesia requires only a few minutes and can be performed in tandem with other steps of patient preparation. In addition to giving general anesthesia, the Anesthesiologist also controls patient monitoring [blood pressure (BP) management, airway management, and anticoagulation], leaving the interventional Neuroradiologist free to concentrate on the technical aspects of the procedure.

A radial arterial line and Foley catheter are placed if time and manpower permit. Alternatively, blood pressure can be monitored via the femoral arterial sheath. Immediately prior to the induction of general anesthesia, the patient's neurological status is re-assessed. If deficits have resolved or are rapidly improving, the procedure should be aborted. Mild induced hypertension (systolic 140–160 mmHg) can maximize cerebral perfusion via leptomeningeal collaterals or through a partial occlusion. However, severe hypertension should be avoided and promptly treated. Sustained systolic BP over 180 mmHg and/or diastolic BP over 110 mmHg is considered a contraindication to thrombolysis. Large bore peripheral access is recommended over central venous catheterization. If central venous access is necessary, a femoral venous catheter can be inserted preferably under fluoroscopy. Both groins should be prepared in standard sterile fashion. The best pulse should be used for arterial access. A micropuncture kit should be used to obtain arterial and venous access in patients who are about to receive or have already received thrombolytics.

12.2.2 Procedural Technique

12.2.2.1 Chemical Thrombolysis

A long flexible sheath should be used to obviate difficult catheterizations in patients with tortuous iliac vessels. Typically, a 5 or 6 French guide catheter with a large inner diameter is used, but if angioplasty or stenting of the cervical vessels is anticipated, an 8 or 9 French catheter may be required. The guide catheter should be placed in the vessel of interest without delay (the Circle of Willis and pial collaterals have been previously evaluated by CTA). After a baseline angiogram confirms the presence and location of vascular occlusion, a wire-guided end hole microcatheter (e.g., Prowler microcatheter – Cordis Neurovascular, Miami Lakes, Fla., USA) is navigated into the face of the clot. The microwire is used to gently traverse the clot. Care must be taken in this essentially blind manipulation to avoid vascular perforation or dissection. Hand injection of a small amount of contrast can be performed to define the distal end of the clot. Once the microcatheter is advanced beyond the clot, thrombolytic infusion begins– the microcatheter is pulled back through the clot while drug is infused. Urokinase (UK) comes in powder form and the dosage is measured in units. It is best to reconstitute the powder (250,000 units per vial) in 5 ml of sterile water solution. This solution is then further diluted in 45 ml of normal saline to obtain a final concentration of 5,000 units/ml. The mixture should be slowly mixed to avoid foaming. UK is injected with 1-ml syringes as the microcatheter is pulled slowly back through the thrombus. This manipulation laces the clot with UK and is repeated several times, crossing the clot with the microcatheter and microwire. After the first pass, the arterial anatomy is better understood and more aggressive manipulations with the microwire can be made to mechanically disrupt the clot. We infuse UK at a rate of approximately 10,000 units/min (600,000 units/h). Rough adjustments are made depending on the clinical circumstances and imaging findings.

The interventional Neuroradiologist should limit the number of angiograms and microcatheter injections performed during the exam. Direct injection of contrast into stagnant vessels, which have injured glial cells, and breakdown of the blood–brain barrier may result in contrast extravasation. Contrast is readily visualized on immediate post-thrombolysis CT as an area of high attenuation in the parenchyma. In some instances, MRI with susceptibility sequence may be necessary to differentiate contrast extravasation from ICH [24]. This may be of particular importance in patients who need early anticoagulation or antiplatelet therapy. The area of contrast stain appears to correlate with the location of eventual infarct.

Despite the direct infusion of UK into the thrombus, clot disintegration requires an average of 90 min with traditional thrombolytic infusion and moderate microwire mechanical manipulation. Recanalization is frequently seen using UK at doses around 750,000 units but the amount of time and thrombolytic needed for recanalization varies according to the age and nature of the thrombus. Freshly formed thrombi usually dissolve easily, but thrombus that has embolized from the heart or from other sources may be older and more resistant to lysis.

Once bulk antegrade flow is restored, it may be necessary to lyse distal emboli in clinically significant territories, which requires repositioning of the microcatheter. Successful recanalization should be based on guide catheter injections rather than microcatheter injections since superselective injections may incorrectly demonstrate antegrade flow even though the vessel is still occluded on guide catheter angiograms. The infusion is terminated when adequate antegrade flow is restored, or the predetermined time limit or maximal dose limit is reached. Ominous signs such as contrast extravasation should prompt immediate termination of drug infusion, followed by the appropriate management steps. Treatment of anterior circulation ischemia should occur within 6 h of ictus or before using more than 1,250,000 units of UK in patients who have not received i.v. t-PA, or before using more than 500,000 units of UK in patients who have received i.v. t-PA. There is no specific time window for posterior circulation ischemia treatment, but dosages of UK are limited to 1,500,000 units.

Fibrinolytic agents have several disadvantages. First, although direct infusion maximizes the local drug concentration, dissolution of a clot takes an extended period of time, and time is critical in preserving the penumbra. Second, fibrinolytics increase

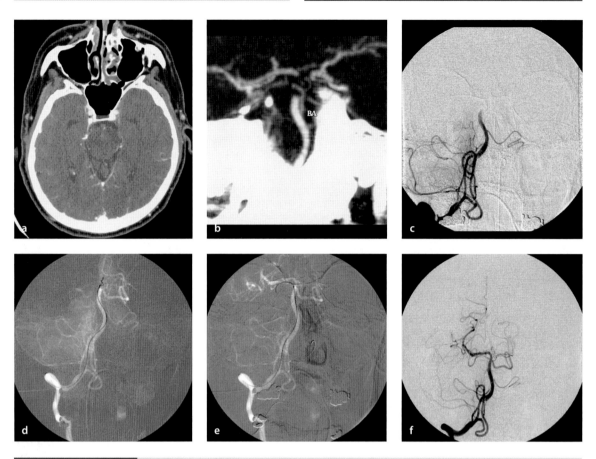

Fig. 12.3 a–f

a–c A 47-year-old male presenting with coma in the setting of left vertebral artery dissection and distal basilar occlusion.
d–f Complete recanalization occurred post-IAT with 3.5 mg of rt-PA and wire manipulation

the risk of hemorrhage locally within the brain or systemically. Lastly, not all thromboembolic occlusions can be lysed with thrombolytic drugs. This resistance to enzymatic degradation may be related to excessive cross-linking in mature embolic clots, or to emboli composed of cholesterol, calcium, or other debris from atherosclerotic lesions. In others, the lack of flow may result in decreased delivery of circulating plasminogen, allowing the high concentration of fibrinolytic to quickly deplete the available plasminogen. This local plasminogen deficiency would result in impaired fibrinolytic activity [25].

12.2.2.2 Mechanical Thrombolysis

Mechanical thrombolysis has several advantages over chemical thrombolysis and may be used as a primary or adjunctive strategy. First, it lessens and may even preclude the use of thrombolytics, in this manner reducing the risk of ICH. Second, by avoiding the use of thrombolytics it may be possible to extend the treatment window beyond 6 h. Third, mechanically fragmenting a clot increases the surface area accessible to fibrinolytic agents and allows inflow of fresh plasminogen, which in turn increases the speed of lysis.

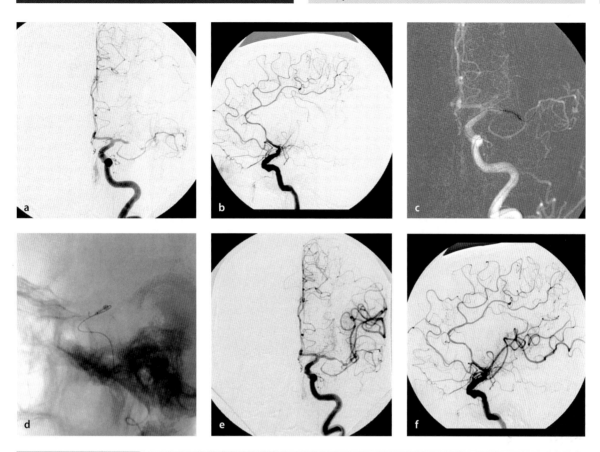

Fig. 12.4 a–f

An 88-year-old male presenting with sudden onset of right hemiparesis, left gaze deviation and aphasia. Angiography demonstrated complete occlusion of the M1 segment of the left MCA (**a, b**). Recanalization of the left MCA (**e, f**) was accomplished after i.a. infusion of 450,000 units of urokinase and angioplasty using a Hyperglide balloon (**c, d**). **d** Note the circumferential "waisting" of the balloon, likely related to a previous existing stenosis. **e** Final angiogram showed mild to moderate residual narrowing at that area

Finally, clot retrieval devices may provide faster recanalization and may be more efficient at coping with material resistant to enzymatic degradation.

Currently, there are several techniques available for mechanical thrombolysis. The most common is the use of probing the thrombus with the microguidewire. This technique useful in facilitating chemical thrombolysis (Fig. 12.3) [7]. Alternatively, a snare (e.g., Amplatz Goose-Neck Microsnare, Microvena, White Bear Lake, Minn., USA) can be used for multiple passes through the occlusion to disrupt the thrombus [26]. A snare can also be used for clot re-

trieval, mostly in situations where the clot has a firm consistency or contains solid material [27]. Inflation of soft balloons in the proximal vessels may reduce or reverse flow and facilitate the clot extraction [9]. Balloon-assisted thrombolysis has gained wide acceptance with the advent of the newer and more compliant balloons (Fig. 12.4). However, the risks of vascular rupture and distal emboli cannot be underestimated and we reserve this technique for patients whose flow cannot be restored by more conservative means. Indeed, when underlying atherosclerotic lesions are found after clot lysis, the need for angio-

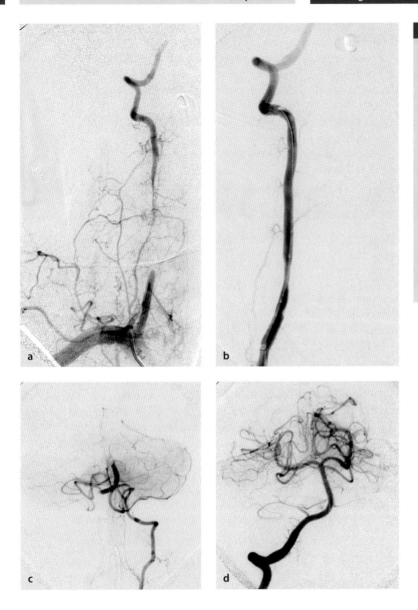

Fig. 12.5 a–d

A 51-year-old male presenting with coma. Angiogram revealed dissection and occlusion of the proximal right vertebral artery with flow reconstitution through muscular collaterals at the level of C4 (a) as well as occlusion of the midbasilar artery (b). The right vertebral artery was successfully recanalized after stent placement across the dissected segment with subsequent balloon angioplasty and i.a. infusion of 4 mg eptifibatide (c). Complete recanalization of the basilar artery was achieved post-IAT with 450,000 units of urokinase and wire manipulation (d)

plasty should be based upon the hemodynamic effects of the stenosis. If antegrade flow can be maintained with anticoagulation alone, angioplasty is not necessary in the acute phase. However, many stenoses reduce flow sufficiently and lead to re-thrombosis [12]. In these patients, angioplasty with or without stenting in concert with thrombolysis can be more effective in maintaining perfusion than thrombolysis alone [28–31]. The angioplasty balloon catheters we have used for mechanical thrombolysis include the Sentry (Boston Scientific, Fremont, Calif., USA) and Hyperglide (Micro Therapeutics, Irvine, Calif., USA). Antegrade flow is essential for the maintenance of vessel patency. This is particularly evident in patients with severe proximal (cervical) stenosis; it is common for these patients to develop re-thrombosis after vessel recanalization. These patients may also benefit from angioplasty and/or stenting of the proximal lesion in addition to thrombolysis of the distal vessels (Fig. 12.5) [10].

The disadvantages of clot removal include the technical difficulty of navigating mechanical devices into the intracranial circulation, excessive trauma to the vasculature, and fragmented thrombus causing distal emboli. Nonetheless, the advantages of mechanical thrombolysis appear to outweigh these disadvantages.

12.2.2.3 New Mechanical Devices

The *Concentric Retriever* (Concentric Medical, Mountain View, Calif., USA), a flexible, tapered Nitinol wire with a helical tip that is used in conjunction with a balloon guide catheter and a microcatheter, is the only device currently approved by the FDA for the endovascular treatment of stroke patients (Fig. 12.6). The Mechanical Embolus Removal in Cerebral Ischemia (MERCI) Trial involved the use of this device in 141 patients with occlusion involving the ICA, the M1 segment of the MCA, or the basilar or vertebral arteries, within 8 h of symptoms onset. None of the patients were eligible for i.v. thrombolysis. Interim data from this trial showed that 47% of patients treated only with the device were successfully revascularized. Of those patients, about half had good functional outcomes measured at 90 days post treatment [8].

The *EKOS MicroLys US infusion catheter* (EKOS, Bothell, Wash., USA) is a 2.5 F standard microinfusion catheter with a 2-mm, 2.1-MHz ring sonography transducer (average power, 0.21–0.45 W) at its distal tip that creates a microenvironment of ultrasonic vibration to facilitate thrombolysis. In a pilot study, where ten patients with anterior-circulation occlusions (mean NIHSS of 18.2) and four with posterior-circulation occlusions (mean NIHSS of 18.75) were treated with this device, TIMI 2–3 flow (for explanation of TIMI see Table 12.2) was achieved in 8 out of the 14 patients in the first hour. Average time to re-

canalization was 46 min. No catheter-related adverse events occurred [32].

The *EPAR* (Endovascular Photoacoustic Recanalization; Endovasix, Belmont, Calif., USA) is a mechanical clot fragmentation device based on laser technology. However, the emulsification of the thrombus is a mechanical thrombolysis and not a direct laser-induced ablation. The photonic energy is converted to acoustic energy at the fiberoptic tip through creation of microcavitation bubbles. In a recent study, where 34 patients (10 ICA, 12 MCA, 1 PCA, and 11 vertebrobasilar occlusions) with a median NIHSS of 19 were treated with EPAR, the overall recanalization rate was 41.1% (14/34). In 18 patients with vessel recanalization, complete EPAR treatment was possible in 11 patients (61.1%). The average lasing time was 9.65 min. Additional treatment with i.a. t-PA occurred in 13 patients. One patient had a vessel rupture resulting in fatal outcome. Symptomatic hemorrhages occurred in 2 patients (5.9%). The overall mortality rate was 38.2% [33].

The *Possis AngioJet system* (Possis Medical, Minneapolis, Minn., USA) is a rheolytic thrombectomy device that uses high-pressure saline jets to create a distal Venturi suction which gently agitates the clot face. The generated clot fragments are then sucked into the access catheter. A 5-French Possis AngioJet catheter has been used in our institution to successfully treat three patients who presented with acute stroke in the setting of ICA occlusion. Patency of the carotid artery was reestablished in two patients. In the third patient, the device was able to create a channel through the column of thrombus, allowing intracranial access [34].

12.2.2.4 Thrombolytic Agents

The thrombolytic drugs act by converting the inactive proenzyme plasminogen into the active enzyme plasmin. Plasmin can degrade fibrinogen, fibrin monomers, and cross-linked fibrin (as is found in thrombus) into fibrin(ogen) degradation products. These agents vary in stability, half-life, and fibrin selectivity. The thrombolytics that have been used for stroke IAT include urokinase (UK), alteplase,

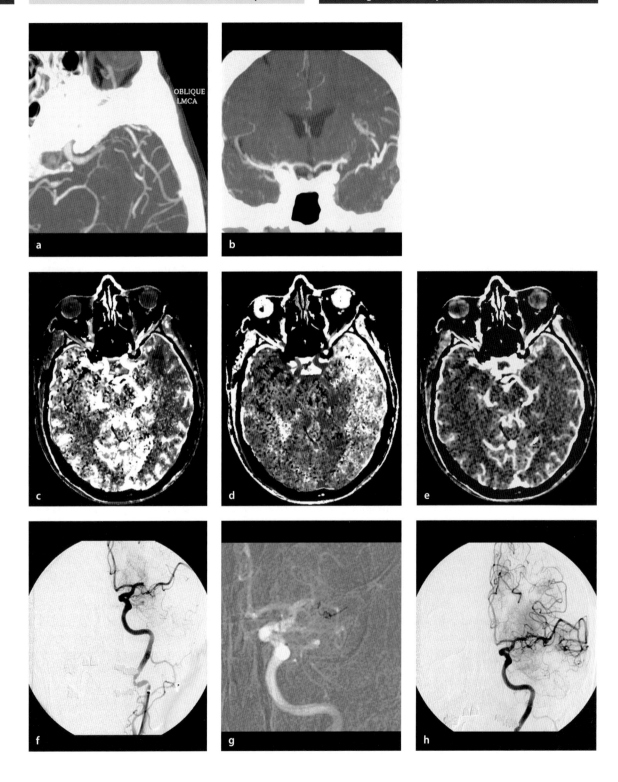

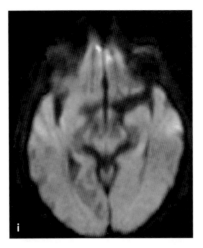
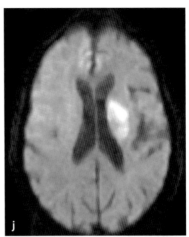

Fig. 12.6 a–j

An 81-year-old female presenting with sudden onset of right hemiparesis, left gaze deviation and aphasia. CTA demonstrated a proximal left MCA cut-off (**a, b**). CT perfusion showed reduction in CBF (**c**) with prolongation of MTT (**d**) and relative preservation of CBV (**e**) in the left MCA territory consistent with a salvable ischemic penumbra (CBF/CBV "mismatch"). Angiogram confirmed proximal MCA occlusion (**f**). Complete recanalization was achieved by using the Concentric Retriever device (**g, h**). Follow-up MRI demonstrated a small deep left MCA infarct sparing the cortex (**i, j**)

reteplase, prourokinase (pro-UK), and streptokinase (SK) [26, 35]. In general, the nonfibrin-selective drugs (e.g., UK and SK) can result in systemic hypofibrinogenemia, whereas the fibrin-selective agents (e.g., rt-PA and rpro-UK) are only active at the site of thrombosis.

First-Generation Agents. *Streptokinase*, a protein derived from group C β-hemolytic streptococci, has a half-life of 16–90 min and low fibrin specificity. This drug is no longer used for stroke IAT. *Urokinase* is a serine protease with a plasma half-life of 14 min and low fibrin specificity. The UK dose used in cerebral IAT has ranged between 0.02×10^6 and 2×10^6 units [35]. UK was withdrawn from the market in 1999 but was approved for lysis of pulmonary embolism in 2003, and has again become the thrombolytic agent of choice for stroke IAT at our institution.

Second-Generation Agents. *Alteplase* (rt-PA) is a serine protease with a plasma half-life of 3.5 min and a high degree of fibrin affinity and specificity. The rt-PA dose used in cerebral IAT has ranged between 20 and 60 mg [35]. The theoretical disadvantages of alteplase include its relatively short half-life and limited penetration in the clot matrix because of strong binding with surface fibrin, which could delay recanalization and increase the risk of recurrent occlusion. *Pro-urokinase* (rpro-UK) is the proenzyme precursor of UK. It has a plasma half-life of 7 min and high fibrin specificity. Despite the favorable results of the PROACT I and II trials, the FDA has not yet approved the use of rpro-UK.

Third-Generation Agents. *Reteplase* is a structurally modified form of alteplase, with a longer half-life (15–18 min). In addition, it does not bind as highly to fibrin; unbound reteplase can then penetrate the clot and potentially improve in vivo fibrinolytic activity. Qureshi et al. [26] have reported the use of low-dose i.a. reteplase (up to 4 units) in conjunction with mechanical thrombolysis [26]. TIMI 2 and 3 recanalization was achieved in 16 out of 19 patients, with no symptomatic ICH. *Tenecteplase* is another modified form of rt-PA with a longer half-life (17 min), greater fibrin specificity, and greater resistance to plasminogen activator inhibitor-1 (PAI-1).

Desmoteplase is a genetically engineered version of the clot-dissolving factor found in the saliva of the vampire bat *Desmodus rotundus*. This drug is more potent and more selective for fibrin-bound plasminogen than any other known plasminogen activator. The i.v. administration of desmoteplase 3–9 h after symptoms onset in stroke patients who demonstrate a PWI–DWI mismatch on MRI is currently being investigated.

No direct comparison between the different thrombolytic agents has been made so far. In a retrospective review of the results for acute stroke IAT performed at our center, we found significantly higher rates of recanalization and good clinical outcome in the era in which i.a. UK was used versus the era in which UK was not available and IAT with rt-PA was the primary treatment [36]. Conversely, in another retrospective study, Eckert et al. [37] found no major difference between the recanalization rates of UK and rt-PA.

12.2.2.5 Adjunctive Therapy

Systemic anticoagulation with i.v. *heparin* during the peri-procedural phase of IAT has several potential advantages, including augmentation of the thrombolytic effect of some agents such as rpro-UK, prevention of acute re-occlusion, and a reduction of the risk of catheter-related embolism. However, these indications are counterbalanced by the potentially increased risk of brain hemorrhage when heparin is combined with a thrombolytic agent. We tend to utilize a regimen similar to the low-dose heparin regimen used in PROACT II (2000 units bolus and 500 units/h for 4 h), aiming for an activated clotting time (ACT) between 200 and 250 s. We avoid using heparin in cases of "bridging" therapy with i.v. rt-PA.

Argatroban and *lepirudin* are direct thrombin inhibitors. These agents should replace heparin in cases where the diagnosis of heparin-induced thrombocytopenia (HIT) type-II is confirmed or even suspected. HIT type II is an immune-mediated disorder characterized by the formation of antibodies against the heparin-platelet factor 4 complex, which results in thrombocytopenia, platelet aggregation, and the potential for arterial and venous thrombosis. The possibility of HIT type II should be raised in patients who demonstrate a platelet count drop to less than 100,000 per milliliter or by more than 50% from baseline, in the setting of heparin therapy (usually 5–12 days after initial exposure).

The use of glycoprotein (GP) IIb/ IIIa antagonists, such as abciximab (*ReoPro®*) or eptifibatide (*Integrilin®*), in ischemic stroke is still investigational. No cases of major ICH were seen in a pilot, randomized, double-blind, placebo-controlled study where 54 patients presenting within 24 h after ischemic stroke onset were randomly allocated to receive escalating doses of abciximab [38]. Similarly, the Abciximab in Emergent Stroke Treatment Trial (AbESTT) demonstrated that intravenous abciximab can be administered with a reasonable degree of safety to patients with acute ischemic stroke within 6 h of symptoms onset. This trial also provided evidence that abciximab may increase the likelihood of a favorable outcome at 3 months. A phase III, multicenter, randomized, double-blind, placebo-controlled trial is currently being performed [39]. In addition, The NIH is currently sponsoring a phase II trial looking at intravenous reteplase in combination with abciximab for the treatment of ischemic stroke 3–24 h from onset. Preliminary analysis of the first 21 patients enrolled has revealed no symptomatic ICH or major hemorrhage [40]. The data for the use of GP IIb/IIIa inhibitors in conjunction with i.a. thrombolysis are even more scant and limited to case reports. Intravenous abciximab has been successfully used as adjunctive therapy to i.a. t-PA or UK in cases of acute stroke [41, 42]. In our institution, we have treated 24 acute stroke patients with i.a. t-PA (mean dosage: 12 mg) in combination with i.v. eptifibatide and found only one case of symptomatic hemorrhage (4.2%), which was related to a rupture during balloon angioplasty. Intra-arterial abciximab has been successfully employed to treated thromboembolic complications encountered during endovascular therapeutic procedures [43, 44]. At MGH, we have used i.a. infusion of eptifibatide at a concentration of 0.75 mg/ml in doses up to 6 mg to treat endovascular

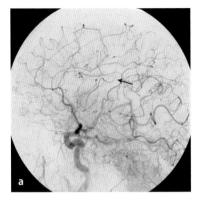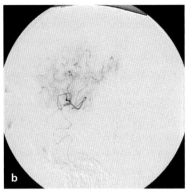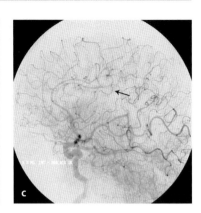

Fig. 12.7 a–c

A 75-year-old man found to have an embolus to a Rolandic branch of the left MCA during catheterization procedure (a). Complete recanalization (c) was obtained after superselective infusion of 250,000 units of urokinase and 3 mg of eptifibatide (b)

complications with good results and no hemorrhagic complications, including a patient who also received 250,000 units of i.a. UK (Fig. 12.7). Depending on the nature of the thrombotic event we may maintain the patient on continuous i.v. infusion of eptifibatide for 24 h. Despite, the promising initial experience with Gp IIb/ IIIa antagonist, we recommend that these drugs should be used judiciously and under close monitoring.

12.3 Intra-arterial Thrombolysis Trials

12.3.1 Background

Similar to the experience with i.v. thrombolysis, the majority of early work on IAT has been reported in nonrandomized case series. Reports of successful IAT go back to the late 1950s, when Sussmann and Fitch [45] described the recanalization of an acutely occluded internal carotid artery with i.a. injection of plasmin. Nonetheless, it was not until the early 1990s that this approach was studied in a more systematic manner.

Lisboa et al. [35] analyzed the safety and efficacy of IAT on the basis of current published data. They found a total of 27 studies (including at least 10 patients in each) with a total of 852 patients who re-

ceived IAT and 100 control subjects. There were more favorable outcomes in the IAT than in the control group (41.5% versus 23%), with a lower mortality rate for IAT (27.2% versus 40%). The IAT group had an odds ratio of 2.4 for a favorable outcome despite a higher frequency of symptomatic ICH (9.5% versus 3%). In addition, they found a trend towards better outcomes with combined i.v. t-PA and IAT than with IAT alone. They also remarked that IAT-treated supratentorial strokes are more likely to have favorable outcomes than the infratentorial ones (42.2% versus 25.6%).

12.3.2 Anterior Circulation Thrombolysis

The safety and efficacy of IAT in the anterior circulation has been evaluated in two randomized, multicenter, placebo-controlled trials. In the Prolyse in Acute Cerebral Thromboembolism (PROACT) I and II trials, patients with proximal MCA (M1 or M2 segment) occlusions within 6 h of symptom onset were treated with recombinant pro-urokinase (rpro-UK) or placebo [46, 47].

In the PROACT I trial, 26 patients with a median NIHSS of 17 were treated with rpro-UK and 14 patients with a median NIHSS of 19 with placebo, at a median of 5.5 h from symptom onset [46]. Patients in the treatment group received 6 mg of i.a. rpro-UK over 2 h, and all patients received high- or low-dose i.v. heparin given as a bolus followed by a 4-h infusion at the time of the angiogram. Mechanical disruption of the clot was not allowed. Both the recanalization rates (TIMI 2 or 3 flow: 57.7% versus 14.3%) and the incidence of symptomatic ICH (15.4% versus 7.1%) were higher in the rpro-UK than in the placebo group. Of note, all patients in the rpro-UK group with early CT changes involving >33% of the MCA territory suffered ICH. In the rpro-UK group, the rates of recanalization were dependent upon the administered dose of heparin. At the end of the 2-h rpro-UK infusion, 81.8% of the patients treated with high-dose heparin (100 IU/kg bolus followed by 1000 IU/h infusion for 4 h) demonstrated recanalization whereas only 40% were recanalized in the low-dose heparin subgroup (2000 IU bolus, followed by a 500 IU/h infusion for 4 h). However, the rate of symptomatic ICH at 24 h was also higher in the high-dose heparin group (27.3% versus 6.7%). The overall 90-day cumulative mortality was 26.9% in the rpro-UK group and 42.9% in the placebo group. While the number of patients in this study was too low to allow any definite conclusions regarding efficacy, its results led to the PROACT II trial.

The PROACT II trial was designed to assess the clinical efficacy and safety of i.a. rpro-UK. In this study, 180 patients were enrolled in a 2:1 randomization scheme to receive either 9 mg i.a. r-proUK plus 4 h of low-dose i.v. heparin or low-dose i.v. heparin alone [47]. The primary clinical outcome, the proportion of patients with slight or no disability at 90 days (modified Rankin Score of ≤2), was achieved in 40% of the 121 patients in the rpro-UK treatment group as compared to 25% of the 59 patients in the control group (absolute benefit 15%, relative benefit 58%, number need = 7; P=0.04). The recanalization rate (TIMI 2 and 3) was 66% for the r-proUK group and 18% for the control group (P<0.001). Symptomatic ICH within 24 h occurred in 10% of r-proUK patients and 2% of control patients (P=0.06). All symptomatic ICH occurred in patients with a baseline NIHSS score of 11 or higher (NIHSS 11–20, 11%; NIHSS >20, 13%). Mortality after symptomatic ICH was 83% (10/12 patients). Blood glucose was significantly as-

sociated with symptomatic ICH in rpro-UK-treated patients (patients with baseline glucose >200 mg/dl experienced a 36% risk of symptomatic ICH compared with 9% for those with ≤200 mg/dl) [48].

Mortality was 25% for the rpro-UK group and 27% for the control group despite the higher incidence of ICH in the rpro-UK patients. Secondary clinical outcomes included the percentage of patients reaching an NIHSS score of <1, the percentage of patients achieving a 50% or greater reduction from baseline NIHSS, and the percentage of patients achieving a Barthel index score of 60 or greater and a Barthel index score of 90 or greater, all measured at 90 days. Despite a trend in favor of the rpro-UK group, none of these secondary functional or neurological outcome measures achieved statistical significance. Although encouraging, the results of PROACT II were not enough to grant the FDA approval of rpro-UK and another larger trial was requested.

Acute strokes due to carotid T occlusion carry a much worse prognosis than MCA occlusions. In a recent analysis of 24 consecutive patients (median NIHSS 19) presenting with T occlusions of the ICA, which was treated by IAT using urokinase at an average of 237 min from symptom onset, only 4 patients (16.6%) had a favorable outcome after 3 months. Partial recanalization of the intracranial ICA was achieved in 15 (63%), of the MCA in 4 (17%), and of the ACA in 8 patients (33%). Complete recanalization did not occur. The presence of good leptomeningeal collaterals and being younger than 60 years were the only predictors of a favorable clinical outcome [49]. New treatment strategies such as the combination of i.v. t-PA and IAT [50] or the use of new mechanical devices [34] may further improve the outcome in these patients.

12.3.3 Posterior Circulation Thrombolysis

No randomized, placebo-controlled studies of IAT for vertebrobasilar occlusion have yet been done and most of the rationale for its use is based on the favorable reports of uncontrolled case series (Table 12.1). Since the first series of IAT for basilar artery occlusion by Zeumer et al. in 1983 [51] approximately 278 cases have been reported, with an overall recanaliza-

Table 12.1. Outcomes in patient series treated with intra-arterial thrombolysis in the vertebrobasilar circulation. (*C* Complete, *N/A* not available, *NR* no recanalization, *P* partial, *Pro-UK* pro-urokinase, *R* recanalized, *SK* streptokinase, *t-PA* tissue plasminogen activator, *UK* urokinase)

Study	Number of patients	Agent	Recanalization (%)	ICH (%)	Time window (h)	Good outcomes (%)
Hacke et al. [64]	43	UK/SK	44	9	6–76	23
Masumoto and Satoh [65]	10	UK	40	N/A	N/A	40
Zeumer et al. [25]	28	t-PA/UK	75	7	≤6	25
Becker et al. [66]	12	UK	83	17	1–48	25
Brandt et al. [67]	51	t-PA/UK	51	14	≤48	20
Wijdicks et al. [68]	9	UK	78	11	2–13	56
Gonner et al. [69]	10	UK	50	10	≤6	50
Cross et al. [70]	20	UK	50	15	N/A	20
Ezaki et al. [71]	26	t-PA/UK/pro-UK	92.3	7.7	≤24	34.6
Arnold et al. [72]	40	UK	80	5	≤11	35

Modified from Phan and Wijdicks [73]

tion rate of 60%, and a mortality rate of 90% in non-recanalized patients and 31% in at least partially recanalized patients [52]. In general, distal occlusions, which are usually embolic, have higher recanalization rates than proximal occlusions, which are more commonly atherothrombotic. Most stroke experts agree that the time window for IAT in the posterior circulation should be longer than the one for strokes in the carotid circulation. The underlying principles for such an approach include not only the extremely poor prognosis of untreated lesions, with a mortality rate as high as 90%, but also a lower rate of hemorrhagic transformation in this vascular territory. In our institution, we typically treat basilar occlusion up to 12 h after symptoms onset. We consider an extension of this window to up to 24 or 48 h for patients with fluctuating symptoms or small infarcts on diffusion MRI.

12.3.4 Combined Intravenous and Intra-arterial Thrombolysis

Four studies have evaluated the feasibility, safety, and efficacy of combined i.v. rt-PA at a dose of 0.6 mg/kg and IAT in patients presenting with acute strokes within 3 h of symptom onset [13, 53–55]. This approach has the potential of combining the advantages of i.v. rt-PA (fast and easy to use) with the advantages of IAT (titrated dosing, mechanical aids to recanalization, and higher rates of recanalization), thus improving the speed and frequency of recanalization.

The Emergency Management of Stroke (EMS) Bridging Trial was a double-blind, randomized, placebo-controlled multicenter Phase I study of i.v. rt-PA or i.v. placebo followed by immediate IAT of rt-PA [53]. Seventeen patients were randomly assigned into the i.v./i.a. group and 18 into the placebo/i.a. group. Clot was found in 22 of 34 patients. TIMI 3 flow recanalization occurred in 6 of 11 i.v./i.a. patients versus 1 of 10 placebo/i.a. patients (*P*=0.03) and correlated to the total dose of rt-PA (*P*=0.05). However, no difference in the 7- to 10-day or the 3-month outcomes was found, and there were more deaths in the i.v./i.a. group. Eight ICHs occurred: all hemorrhagic infarctions. Symptomatic ICH occurred in one placebo/i.a. patient and two i.v./i.a. patients. Life-threatening bleeding complications occurred in two patients, both in the i.v./i.a. group.

The Interventional Management of Stroke (IMS) Study was a multicenter, open-labeled, single-arm pilot study where 80 patients (median NIHSS 18) were enrolled to receive i.v. rt-PA (0.6 mg/kg, 60 mg maximum, 15% of the dose as a bolus with the remainder administered over 30 min) within 3 h of stroke onset (median time to initiation: 140 min) [13]. Additional rt-PA was subsequently administered via a microcatheter at the site of the thrombus up to a total dose of 22 mg over 2 h of infusion or until thrombolysis in 62 of the 80 patients. Primary comparisons were with similar subsets of placebo- and rt-PA-treated subjects from the NINDS rt-PA Stroke Trial. The 3-month mortality in Interventional Management Study (IMS) subjects (16%) was numerically lower but not statistically different than the mortality of placebo (24%) and rt-PA-treated subjects (21%) in the NINDS rt-PA Stroke Trial. The rate of symptomatic ICH (6.3%) in IMS subjects was similar to that of rt-PA-treated subjects (6.6%) but higher than the rate in placebo-treated subjects (1.0%, $P=0.018$) in the NINDS rt-PA Stroke Trial. IMS subjects had a significantly better outcome at 3 months than NINDS placebo-treated subjects for all outcome measures (odds ratios ≥2). For the 62 subjects who received i.a. rt-PA in addition to i.v. t-PA, the rate of complete recanalization (TIMI 3 flow) was 11% (7/62) and the rate of partial or complete recanalization (TIMI 2 or 3 flow) was 56% (35/62).

Ernst et al. [54] performed a retrospective analysis of 20 consecutive patients (median NIHSS 21) who presented within 3 h of stroke symptoms and were treated using i.v. rt-PA (0.6 mg/kg) followed by i.a. rt-PA (up to 0.3 mg/kg or 24 mg whichever is less, over a maximum of 2 h) in 16 of the 20 patients. Despite a high number of ICA occlusions (8/16), TIMI 2 and 3 recanalization rates were obtained in 50% (8/16) and 19% (3/16) of the patients, respectively. One patient (5%) developed a fatal ICH. Ten patients (50%) recovered to a modified Rankin Scale (mRS) of 0 or 1; three patients (15%), to an mRS of 2; and five patients (25%), to an mRS of 4 or 5.

Suarez et al. [55] studied "bridging" therapy in 45 patients using i.v. t-PA at 0.6 mg/kg within 3 h of stroke onset. Patients exhibiting evidence of PWI–DWI mismatches on MRI underwent subsequent IAT. Eleven patients received IAT with rt-PA (maximal dose 0.3 mg/kg) and 13 patients received IAT with UK

(maximal dose 750,000 units). Symptomatic ICH occurred in 2 of the 21 patients in the i.v. rt-PA-only group, but in none of the patients in the i.v. rt-PA/IAT group. Out of the 24 patients in the i.v. rt-PA/IAT group, 21 had MCA occlusions, 2 had ACA occlusions and 1 had PCA occlusion. Complete recanalization occurred in 5 of the 13 patients treated with i.v. rt-PA/i.a. UK and 4 of the 11 patients treated with i.v. rt-PA/i.a. rt-PA. Partial recanalization also occurred in 5 of the 13 patients treated with i.v. rt-PA/i.a. UK and 4 of the 11 treated with i.v. rt-PA/i.a. rt-PA. Favorable outcomes (Barthel index 95) were seen in 92%, 64%, and 66% of the i.v. rt-PA/i.a. UK, i.v. rt-PA/i.a. rt-PA, and i.v. rt-PA-only groups, respectively.

A "reversed bridging" approach has been proposed by Keris et al. [56]. In this study, 12 patients (3 ICA occlusions and 9 MCA occlusions) out of the 45 enrolled patients (all with NIHSS >20) were randomized to receive an initial i.a. infusion of 25 mg rt-PA over 5–10 min followed by i.v. infusion of another 25 mg over 60 min, within 6 h of stroke onset (total combined dose 50 mg with a maximal dose of 0.7 mg/kg). The remaining 33 patients were assigned to a control group and did not undergo any thrombolysis. TIMI 2 and 3 recanalization occurred in 1/12 and 5/12 of the patients, respectively. None had symptomatic ICH. At 12 months, 83% of the patients in the thrombolysis group were functionally independent whereas only 33% of the control subjects had a good outcome.

In a prospective, open-label study, Hill et al. [57] assessed the feasibility of a "bridging" approach using full-dose i.v. rt-PA [57]. Following i.v. infusion of 0.9 mg/kg rt-PA, six patients underwent IAT with rt-PA (maximum 20 mg) and one underwent intracranial angioplasty. TIMI 2 or 3 recanalization was achieved in three of these patients. None had symptomatic ICH.

At our institution, we have treated 18 patients (mean NIHSS 17.4) with a full (0.9 mg/kg) i.v. rt-PA dose followed by IAT with rt-PA (mean dose 6 mg) [58]. We have achieved TIMI 2 or 3 recanalization in 72% of these patients with a symptomatic ICH rate of 16.7%. In our current "bridging" protocol, i.a. rt-PA has been replaced by i.a. UK.

Table 12.2. Modified Thrombolysis in Myocardial Infarction (*TIMI*) grading system [59, 60]

Grade 0	No flow
Grade 1	Some penetration past the site of occlusion, but no flow distal to the occlusion
Grade 2	Distal perfusion, but delayed filling in all vessels
Grade 3	Distal perfusion with adequate perfusion in less than half of the distal vessels
Grade 4	Distal perfusion with adequate perfusion in more than half of the distal vessels

Table 12.3. Thrombolysis in Cerebral Infarction (*TICI*) perfusion categories [61]

Grade 0	**No perfusion.** No antegrade flow beyond the point of occlusion
Grade 1	**Penetration with minimal perfusion.** The contrast material passes beyond the area of obstruction but fails to opacify the entire cerebral bed distal to the obstruction for the duration of the angiographic run
Grade 2	**Partial perfusion.** The contrast material passes beyond the obstruction and opacifies the arterial bed distal to the obstruction. However, the rate of entry of contrast into the vessel distal to the obstruction and/or its rate of clearance from the distal bed are perceptibly slower than its entry into and/or clearance from comparable areas not perfused by the previously occluded vessel, e.g., the opposite cerebral artery or the arterial bed proximal to the obstruction
Grade 2a	Only partial filling (<2/3) of the entire vascular territory is visualized
Grade 2b	Complete filling of all of the expected vascular territory is visualized, but the filling is slower than normal
Grade 3	**Complete perfusion.** Antegrade flow into the bed distal to the obstruction occurs as promptly as into the obstruction *and* clearance of contrast material from the involved bed is as rapid as from an uninvolved bed of the same vessel or the opposite cerebral artery

12.4 Grading Systems

Several grading systems have been developed as an attempt to quantify recanalization rates. The Thrombolysis in Myocardial Infarction (TIMI) [59] grading system, either in its original or modified form (Table 12.2) [60], has been widely used. Another modification of the TIMI grading scheme was recently proposed by an Assessment Committee of the American Society of Interventional and Therapeutic Neuroradiology (Table 12.3) [61]. However, the aforementioned, classification systems are limited because they do not account for occlusion location or collateral circulation. Qureshi [62] has proposed a scheme based primarily on the occlusion site and degree of collateralization (Table 12.4). This scheme appears to have a strong correlation with the initial severity and in-hospital outcome of acute ischemic stroke [63].

12.5 Conclusion

The efficacy of i.v. thrombolysis is restricted by several factors including the relatively short therapeutic window, increased hemorrhagic rate, and poor recanalization rates as the clot burden is increased. IAT improves the rates of recanalization and good functional outcome in patients presenting with proximal occlusion of the intracranial arteries. Intravenous thrombolysis with rt-PA should be considered in patients presenting within 3 h of stroke onset as a "bridging" therapy to IAT. Mechanical thrombolysis has become a powerful adjunct to i.a. infusion of thrombolytics and should be considered as primary therapy in patients who have contraindications to thrombolytics or have late presentation (up to 8 h in the anterior circulation). The time window for IAT in the posterior circulation has not been well estab-

Table 12.4. Grades of increasing severity of arterial occlusion according to a new classification scheme. (*ACA* Anterior cerebral artery, *BA* basilar artery, *ICA* internal carotid artery, *MCA* middle cerebral artery, *VA* vertebral artery)

Grade	Type of occlusion		
0		No occlusion	
1	MCA occlusion (M3 segment)	ACA occlusion (A2 or distal segments)	1 BA and/or VA branch occlusion
2	MCA occlusion (M2 segment)	ACA occlusion (A1 and A2 segments)	≥2 BA and/or VA branch occlusions
3		MCA occlusion (M1 segment)	
3A		Lenticulostriate arteries spared and/or leptomeningeal collaterals visualized	
3B		No sparing of lenticulostriate arteries, and no leptomeneningeal collaterals visualized	
4	ICA occlusion (collaterals present)		BA occlusion (partial filling direct or via collaterals)
4A	Collaterals fill MCA		Anterograde filling[a]
4B	Collaterals fill ACA		Retrograde filling[a]
5	ICA occlusion (no collaterals)		BA occlusion (complete)

[a] Predominant pattern of filling
From Qureshi [62]

lished and, at this point, a judicious decision should be made on a case-by-case basis. The new neuroimaging techniques, including CT perfusion and MRI with DWI/PWI, have become essential in the decision-making process of thrombolysis. These methods may eventually define a subgroup of patients who will benefit from late thrombolysis.

Appendix: MGH Protocols for Intra-arterial Thrombolytics (Chemical and/or Mechanical) for Acute Stroke

Intra-arterial Inclusion Criteria

– A significant neurologic deficit expected to result in long-term disability, and attributable to large vessel occlusion (basilar, vertebral, internal carotid or middle cerebral artery M1 or M2 branches).
– Noncontrast CT scan without hemorrhage or well-established infarct. If MRI obtained, DWI–PWI mismatch with relatively small DWI abnormality (for example, less than one-third MCA territory).
– Acute ischemic stroke symptoms with onset or last known well clearly defined. Treatment within 6 h of established, nonfluctuating deficits due to anterior circulation (carotid/MCA) stroke. Treatment with mechanical thrombolysis using the Concentric Retriever device is a consideration in patients between 6 and 8 h of stroke symptom onset. The window of opportunity for treatment is less well defined in posterior circulation (vertebral/basilar) ischemia, and patients may have fluctuating, reversible ischemic symptoms over many hours or even days and still be appropriate candidates for therapy.

Absolute Exclusion Criteria

– Hemorrhage or well-established acute infarct on CT involving greater than one-third of the affected vascular territory.

- CNS lesion with high likelihood of hemorrhage status post chemical thrombolytic agents (e.g., brain tumors, abscess, vascular malformation, aneurysm, contusion).
- Established bacterial endocarditis.

Relative Contraindications

- Mild or rapidly improving deficits.
- Significant trauma within 3 months.*
- CPR with chest compressions within past 10 days.*
- Stroke within 3 months.
- History of intracranial hemorrhage; or symptoms suspicious for subarachnoid hemorrhage.
- Major surgery within past 14 days.*
- Minor surgery within the past 10 days, including liver and kidney biopsy, thoracocentesis, lumbar puncture.*
- Arterial puncture at a noncompressible site within past 14 days (see below for femoral artery puncture).*
- Pregnant (up to 10 days postpartum) or nursing woman.*
- Suspected bacterial endocarditis.
- Gastrointestinal, urologic, or respiratory hemorrhage within past 21 days.*
- Known bleeding diathesis (includes renal and hepatic insufficiency).*
- Life expectancy <1 year from other causes.
- Peritoneal dialysis or hemodialysis.*
- PTT >40 s; platelet count <100,000/ml.*
- INR >1.7 (PT>15 if no INR available) with or without chronic oral anticoagulant use.*
- Seizure at onset of stroke. (This relative contraindication is intended to prevent treatment of patients with a deficit due to postictal Todd's paralysis or with seizure due to some other CNS lesion that precludes thrombolytic therapy. If rapid diagnosis of vascular occlusion can be made, treatment may be given.)

---

* Items marked with an asterisk may not be exclusions for mechanical thrombolysis with or without limited dose chemical agents.

- Glucose <50 or >400 mg/dl. (This relative contraindication is intended to prevent treatment of patients with focal deficits due to hypo- or hyperglycemia. If the deficit persists after correction of the serum glucose, or if rapid diagnosis of vascular occlusion can be made, treatment may be given.)

Pre-Thrombolysis Work-up

- Temperature, pulse, BP, respiratory rate.
- Physical exam/neurologic exam including NIHSS.
- 12-lead EKG.
- Complete blood count (CBC) with platelets, basic metabolic [electrolytes, blood urea nitrogen (BUN)/creatinine, glucose] and hepatic function panel, prothrombin time (PT, INR), partial thromboplastin time (PTT), erythrocyte sedimentation rate (ESR), fibrinogen. Blood for type and screen.
- Urine or blood pregnancy test in women of childbearing potential.
- Consider hypercoagulable panel in young patients without apparent stroke risk factors.

Pre-Thrombolysis Management

- Start supplementary oxygen. Treat any fever with acetaminophen. Nil by mouth (NPO) except medications.
- Do not place Foley, nasogastric tube, arterial line or central venous line unless it is absolutely necessary for patient safety.
- Do not lower blood pressure unless it is causing myocardial ischemia or exceeds 220/120 mmHg. Use labetolol i.v. (5–20 mg i.v. q 10–20 min) or, if necessary, sodium nitroprusside i.v. (0.5–10 µg/kg per min). Monitor with noninvasive cuff pressures q 15 min or continuous arterial pressure monitoring.
- Do not administer heparin unless recommended by the Acute Stroke Team.
- STAT head CT/CTA/CTP and possible MRI with DWI/PWI.
- Consider bypassing CTA if renal failure, diabetes, congestive heart failure. Hold metformin 48 h after iodinated contrast.

- Check patency of 16–18 gauge forearm i.v.
- Consider chest radiograph to exclude acute congestive heart failure or aortic dissection if clinical suspicion.
- Check MRI exclusions (e.g., severe claustrophobia, implanted pacemaker, metal fragments, shrapnel).
- Review CT/CTA with Interventionalist and Stroke Team.
- Obtain consent for procedure and general anesthesia in writing from patient or family.
- If time permits, obtain STAT DWI MR imaging but do not delay time to treatment.

Peri-Thrombolysis Management

- Confirm case with Anesthesia and consider starting heparin 3000-unit bolus and 800 units/h.
- Request orogastric or nasogastric tube placement prior to thrombolytic drug infusion.
- Induce moderate hypothermia (33–34 °C) during the case with cooling blanket.
- Consider induced hypertension until patency restored in patients with poor collateral flow.
- Consider terminating infusion of thrombolytic by 6 h in anterior circulation stroke. Consider early angioplasty at common carotid bifurcation or distal internal carotid bifurcation in selected cases.
- To prevent or treat acute re-occlusion or after angioplasty or stenting, consider i.v. eptifibatide.
- Call for CT scan to be done post thrombolysis en route to Neuro ICU. Repeat CT 6 h later, consider CTA if renal and cardiovascular function permits.
- Begin passive rewarming in Neuro ICU. Do not apply extra blankets or heating devices.
- If considering antiplatelet or anticoagulant agents, check fibrinogen >100 mg/dl and PTT <80 s.

Pre- and Post-Treatment Management

ICU admission for monitoring during first 24 h:
- Vital signs q 15 min for 2 h, then q 30 min for 6 h, then q 1 h for 16 h.
- Strict control of BP for 24 h per protocol.
- Neuro checks q 1 h for 24 h.
- Pulse oximeter; oxygen cannula or mask to maintain O_2 saturation >95%.

- Acetaminophen 650 mg p.o./p.r. q 4 h p.r.n. T >37 °C (99.4 °F); cooling blanket p.r.n. T >39 °C (102 °F), set to avoid shivering.
- No antiplatelet agents or anticoagulants in first 24 h.
- No Foley catheter, nasogastric tube, arterial catheter or central venous catheter for 24 h, unless absolutely necessary.
- STAT head CT for any worsening of neurologic condition.

Protocol for Blood Pressure Control After Thrombolysis

Patients will be admitted to the ICU for hemodynamic monitoring for a minimum of 24 h. A noninvasive blood pressure (BP) cuff is recommended unless sodium nitroprusside is required. BP will be strictly controlled according to the guidelines used in the NINDS trial as listed below. Clinical deterioration associated with acute reduction in BP should be evaluated immediately.

Monitor arterial BP during the first 24 h after starting treatment:
- Every 15 min for 2 h after starting the infusion, then
- Every 30 min for 6 h, then
- Every 60 min for 24 h after starting treatment.

If systolic BP is 180–230 mmHg or if diastolic BP is 105–120 mmHg for two or more readings 5–10 min apart:
- Give intravenous labetolol 10 mg over 1–2 min. The dose may be repeated or doubled every 10–20 min up to a total dose of 150 mg.
- Monitor BP every 15 min during labetolol treatment and observe for development of hypotension.

If systolic BP is >230 mmHg or if diastolic BP is in the range of 121–140 mmHg for two or more readings 5–10 min apart:
- Give i.v. labetolol 10 mg over 1–2 min. The dose may be repeated or doubled every 10 min up to a total dose of 150 mg.

- Monitor BP every 15 min during the labetolol treatment and observe for development of hypotension.
- If no satisfactory response, infuse sodium nitroprusside (0.5–10 µg/kg per min).

If diastolic BP is >140 mmHg for two or more readings 5–10 min apart:

- Infuse sodium nitroprusside (0.5–10 µg/kg per minute).
- Monitor BP every 15 min during infusion of sodium nitroprusside and observe for development of hypotension.
- Continuous arterial monitoring is advised if sodium nitroprusside is used. The risk of bleeding secondary to an arterial puncture should be weighed against the possibility of missing dramatic changes in pressure during infusion.

Management of Symptomatic Hemorrhage After Thrombolysis

- STAT head CT, if ICH suspected.
- Consult Neurosurgery for ICH.
- Check CBC, PT, PTT, platelets, fibrinogen and D-dimer. Repeat q 2 h until bleeding is controlled.
- Give fresh frozen plasma 2 units every 6 h for 24 h after dose.
- Give cryoprecipitate 20 units. If fibrinogen level <200 mg/dl at 1 h, repeat cryoprecipitate dose.
- Give platelets 4 units.
- Give protamine sulfate 1 mg/100 units heparin received in last 3 h (give initial 10 mg test dose i.v. slowly over 10 min and observe for anaphylaxis; if stable give entire calculated dose slow i.v.; maximum dose 100 mg).
- Institute frequent neurochecks and therapy of acutely elevated intracranial pressure (ICP), as needed.
- May give aminocaproic acid (Amicar®) 5 g in 250 ml normal saline i.v. over 1 h as a last resort.

References

1. WHO Task Force on Stroke and other Cerebrovascular Disorders (1989) Recommendations on stroke prevention, diagnosis, and therapy. Stroke 20(10):1407–1431
2. The National Institute of Neurological Disorders and Stroke rt-PA Stroke Study Group (1995) Tissue plasminogen activator for acute ischemic stroke. N Engl J Med 333(24):1581–1587
3. Wardlaw JM et al (2003) Thrombolysis for acute ischaemic stroke. Cochrane Database Syst Rev 3:CD000213
4. Wolpert SM et al (1993) Neuroradiologic evaluation of patients with acute stroke treated with recombinant tissue plasminogen activator. The rt-PA Acute Stroke Study Group. Am J Neuroradiol 14(1):3–13
5. Caplan LR et al (1997) Should thrombolytic therapy be the first-line treatment for acute ischemic stroke? Thrombolysis – not a panacea for ischemic stroke. N Engl J Med 337(18):1309–1310; discussion 1313
6. Haley EC Jr, Lewandowski C, Tilley BC (1997) Myths regarding the NINDS rt-PA Stroke Trial: setting the record straight. Ann Emerg Med 30(5):676–682
7. Barnwell SL et al (1994) Safety and efficacy of delayed intraarterial urokinase therapy with mechanical clot disruption for thromboembolic stroke. Am J Neuroradiol 15(10):1817–1822
8. Starkman S, The MERCI Investigators. Results of the Combined MERCI® I-II (Mechanical Embolus Removal in Cerebral Ischemia) Trials. 29th International Stroke Conference, February 2004, San Diego, Calif., USA
9. Mayer TE, Hamann GF, Brueckmann H (2002) Mechanical extraction of a basilar-artery embolus with the use of flow reversal and a microbasket. N Engl J Med 347(10):769–770
10. Yu W et al (2003) Endovascular embolectomy of acute basilar artery occlusion. Neurology 61(10):1421–1423
11. Ueda T et al (1997) Endovascular treatment for acute thrombotic occlusion of the middle cerebral artery: local intra-arterial thrombolysis combined with percutaneous transluminal angioplasty. Neuroradiology 39(2):99–104
12. Qureshi AI et al (2004) Reocclusion of recanalized arteries during intra-arterial thrombolysis for acute ischemic stroke. Am J Neuroradiol 25(2):322–328
13. Investigators IS (2004) Combined intravenous and intra-arterial recanalization for acute ischemic stroke: the Interventional Management of Stroke Study. Stroke 35(4):904–911
14. Lev MH et al (1999) Acute stroke: improved nonenhanced CT detection – benefits of soft-copy interpretation by using variable window width and center level settings. Radiology 213(1):150–155
15. Hacke W et al (1995) Intravenous thrombolysis with recombinant tissue plasminogen activator for acute hemispheric stroke. The European Cooperative Acute Stroke Study (ECASS). J Am Med Assoc 274(13):1017–1025

16. Hunter GJ et al (2003) Whole-brain CT perfusion measurement of perfused cerebral blood volume in acute ischemic stroke: probability curve for regional infarction. Radiology 227(3):725–730

17. Wintermark M et al (2002) Prognostic accuracy of cerebral blood flow measurement by perfusion computed tomography, at the time of emergency room admission, in acute stroke patients. Ann Neurol 51(4):417–432

18. Selim M et al (2002) Seizure at stroke onset: should it be an absolute contraindication to thrombolysis? Cerebrovasc Dis 14(1):54–57

19. Ay H et al (1999) Normal diffusion-weighted MRI during stroke-like deficits. Neurology 52(9):1784–1792

20. Schaefer PW et al (2004) Characterization and evolution of diffusion MR imaging abnormalities in stroke patients undergoing intra-arterial thrombolysis. Am J Neuroradiol 25(6):951–957

21. Kidwell CS, Alger JR, Saver JL (2003) Beyond mismatch: evolving paradigms in imaging the ischemic penumbra with multimodal magnetic resonance imaging. Stroke 34(11):2729–2735

22. Schellinger PD, Fiebach JB, Hacke W (2003) Imaging-based decision making in thrombolytic therapy for ischemic stroke: present status. Stroke 34(2):575–583

23. Stephen Davis GD, Butcher K, Parsons M, Barber A, Gerraty R, Frayne J, Talman P, Bladin C, Levi C, Herkes G, Watson J, Hankey G, Chalk J, Schultz D, Kimber T, Fink J, Muir K (2003) Echoplanar imaging thrombolysis evaluation trial: EPITHET. 28th International Stroke Conference, February 2003, Phoenix, Ariz., USA

24. Greer DM et al (2004) Magnetic resonance imaging improves detection of intracerebral hemorrhage over computed tomography after intra-arterial thrombolysis. Stroke 35(2):491–495

25. Zeumer H et al (1993) Local intra-arterial fibrinolytic therapy in patients with stroke: urokinase versus recombinant tissue plasminogen activator (r-TPA). Neuroradiology 35(2):159–162

26. Qureshi AI et al (2002) Aggressive mechanical clot disruption and low-dose intra-arterial third-generation thrombolytic agent for ischemic stroke: a prospective study. Neurosurgery 51(5):1319–1327; discussion 1327–1329

27. Kerber CW et al (2002) Snare retrieval of intracranial thrombus in patients with acute stroke. J Vasc Interv Radiol 13(12):1269–1274

28. Ueda T et al (1998) Angioplasty after intra-arterial thrombolysis for acute occlusion of intracranial arteries. Stroke 29(12):2568–2574

29. Nakayama T et al (1998) Thrombolysis and angioplasty for acute occlusion of intracranial vertebrobasilar arteries. Report of three cases. J Neurosurg 88(5):919–922

30. Ringer AJ et al (2001) Angioplasty of intracranial occlusion resistant to thrombolysis in acute ischemic stroke. Neurosurgery 48(6):1282–1288; discussion 1288–1290

31. Ramee SR et al (2004) Catheter-based treatment for patients with acute ischemic stroke ineligible for intravenous thrombolysis. Stroke 35(5):e109–e111

32. Mahon BR et al (2003) North American clinical experience with the EKOS MicroLysUS infusion catheter for the treatment of embolic stroke. Am J Neuroradiol 24(3):534–538

33. Berlis A et al (2004) Mechanical thrombolysis in acute ischemic stroke with endovascular photoacoustic recanalization. Stroke 35(5):1112–1116

34. Bellon RJ et al (2001) Rheolytic thrombectomy of the occluded internal carotid artery in the setting of acute ischemic stroke. Am J Neuroradiol 22(3):526–530

35. Lisboa RC, Jovanovic BD, Alberts MJ (2002) Analysis of the safety and efficacy of intra-arterial thrombolytic therapy in ischemic stroke. Stroke 33(12):2866–2871

36. Hoh BL, Nogueira RG, O'Donnell J, Pryor JC, Rabinov JD, Hirsch JA, Rordorf GA, Buonanno FS, Koroshetz WJ, Schwamm LH (2004) Intra-arterial thrombolysis for acute stroke: comparison of era using urokinase versus era not using urokinase at a single center. Seventh Joint Meeting of the AANS/CNS Section on Cerebrovascular Surgery and the American Society of Interventional and Therapeutic Neuroradiology, February 2004, San Diego, Calif., USA

37. Eckert B et al (2003) Local intra-arterial fibrinolysis in acute hemispheric stroke: effect of occlusion type and fibrinolytic agent on recanalization success and neurological outcome. Cerebrovasc Dis 15(4):258–263

38. The Abciximab in Ischemic Stroke Investigators (2000) Abciximab in acute ischemic stroke: a randomized, double-blind, placebo-controlled, dose-escalation study. Stroke 31(3):601–609

39. Adams H Jr, tA-I Investigators (2004) Abciximab in emergent stroke treatment trial. II. 29th International Stroke Conference, February 2004, San Diego, Calif., USA

40. Warach S, tA-I Investigators (2004) ReoPro Retavase Reperfusion of Stroke Safety Study Imaging Evaluation (ROSIE). 29th International Stroke Conference, February 2004, San Diego, Calif., USA

41. Eckert B et al (2002) Acute basilar artery occlusion treated with combined intravenous Abciximab and intra-arterial tissue plasminogen activator: report of 3 cases. Stroke 33(5):1424–1427

42. Lee DH et al (2002) Local intraarterial urokinase thrombolysis of acute ischemic stroke with or without intravenous abciximab: a pilot study. J Vasc Interv Radiol 13(8):769–774

43. Fiorella D et al (2004) Strategies for the management of intraprocedural thromboembolic complications with abciximab (ReoPro). Neurosurgery 54(5):1089–1097; discussion 1097–1098

44. Song JK et al (2004) Thrombus formation during intracranial aneurysm coil placement: treatment with intra-arterial abciximab. Am J Neuroradiol 25(7):1147–1153

45. Sussman BJ, Fitch TS (1958) Thrombolysis with fibrinolysin in cerebral arterial occlusion. J Am Med Assoc 167(14):1705–1709

46. Del Zoppo GJ et al (1998) PROACT: a phase II randomized trial of recombinant pro-urokinase by direct arterial delivery in acute middle cerebral artery stroke. PROACT investigators. Prolyse in acute cerebral thromboembolism. Stroke 29(1):4–11

47. Furlan A et al (1999) Intra-arterial prourokinase for acute ischemic stroke. The PROACT II study: a randomized controlled trial. Prolyse in acute cerebral thromboembolism. J Am Med Assoc 282(21):2003–2011

48. Kase CS et al (2001) Cerebral hemorrhage after intra-arterial thrombolysis for ischemic stroke: the PROACT II trial. Neurology 57(9):1603–1610

49. Arnold M et al (2003) Intra-arterial thrombolysis in 24 consecutive patients with internal carotid artery T occlusions. J Neurol Neurosurg Psychiatry 74(6):739–742

50. Zaidat OO et al (2002) Response to intra-arterial and combined intravenous and intra-arterial thrombolytic therapy in patients with distal internal carotid artery occlusion. Stroke 33(7):1821–1826

51. Zeumer H, Hacke W, Ringelstein EB (1983) Local intraarterial thrombolysis in vertebrobasilar thromboembolic disease. Am J Neuroradiol 4(3):401–404

52. Furlan A, Higashida R (2004) Intra-arterial thrombolysis in acute ischemic stroke. In: Mohr JP et al (eds) Stroke: pathophysiology, diagnosis, and management. Churchill Livingstone, Philadelphia, Pa., pp 943–951

53. Lewandowski CA et al (1999) Combined intravenous and intra-arterial r-TPA versus intra-arterial therapy of acute ischemic stroke: Emergency Management of Stroke (EMS) Bridging Trial. Stroke 30(12):2598–2605

54. Ernst R et al (2000) Combined intravenous and intra-arterial recombinant tissue plasminogen activator in acute ischemic stroke. Stroke 31(11):2552–2557

55. Suarez JI et al (2002) Endovascular administration after intravenous infusion of thrombolytic agents for the treatment of patients with acute ischemic strokes. Neurosurgery 50(2):251–259; discussion 259–260

56. Keris V et al (2001) Combined intraarterial/intravenous thrombolysis for acute ischemic stroke. Am J Neuroradiol 22(2):352–358

57. Hill MD et al (2002) Acute intravenous – intra-arterial revascularization therapy for severe ischemic stroke. Stroke 33(1):279–282

58. Nogueira RG, Hoh BL, O'Donnell J, Pryor JC, Rabinov JD, Hirsch JA, Rordorf GA, Buonanno FS, Koroshetz WJ, Schwamm LH (2004) Safety of combined standard dose i.v. tPA (0.9 mg/Kg) followed by i.a. tPA vs. i.a. tPA alone in acute ischemic stroke: is dose reduction in bridging therapy necessary? Seventh Joint Meeting of the AANS/CNS Section on Cerebrovascular Surgery and the American Society of Interventional and Therapeutic Neuroradiology, February 2004, San Diego, Calif., USA

59. Sheehan FH et al (1987) The effect of intravenous thrombolytic therapy on left ventricular function: a report on tissue-type plasminogen activator and streptokinase from the Thrombolysis in Myocardial Infarction (TIMI Phase I) trial. Circulation 75(4):817–829

60. Qureshi AI et al (2001) Intra-arterial third-generation recombinant tissue plasminogen activator (reteplase) for acute ischemic stroke. Neurosurgery 49(1):41–48; discussion 48–50

61. Higashida RT et al (2003) Trial design and reporting standards for intra-arterial cerebral thrombolysis for acute ischemic stroke. Stroke 34(8):e109–e137

62. Qureshi AI (2002) New grading system for angiographic evaluation of arterial occlusions and recanalization response to intra-arterial thrombolysis in acute ischemic stroke. Neurosurgery 50(6):1405–1414; discussion 1414–1415

63. Mohammad Y et al (2004) Qureshi grading scheme for angiographic occlusions strongly correlates with the initial severity and in-hospital outcome of acute ischemic stroke. J Neuroimaging 14(3):235–241

64. Hacke W et al (1988) Intra-arterial thrombolytic therapy improves outcome in patients with acute vertebrobasilar occlusive disease. Stroke 19(10):1216–1222

65. Matsumoto K, Satoh N (1991) Topical intra-arterial urokinase infusion for acute stroke. In: Hacke W, del Zoppo GJ, Hirshberg M (eds) Thrombolytic therapy in acute ischemic stroke. Springer, Berlin Heidelberg New York, pp 207–212

66. Becker KJ et al (1996) Intraarterial thrombolysis in vertebrobasilar occlusion. Am J Neuroradiol 17(2):255–262

67. Brandt T et al (1996) Thrombolytic therapy of acute basilar artery occlusion. Variables affecting recanalization and outcome. Stroke 27(5):875–881

68. Wijdicks EF et al (1997) Intra-arterial thrombolysis in acute basilar artery thromboembolism: the initial Mayo Clinic experience. Mayo Clin Proc 72(11):1005–1013

69. Gonner F et al (1998) Local intra-arterial thrombolysis in acute ischemic stroke. Stroke 29(9):1894–1900

70. Cross DT 3rd et al (1997) Relationship between clot location and outcome after basilar artery thrombolysis. Am J Neuroradiol 18(7):1221–1228

71. Ezaki Y et al (2003) Retrospective analysis of neurological outcome after intra-arterial thrombolysis in basilar artery occlusion. Surg Neurol 60(5):423–429; discussion 429–430

72. Arnold M et al (2004) Clinical and radiological predictors of recanalisation and outcome of 40 patients with acute basilar artery occlusion treated with intra-arterial thrombolysis. J Neurol Neurosurg Psychiatry 75(6):857–862

73. Phan TG, Wijdicks EF (1999) Intra-arterial thrombolysis for vertebrobasilar circulation ischemia. Crit Care Clin 15(4):719–742, vi

Epilogue: CT versus MR in Acute Ischemic Stroke

R. Gilberto González

This book reviews the merits and describes the technical details for using CT and MRI to rapidly evaluate the patient who presents with symptoms of acute stroke. Both modalities are widely available and provide information on the state of the brain parenchyma, the vessels, and brain tissue perfusion. Since many have the capability to perform either or both, the question arises as what to use. The question is practical, but the answer is complex and depends on many factors including the state of the patient, the time since stroke onset, the logistical constraints of using one or the other modality, and the capability of a facility to perform advanced therapy such as intra-arterial thrombolysis.

In clarifying this issue, it is important to consider the fundamental questions that require rapid answers in the clinical setting we are considering. There are four key questions including: (1) is there a hemorrhage?, (2) is a large vessel occluded?, (3) what part of the brain is irreversibly injured?, and (4) is there a part of the brain that is viable but underperfused and in danger of infarcting? Both CT and MR provide information to answer each of these questions. However, they are not equal, and it is illuminating to consider the relative strengths of each modality. Let us consider each question in turn, and, assuming state-of-the-art CT and MRI instruments, estimate which modality is superior.

1. Is there a hemorrhage? CT is superior. Both can detect clinically significant parenchymal hemorrhages; however, CT remains superior in detecting acute subarachnoid hemorrhage, which is an important consideration in the acute stroke patient. MRI is less sensitive because the high oxygen levels in cerebrospinal fluid results in erythrocytes maintaining near-normal levels oxyhemoglobin.

2. Is a large vessel occluded? CTA is superior. The question of whether the internal carotid artery (ICA), middle cerebral artery (MCA) M1 or M2 branch or the basilar artery is occluded is extremely important especially if the capability exists for intra-arterial intervention. Under optimal conditions, MR angiography (MRA) is equivalent to CT angiography (CTA), but conditions are seldom optimal when dealing with the acute stroke patient. The longer time required for MRA is an important consideration, but of greater importance is the vulnerability of MRA to motion artifact that commonly results in an MRA of poor quality. CTA more reliably produces high-quality angiographic information of both the head and neck vessels in less than 2 min.

3. What part of the brain is irreversibly injured? Diffusion MRI is superior. CTA source images provide an estimate of irreversible injury, but are less sensitive than diffusion-weighted images.

4. Is there a part of the brain that is viable but underperfused and in danger of infarcting? Perfusion MRI is superior. Both methods provide information of similar quality. However, MRI systems can evaluate a larger proportion of the brain. These last two questions together are estimating the infarct core and the operational penumbra, a clinically highly relevant determination well illustrated by the success of the Desmoteplase in Acute Ischemic Stroke (DIAS) Trial discussed elsewhere in this book.

The answers to each question are based on review of the literature detailed in the six chapters on CT and MRI found in this book, and the practical, everyday clinical experience of dealing with stroke patients

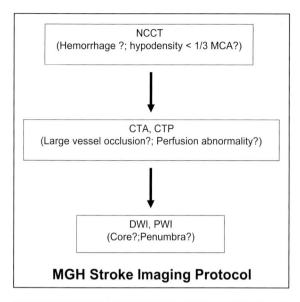

MGH Stroke Imaging Protocol

Fig. 13.1

MGH stroke imaging protocol

that come to Massachusetts General Hospital (MGH). So what do we use at the MGH? The answer is both whenever possible. The imaging triage of patients is shown in Fig. 13.1.

We will perform both in the majority of cases because we are fortunate to have in our emergency department state-of-the-art CT and MRI systems that are located close to each other. The studies are also rapid with CT/CTA/CTP requiring 10 min or less and the MRI restricted to diffusion, perfusion and perhaps one additional sequence taking no more than 10 min of imaging time. Many institutions will have CT and MRI scanners in different locations, raising logistical issues. The optimal solution will obviously vary from institution to institution, and from patient to patient. It is our hope that this book will help each institution to develop the optimal solutions to maximize the number of good clinical outcomes in the acute stroke patient.

Subject Index